D0521366

American Heart Association®
Learn and Live℠

PALS
PROVIDER MANUAL

Editors
Mark Ralston, MD
Oversight Editor
Mary Fran Hazinski, RN, MSN
Senior Science Editor
Arno L. Zaritsky, MD
Stephen M. Schexnayder, MD
Monica E. Kleinman, MD

Special Contributors
Louis Gonzales, NREMT-P, *Senior Oversight Editor*
Brenda Drummonds, *PALS Writer*
Ulrik Christensen, MD
Frank Doto, MS, *Senior Oversight Editor*
Alan J. Schwartz, MD

American Academy of Pediatrics Reviewers
Susan Fuchs, MD
Wendy Simon, MA

PALS Subcommittee 2006-2007
Arno L. Zaritsky, MD, Chair
Stephen M. Schexnayder, MD, Immediate Past Chair, 2005-2006
Robert A. Berg, MD
Douglas S. Diekema, MD
Diana G. Fendya, RN, MSN
Mary Jo Grant, RN, PNP, PhD
George W. Hatch, Jr, EdD, EMT-P
Monica E. Kleinman, MD
Lester Proctor, MD
Faiqa A. Qureshi, MD
Ricardo A. Samson, MD
Elise W. van der Jagt, MD, MPH
Dianne L. Atkins, MD
Marc D. Berg, MD
Allan R. de Caen, MD
Michael J. Gerardi, MD
Jeffrey Perlman, MD
L. R. "Tres" Scherer III, MD, HSc
Wendy Simon, MA

ISBN 0-87493-528-8

PALS Subcommittee 2005-2006

Arno L. Zaritsky, MD, Chair
Stephen M. Schexnayder, MD, Immediate Past Chair, 2004-2005
Robert A. Berg, MD
Douglas S. Diekema, MD
Diana G. Fendya, RN, MSN
Mary Jo Grant, RN, PNP, PhD
George W. Hatch, Jr, EdD, EMT-P
Monica E. Kleinman, MD
Lester Proctor, MD
Faiqa A. Qureshi, MD
Ricardo A. Samson, MD
Elise W. van der Jagt, MD, MPH
Dianne L. Atkins, MD
Marc D. Berg, MD
Allan R. de Caen, MD
Jeffrey Perlman, MD
Melinda Fiedor, MD, HSc
Michael J. Gerardi, MD
Dianne Molsberry, RN-C, BSN, MA
L. R. "Tres" Scherer III, MD, HSc
Wendy Simon, MA
Mark Terry, EMT-P
Michael G. Tunik, MD

Content Experts

Anthony Busti, PharmD
David Gilmore, MD
Robert W. Hickey, MD
Vinay Nadkarni, MD
Anthony J. Scalzo, MD

Medical Illustrators

Anne Jorunn Johnsen
Pierce Goetz

To find out about any updates or corrections to this text, visit *www.americanheart.org/cpr* and click on the "Course Materials" button.

Contents

Chapter 1:
Pediatric Assessment **1**

Overview 1
Approach to Pediatric Assessment 4
General Assessment 6
Primary Assessment 7
Life-threatening Conditions 25
Secondary Assessment 25
Assessment of Circulatory Abnormalities 29
References 32

Chapter 2:
Recognition of Respiratory Distress and Failure **33**

Overview 33
Impairment of Oxygenation and Ventilation in Respiratory Problems 34
Physiology of Breathing in Respiratory Problems 37
Categorization of Respiratory Problems by Severity 40
Classification of Respiratory Problems by Type 41
References 43

Chapter 3:
Management of Respiratory Distress and Failure **45**

Overview 45
Initial Management of Respiratory Distress and Failure 46
Management of Upper Airway Obstruction 47
Specific Management Recommendations for Upper Airway Obstruction by Etiology 48
Management of Lower Airway Obstruction 50
Specific Management Recommendations for Lower Airway Obstruction by Etiology 51
Management of Lung Tissue Disease 53
Specific Management Recommendations for Lung Tissue Disease by Etiology 54

Management of Disordered Control of Breathing 57

References 58

Chapter 4: Recognition of Shock **61**

Overview 61

Physiology of Shock 64

Categorization of Shock by Severity (Effect on Blood Pressure) 66

Categorization of Shock by Type 68

Hypovolemic Shock 69

Distributive Shock 70

Septic Shock 72

Anaphylactic Shock 75

Neurogenic Shock 75

Cardiogenic Shock 76

Obstructive Shock 78

References 80

Chapter 5: Management of Shock **81**

Overview 81

Goals of Shock Management 81

Fundamentals of Shock Management 82

General Management of Shock 85

Advanced Management of Shock 91

Fluid Therapy 92

Glucose 96

Management of Specific Categories of Shock 97

Management of Hypovolemic Shock 97

Management of Distributive Shock 101

Management of Septic Shock 102

Management of Anaphylactic Shock 106

Management of Neurogenic Shock 107

Management of Cardiogenic Shock 107

Management of Obstructive Shock 109

References 111

Chapter 6:
Recognition and Management of Bradyarrhythmias and Tachyarrhythmias 115

Overview 115

Bradyarrhythmias 116

Recognition of Bradyarrhythmias 117

Management of Bradyarrhythmias: Pediatric Bradycardia With a Pulse Algorithm 122

Tachyarrhythmias 126

Sinus Tachycardia 127

Supraventricular Tachycardia 128

Comparison of ST and SVT 131

Atrial Flutter 132

Ventricular Tachycardia 132

Management of Tachyarrhythmias 134

Emergency Interventions 135

Pharmacologic Therapy 137

Summary 140

Pediatric Tachycardia With Adequate Perfusion Algorithm 141

Pediatric Tachycardia With Pulses and Poor Perfusion Algorithm 144

References 147

Chapter 7:
Recognition and Management of Cardiac Arrest 153

Overview 153

Presentations of Cardiac Arrest 154

Causes of Cardiac Arrest 155

Recognition of Cardiac Arrest 157

Management of Cardiac Arrest 160

Basic Life Support 161

Pediatric Advanced Life Support in Cardiac Arrest 163

Pediatric Pulseless Arrest Algorithm 167

Pediatric Cardiac Arrest: Special Circumstances 178

Social Issues and Ethics in Resuscitation 182

Predictors of Outcomes After Cardiac Arrest 183

References 184

Chapter 8: Postresuscitation Management **191**

Overview 191
Postresuscitation Management 192
Respiratory System 193
Cardiovascular System 196
PALS Postresuscitation of Shock Algorithm 199
Administration of Maintenance Fluids 203
Neurologic System 204
Renal System 206
Gastrointestinal System 208
Hematologic System 209
Postresuscitation Transport 210
Mode of Transport and Transport Team Composition 214
Summary: Transport Checklist 216
References 217

Chapter 9: Pharmacology

Overview 221
Adenosine 222
Albumin 223
Albuterol 224
Alprostadil (PGE_1) 225
Amiodarone 226
Atropine 228
Calcium Chloride 229
Dexamethasone 230
Dextrose (Glucose) 232
Diphenhydramine 232
Dobutamine 233
Dopamine 234
Epinephrine 236
Furosemide 238
Hydrocortisone 239

Inamrinone 240

Ipratropium Bromide 241

Lidocaine 242

Magnesium Sulfate 244

Methylprednisolone 245

Milrinone 246

Naloxone 247

Nitroglycerin 248

Norepinephrine 249

Oxygen 250

Procainamide 251

Sodium Bicarbonate 252

Sodium Nitroprusside 253

Terbutaline 255

Chapter 1

Pediatric Assessment

Overview

Introduction

For the PALS provider the best approach to the assessment and treatment of a seriously ill or injured child is a systematic one. In the past various pediatric life support training programs used different terminologies to teach assessment and treatment approaches. These differences in terminology and approach caused confusion among pediatric providers, complicated instructor training, and interfered with the goal shared by all of these training programs: to improve the recognition, treatment, and outcomes of seriously ill and injured children. A consensus has now been reached to standardize definitions, assessment, and treatment approaches used in pediatric resuscitation.

Standardized Approach to Pediatric Assessment

The recommended assessment model for all pediatric life support courses consists of a general assessment (an initial brief observation of the child represented by the pediatric assessment triangle), primary assessment, secondary assessment, and tertiary assessment. The hope is that this consistent approach to pediatric assessment will facilitate training and communication among healthcare providers and improve outcomes for seriously ill and injured children.

The purpose of a standardized approach to assessment is to enable you to recognize signs of respiratory distress, respiratory failure, and shock so that you can provide life-saving interventions. If not adequately treated, pediatric patients with respiratory failure and shock can quickly progress to the final pathway of cardiopulmonary failure leading to cardiac arrest (Figure 1).

Figure 1. Pathway to pediatric cardiac arrest.

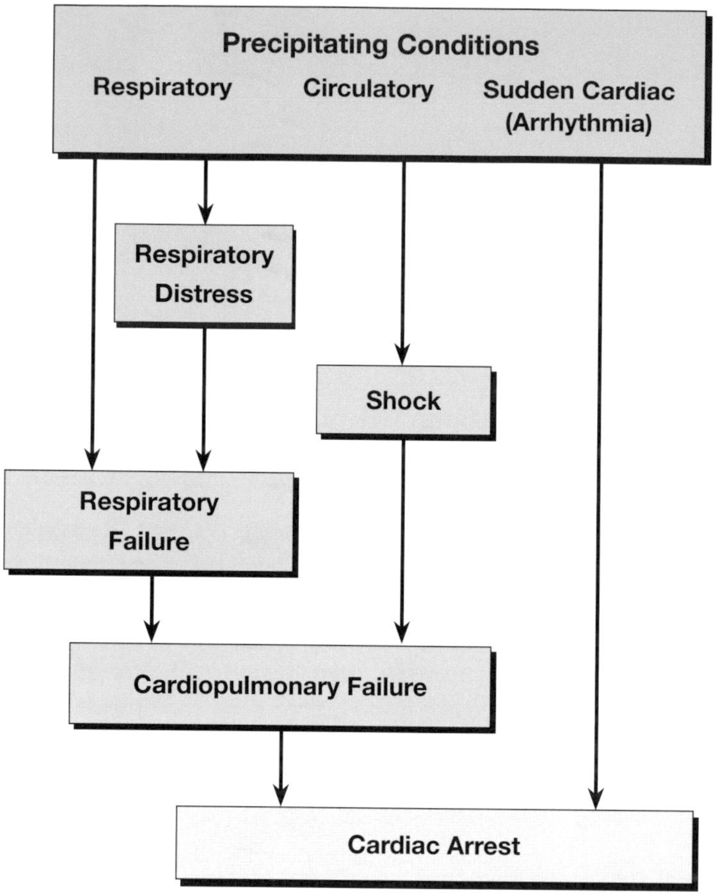

Note that respiratory conditions may progress to respiratory failure with or without signs of respiratory distress. Respiratory distress occurs when the child fails to maintain an open airway or adequate respiratory effort and is typically associated with altered level of consciousness. Sudden cardiac arrest in children is less common than in adults and typically results from arrhythmias, such as ventricular fibrillation or ventricular tachycardia.

Timely Intervention to Prevent Cardiac Arrest

Cardiac arrest, also referred to as cardiopulmonary arrest, is the cessation of clinically detectable cardiac mechanical activity. It is characterized by unresponsiveness, apnea, and the absence of detectable central pulses. *In infants and children, most cardiac arrests result from progressive respiratory failure or shock, or both.* Less commonly, pediatric cardiac arrests can occur without warning (ie, with sudden collapse) secondary to an arrhythmia (ventricular fibrillation or ventricular tachycardia).

Once cardiac arrest occurs, even with optimal efforts at resuscitation the outcome is generally poor. In the out-of-hospital setting only 5% to 12% of children who experience cardiac arrest survive to hospital discharge. The outcome is better for children who experience cardiac arrest in the in-hospital setting, yet only about 27% of those patients survive to hospital discharge.[1] For this reason it is important to learn how to perform and interpret the elements of pediatric assessment taught in this chapter so that you can recognize signs of respiratory failure and shock and treat these problems before they cause cardiac arrest.

Timely intervention in seriously ill or injured children is the key to preventing progression toward cardiac arrest and to saving lives.

Learning Objectives

After completing this chapter you should be able to

- discuss the "assess-categorize-decide-act" approach
- explain the purpose and components of the general assessment (pediatric assessment triangle)
- summarize the ABCDE components of the primary assessment
- explain the implications of clinical findings during the general and primary assessments
- evaluate respiratory or circulatory problems using the ABCDE model
- categorize the clinical condition of a seriously ill or injured child by type and severity
- summarize the life-saving interventions you should institute if a life-threatening condition is identified
- recall the components of the secondary and tertiary assessments

Detailed and Advanced Concepts

This symbol is used to indicate more detailed or advanced concepts. Many of these concepts were provided by the members of the Subcommittee on Pediatric Resuscitation and result from years of research and experience in the field of pediatric advanced life support.

Approach to Pediatric Assessment

Introduction

Use the "assess-categorize-decide-act" model to evaluate and treat a seriously ill or injured child. Initial and repeated *assessment* allows you to determine the best treatment or intervention at any point in time. From the information gathered during assessment, you *categorize* the clinical condition of the child by type and severity, *decide* what needs to be done, and *act* to implement appropriate treatment. Then you reassess and repeat the process. This process is iterative (Figure 2).

Figure 2. Assess-Categorize-Decide-Act.

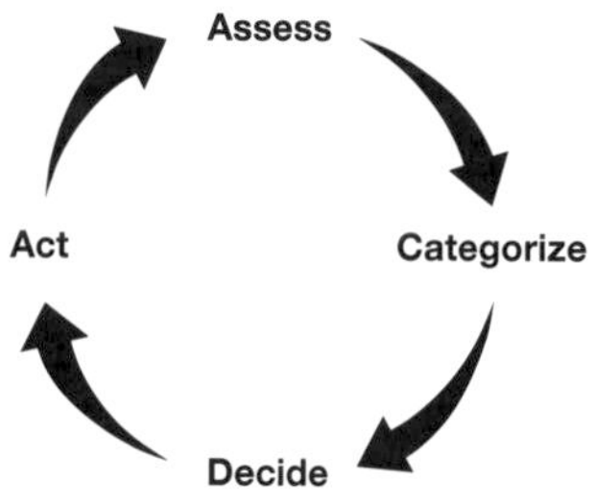

> *If at any point you identify a life-threatening problem, start life-saving interventions immediately and get help by activating the emergency response system (ERS).*

Assess

Assess the child using a systematic approach. There are 4 parts to pediatric assessment. The *general assessment* is an initial quick visual and auditory observation.[2] The pediatric assessment triangle (PAT) illustrates this assessment. The *primary assessment* is next. Then depending on the child's condition and the available resources, evaluation may continue with the *secondary* and *tertiary assessments.*

Clinical Assessment	Brief Description
General assessment (Pediatric assessment triangle)	A rapid visual and auditory assessment of the child's overall appearance, work of breathing, and circulation completed within the first few seconds of patient encounter
Primary assessment	A rapid, hands-on ABCDE approach to evaluate cardiopulmonary and neurologic function; this step includes assessment of vital signs and pulse oximetry
Secondary assessment	A focused medical history using the SAMPLE mnemonic and a thorough head-to-toe physical exam
Tertiary assessment	Laboratory, radiographic, and other advanced tests that help to establish the child's physiologic condition and diagnosis

Note: In out-of-hospital settings, always assess the scene before you assess the patient. See "Scene Assessment for Out-of-Hospital Providers" on the student CD.

Categorize

Attempt to categorize the clinical condition by type and severity:

Type		Severity
Respiratory	— Upper airway obstruction — Lower airway obstruction — Lung tissue (parenchymal) disease — Disordered control of breathing	– Respiratory distress – Respiratory failure
Circulatory	— Hypovolemic shock — Distributive shock — Cardiogenic shock — Obstructive shock	– Compensated shock – Hypotensive shock

The clinical condition can also be a combination of respiratory and circulatory problems. As a seriously ill or injured child deteriorates, one category of problems may lead to others. Note that in the initial phase of your evaluation, you may be uncertain about the type or severity of problems, or both.

This categorization will help you determine the best course of action. Recognition and management of these conditions are discussed in detail later in this book.

Decide

Decide what to do based on your assessment and initial categorization of the clinical condition. Base these decisions on your scope of practice.

Act

Initiate treatment (actions) appropriate for the child's clinical condition and severity. An action may be simple, such as positioning the child for airway protection or administering oxygen.

Actions for PALS providers may include

- activating the ERS
- starting CPR
- obtaining the code cart and monitor/defibrillator
- placing the patient on a monitor and a pulse oximeter
- giving oxygen
- starting treatments (eg, nebulizer treatment, IV fluid bolus)

Transition of Care

If you anticipate transition of care, it is important to continue your life-saving interventions until other rescuers are in position to care for the child. When help arrives, provide a summary of what happened and what you and others have done.

Reassess

The process of assess-categorize-decide-act is ongoing. Reassess the patient as you are providing interventions. For example, if you give oxygen, then reassess the patient. Is breathing a little easier? Are the color and mental status improving? After you give a fluid bolus to a child in hypovolemic shock, does the child's perfusion improve? Is another bolus needed?

> *Remember to repeat the assess-categorize-decide-act cycle as you provide interventions.*

General Assessment

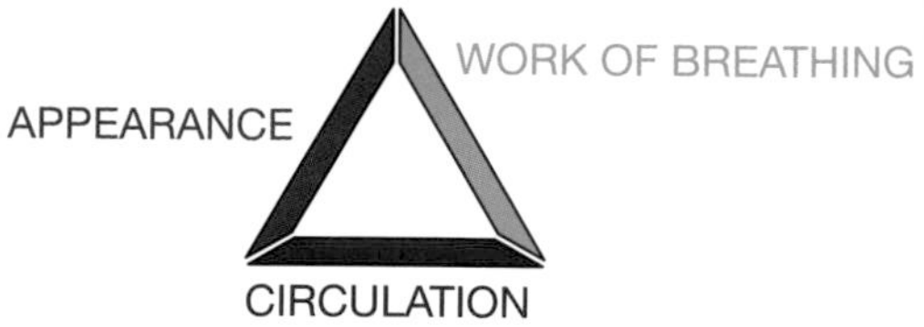

General Assessment

The general assessment using the pediatric assessment triangle (PAT) represents the initial visual and auditory assessment of the seriously ill or injured child, which is instinctively accomplished by the experienced healthcare provider within the first seconds of patient contact. You should quickly process visual and auditory clues to simultaneously assess a child's *appearance, work of breathing,* and *circulation* as summarized in the table below.

PAT	General Assessment
Appearance	Muscle tone, interaction, consolability, look/gaze, or speech/cry
Work of Breathing	Increased work of breathing (eg, nasal flaring, retractions), decreased or absent respiratory effort, or abnormal sounds (eg, wheezing, grunting, stridor)
Circulation	Abnormal skin color (eg, pallor or mottling) or bleeding

Decreases in interaction, speech or cry, look or gaze, and muscle tone usually suggest a serious underlying illness or injury. Abnormalities in work of breathing include use of accessory muscles, extra sounds of breathing, or abnormal breathing patterns. Pale, mottled, bluish/gray skin color suggests poor perfusion, poor oxygenation, or both. A flushed appearance suggests fever or toxicity. Diaphoresis (sweating) suggests significant distress, which may be related to a cardiac problem or hyperthermia.

Determine if Life Threatening

Based on this initial crucial information, determine if the condition is

- life threatening
- not life threatening

If the condition is life threatening, start life-saving interventions and activate the ERS. If the condition is not life threatening, continue with the systematic assessment. (See "Life-threatening Conditions" later in this chapter.)

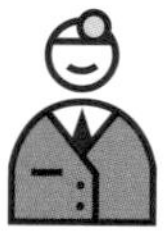

There are some cases in which a child's appearance might seem normal, yet the child has a potentially life-threatening problem. Examples include a child who has ingested a toxin but is not yet showing effects or a trauma victim with internal bleeding who is temporarily maintaining blood pressure by increasing heart rate and systemic vascular resistance.[2]

Primary Assessment

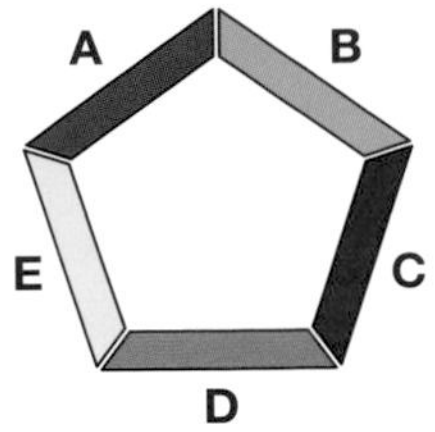

Overview

The primary assessment uses an ABCDE approach:

- **A**irway
- **B**reathing
- **C**irculation
- **D**isability
- **E**xposure

In contrast to the general assessment (PAT), which uses only visual and auditory clues, the primary assessment is a hands-on evaluation. Here you assess cardiopulmonary and neurologic function to categorize the child's condition. Based on that categorization, you can then decide what you need to do and implement the action or treatment needed. This assessment includes evaluation of vital signs and oxygen saturation by pulse oximetry.

> *Important:* During each step of the primary assessment, *watch for any life-threatening abnormality.* If one is present, treat it before you complete the rest of the assessment.

Once the primary assessment is completed, life-threatening problems are addressed, and appropriate actions are implemented, proceed to the secondary and tertiary assessments.

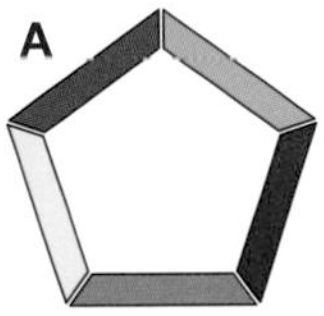

Airway

Airway Assessment

Assessment of the airway is essential to determine if it is patent (open or unobstructed). To assess upper airway patency:

- look for movement of the chest or abdomen
- listen for breath sounds and air movement
- feel the movement of air at the nose and mouth

You must establish if the upper airway is clear, maintainable, or not maintainable as described below:

Status	Description
Clear	Airway is open and unobstructed for normal breathing
Maintainable	Airway can be maintained by *simple measures*
Not maintainable	Airway cannot be maintained without *advanced interventions*

The following signs suggest that the upper airway is obstructed:

- Increased inspiratory effort with retractions
- Abnormal inspiratory sounds (snoring or high-pitched stridor)
- Episodes where no airway or breath sounds are produced despite respiratory effort (ie, complete upper airway obstruction)

If the upper airway is obstructed, the next step is to determine if you can open and maintain the airway with *simple measures* or if you need *advanced interventions.*

Simple Measures

Simple measures to restore upper airway patency may include one or more of the following:

- Allow child to assume a position of comfort or position the child to improve airway patency
- Use head tilt–chin lift to open the airway unless cervical spine injury is suspected. If *cervical spine injury is suspected*, open the airway using a jaw thrust without neck extension. If this maneuver does not open the airway, use head tilt–chin lift or jaw thrust with neck extension because opening the airway is a priority. During CPR manually stabilize the head and neck rather than use immobilization devices. (Note that the jaw thrust may be used in children without trauma as well.)
- Suction the nose and oropharynx
- Perform foreign-body airway obstruction (FBAO) relief techniques if the child is responsive:
  - <1 year of age: back slaps and chest thrusts
  - ≥ 1 year of age: abdominal thrusts
- Use airway adjuncts (eg, nasopharyngeal or oral airway)

Advanced Interventions

Advanced interventions used to maintain airway patency may include one or more of the following:

- Endotracheal (ET) intubation
- Removal of foreign body; this intervention may require direct laryngoscopy (ie, visualizing the larynx with a laryngoscope)
- Application of continuous positive airway pressure (CPAP)
- Cricothyrotomy (a needle puncture or surgical opening through the skin and cricothyroid membrane)

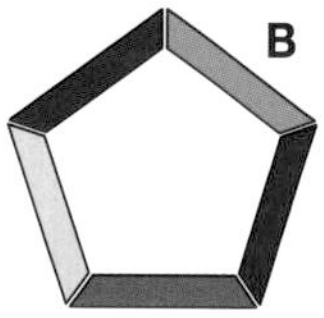

Breathing

Breathing Assessment

Assessment of breathing includes evaluation of

- respiratory rate
- respiratory effort
- tidal volume
- airway and lung sounds
- pulse oximetry

Respiratory Rate (Normal)

Normal spontaneous ventilation is accomplished with minimal work, resulting in quiet breathing with easy inspiration and passive expiration. The normal respiratory rate is inversely related to age. It is rapid in the neonate, then decreases in older infants and children.

Table 1. Normal Respiratory Rates by Age[3]

Age	Breaths per Minutes
Infant (<1 year)	30 to 60
Toddler (1 to 3 years)	24 to 40
Preschooler (4 to 5 years)	22 to 34
School age (6 to 12 years)	18 to 30
Adolescent (13 to 18 years)	12 to 16

A respiratory rate consistently greater than 60 breaths per minute in a child of any age is abnormal and is a "red flag."

Respiratory rate is often best evaluated before your hands-on assessment because anxiety and agitation commonly alter the baseline rate. If the child has any condition that causes an increase in metabolic demand (eg, excitement, anxiety, exercise, pain, or fever), you can expect the respiratory rate to be higher than normal.

Determine the respiratory rate by doubling the number of chest rises in 30 seconds. (Be aware that normal sleeping infants may start and stop breathing in intervals lasting up to 10 to 15 seconds. If you count chest rises for less than 30 seconds, you may interpret the respiratory rate inaccurately.) Count the respiratory rate several times as you assess and reassess the child to detect changes. Alternatively, the respiratory rate may be continuously monitored using a cardiorespiratory monitor.

A decrease in respiratory rate from a rapid to a more "normal" rate may indicate overall improvement if it is associated with a better level of consciousness and reduced signs of air hunger and work of breathing. A decreasing or irregular respiratory rate in a child with a deteriorating level of consciousness, however, often indicates a worsening of the child's clinical condition.

Respiratory Rate (Abnormal)

Abnormal respiratory rates are classified as

- tachypnea
- bradypnea
- apnea

Tachypnea

Tachypnea is a breathing rate that is more rapid than normal for age. It is often the first sign of respiratory distress in infants. Tachypnea can also be a physiologic response to stress.

Tachypnea with respiratory distress is by definition associated with other signs of increased respiratory effort. "Quiet tachypnea" is the term used if tachypnea is present without signs of increased respiratory effort (ie, without respiratory distress). This condition often results from an attempt to maintain normal blood pH by increasing the amount of air moved in and out of the lungs, which decreases carbon dioxide levels in the blood and increases blood pH.

Quiet tachypnea commonly results from nonpulmonary conditions, including

- high fever
- pain
- mild metabolic acidosis associated with dehydration
- sepsis (without pneumonia)

Bradypnea

Bradypnea is a breathing rate that is slower than normal for age. Frequently the breathing is both slow and irregular. Possible causes include fatigue, central nervous system injury or infection, hypothermia, or medications that depress respiratory drive.

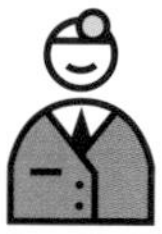

Bradypnea or an irregular respiratory rate in an acutely ill infant or child is an ominous clinical sign because it often signals impending arrest.

Apnea

Apnea is the cessation of inspiratory airflow for 20 seconds or for a shorter period of time if accompanied by bradycardia, cyanosis, or pallor.

Apnea is classified into the following 3 types depending on whether inspiratory muscle activity is present:

- *Central apnea* is characterized by absence of inspiratory muscle activity, usually from abnormalities in or suppression of the brain or spinal cord (ie, there is no respiratory effort or attempt).
- *Obstructive apnea* is characterized by inspiratory muscle activity without airflow (ie, airflow is blocked or impeded).
- *Mixed apnea* is characterized by mixed central and obstructive apnea.

Respiratory Effort

Signs of increased respiratory effort reflect the child's attempt to improve oxygenation, ventilation, or both. Use the presence or absence of these signs to assess the severity of the condition and the urgency for intervention. Signs of increased respiratory effort include

- nasal flaring
- chest retractions
- head bobbing or seesaw respirations

Other signs of increased respiratory effort are prolonged inspiratory or expiratory times, open-mouth breathing, gasping, and use of accessory muscles. Grunting is a serious sign and may indicate respiratory distress or respiratory failure. See "Grunting" later in this chapter.

Increased breathing effort results from conditions that increase resistance to airflow (eg, asthma or bronchiolitis) or that cause the lungs to be stiffer and difficult to inflate (eg, pneumonia, pulmonary edema, and pleural effusion). Nonpulmonary conditions that result in severe metabolic acidosis (eg, diabetic ketoacidosis, salicylate ingestion, inborn errors of metabolism) can also cause increased respiratory rate and effort.

Nasal Flaring

Nasal flaring is the enlargement of the nostrils with each inspiratory breath. The nostrils enlarge to maximize airflow during breathing. Nasal flaring is most commonly observed in infants and younger children. It is usually a sign of respiratory distress.

Chest Retractions

Chest retractions are inward movement of the soft tissues of the chest wall or sternum during inspiration. Chest retractions are a sign that the child is trying to move air into the lungs by increased use of the chest muscles. But air movement is impaired by increased airway resistance or by noncompliant lungs. Retractions may occur in several areas of the chest. The severity of the retractions generally corresponds with the severity of the child's breathing difficulty.

The table below describes the location of retractions commonly associated with each level of breathing difficulty:

Breathing Difficulty	Location of Retraction	Description
Mild to moderate	Subcostal	Retraction of the abdomen, just below the rib cage
	Substernal	Retraction of the abdomen, at the bottom of the breastbone
	Intercostal	Retraction between the ribs
Severe *(may include the same retractions as seen with mild to moderate breathing difficulty)*	Supraclavicular	Retraction in the neck, just above the collarbone
	Suprasternal	Retraction in the chest, just above the breastbone
	Sternal	Retraction of the sternum toward the anterior spine

Retractions accompanied by stridor or an inspiratory snoring sound suggest upper airway obstruction. Retractions accompanied by expiratory wheezing suggest marked lower airway obstruction (asthma or bronchiolitis) causing obstruction during both inspiration and expiration. Retractions accompanied by grunting or labored respirations suggest lung tissue (parenchymal) disease. Severe retractions may also be accompanied by head bobbing or seesaw respirations.

Head Bobbing or Seesaw Respirations

Be alert for other signs of increased respiratory effort. Two of these signs, head bobbing and seesaw respirations, often indicate increased patient risk for deterioration.

- Head bobbing is the use of the neck muscles to assist breathing. The child lifts the chin and extends the neck during inspiration and allows the chin to fall forward during expiration. Head bobbing is most frequently seen in infants and can be a sign of respiratory failure.

- Seesaw respirations (abdominal breathing) are present when the chest retracts and the abdomen expands during inspiration. During expiration the movement reverses: the chest expands and the abdomen moves inward. Seesaw respirations usually indicate upper airway obstruction. But they may also be observed in severe lower airway obstruction, lung tissue disease, and states of disordered control of breathing. Seesaw respirations are characteristic of infants and children with neuromuscular weakness. This inefficient form of ventilation can quickly lead to fatigue.

  The cause of seesaw breathing in most children with neuromuscular disease is weakness of the abdominal and chest wall muscles. Movement of the weaker abdominal and chest wall muscles is largely determined by the relatively stronger diaphragm.

Tidal Volume

Tidal volume is the volume of each breath. Normal tidal volume is approximately 5 to 7 milliliters per kilogram of body weight and remains fairly constant throughout life. Tidal volume is difficult to measure unless a patient is intubated. To assess tidal volume clinically, you should

- observe magnitude of chest wall excursion
- auscultate for distal air movement

Observation of Chest Wall Excursion

Chest expansion (chest rise) during inspiration should be symmetric. Expansion may be subtle during spontaneous quiet breathing when the chest is covered by clothing. But it should be readily seen when the chest is uncovered. In normal infants the abdomen may move more than the chest. Decreased or asymmetric chest expansion may result from inadequate effort, airway obstruction, atelectasis, pneumothorax, hemothorax, pleural effusion, mucous plug, or foreign-body aspiration.

Auscultation of Air Movement

This component of the exam is critical. Note the intensity of breath sounds and quality of air movement, particularly in the distal lung fields. The areas below the axillae are the best location for evaluating distal air entry. Because these areas are farthest from the larger conducting airways, upper airway sounds are less likely to be transmitted. Normally the inspiratory sounds should be heard distally as a soft, quiet noise occurring simultaneously with the observed inspiratory effort. The expiratory breath sounds are often short and quieter, or they may be absent.

You should also auscultate for lung and airway sounds over the anterior and posterior chest. Because the chest is small and the chest wall thin in an infant or child, breath sounds are readily transmitted and heard from one hemithorax to the other. Breath sounds also may be transmitted from the upper airway.

Decreased chest excursion or decreased air movement on lung auscultation often accompanies poor respiratory effort. In the child with apparently normal or increased respiratory effort, diminished distal air entry suggests airflow obstruction or lung tissue disease. If the child's work of breathing and coughing suggest lower airway obstruction but no wheezes are heard, the amount and rate of air flow may be insufficient to cause wheezing.

Distal air entry may be difficult to hear in the obese child, in whom significant airway abnormalities may be missed.

Minute Ventilation

Minute ventilation is the volume of air that moves into and out of the lungs each minute. It is the product of the frequency of breathing per minute (respiratory rate) and the volume of each breath (tidal volume).

$$\text{Minute Ventilation} = \text{Respiratory Rate} \times \text{Tidal Volume}$$

Low minute ventilation (hypoventilation) may result from

- slow respiratory rate
- small tidal volume (ie, shallow breathing, high airway resistance, stiff lungs)
- rapid respiratory rate (if tidal volumes are sufficiently small)

Abnormal Lung and Airway Sounds

During the primary assessment you should evaluate the child for abnormal lung and airway sounds. Abnormal sounds include stridor, grunting, gurgling, wheezing, and crackles.

Stridor

Stridor is a coarse, usually higher-pitched breathing sound typically heard on inspiration. It may, however, be present on both inspiration and expiration. Stridor is a sign of upper airway (extrathoracic) obstruction and may indicate critical airway obstruction requiring immediate intervention.

There are many causes of stridor, such as foreign-body airway obstruction (FBAO) and infection (eg, croup). Congenital airway abnormalities (eg, laryngomalacia) and acquired airway abnormalities (eg, tumor or cyst) also can cause stridor. Upper airway edema (eg, allergic reaction or swelling after a medical procedure) is another cause of this abnormal breathing sound.

Grunting

Grunting is typically a short, low-pitched sound heard during expiration. Sometimes it is misinterpreted as a small cry. Grunting occurs as the child exhales against a partially closed glottis. Although grunting may accompany the child's response to pain or fever, infants and children often grunt to help keep the small airways and alveolar sacs in the lungs open in an attempt to optimize oxygenation and ventilation.

Grunting is often a sign of lung tissue disease resulting from small airway collapse, alveolar collapse, or both. Grunting may indicate progression of respiratory distress to respiratory failure. Pulmonary conditions that cause grunting include pneumonia, pulmonary contusion, and acute respiratory distress syndrome. Grunting may be caused by cardiac conditions causing pulmonary edema, such as myocarditis and congestive heart failure. It may also be a sign of abdominal pathology causing pain and abdominal splinting (eg, bowel obstruction, perforated viscus, appendicitis, or peritonitis).[4]

Grunting is typically a sign of severe respiratory distress or failure from lung tissue disease. You should identify and treat the cause as quickly as possible.

Gurgling

Gurgling is a bubbling sound heard during inspiration or expiration. It results from upper airway obstruction due to airway secretions, vomit, or blood.

Wheezing

Wheezing is a high-pitched or low-pitched whistling or sighing sound heard most often during expiration. It occurs less frequently during inspiration. This sound indicates lower (intrathoracic) airway obstruction, especially of the smaller airways. Common causes of wheezing are bronchiolitis and asthma. Inspiratory wheezing suggests a foreign body or other cause of obstruction in the trachea or upper airway.

Crackles

Crackles, also known as rales, are sharp, crackling sounds heard on inspiration. Crackles may be described as moist or dry. Moist crackles indicate accumulation of alveolar fluid, such as with pneumonia. The sound of dry crackles can be described as the sound made when you rub your hair together close to your ear. Dry crackles are heard more often with atelectasis (small airway collapse) and interstitial lung diseases. Crackles are typically associated with lung tissue disease (eg, pneumonia and pulmonary edema) or interstitial lung disease.

Pulse Oximetry

Pulse oximetry is a tool to monitor the percentage of the child's hemoglobin that is saturated with oxygen. This noninvasive method can detect low oxygen saturation (hypoxemia) in a child before it becomes clinically apparent by the appearance of cyanosis or bradycardia.

The pulse oximeter consists of a probe attached to the child's finger, toe, or ear lobe. The probe is linked to a unit that displays the calculated percent of hemoglobin that is saturated with oxygen. An audible signal for each pulse beat and a heart rate are usually displayed. Some models display the quality of the pulse signal as a waveform.

Oxygen saturation readings at or above 94% while breathing room air usually indicate adequate oxygenation. Consider oxygen administration for oxyhemoglobin saturations below this value, Additional intervention is likely to be required if the oxygen saturation is below 90% in a child receiving 100% oxygen by a nonrebreathing mask.

Interpreting Pulse Oximetry Readings

Be careful to interpret pulse oximetry readings in conjunction with your clinical assessment and other signs, such as respiratory rate, respiratory effort, and level of consciousness. A child may be in respiratory distress yet maintain normal oxygen saturation by increased respiratory rate and effort, especially if supplementary oxygen is administered. If the heart rate displayed by the pulse oximeter is not the same as the heart rate determined by ECG monitoring, the oxygen saturation reading is not reliable. When the pulse oximeter does not detect a consistent pulse or there is an irregular or poor waveform, you should suspect that the child has poor distal perfusion and that the pulse oximeter reading may not be accurate.

The pulse oximeter does not accurately recognize methemoglobin or hemoglobin saturated with carbon monoxide. If carboxyhemoglobin (from carbon monoxide) is present, the pulse oximeter will reflect a *falsely high* oxyhemoglobin saturation. If methemoglobin concentrations are increased above 5%, the pulse oximeter will read ~85% regardless of the degree of methemoglobinemia. If either of these conditions is suspected, you should obtain an oxyhemoglobin saturation measurement with a co-oximeter.

It is important to recognize that pulse oximetry calculates only the oxygen saturation of hemoglobin. It does not evaluate oxygen content of the blood or oxygen delivery to the tissues. For example, if the child is profoundly anemic, saturation may be 100% but oxygen delivery may be low.

If the heart rate displayed by the pulse oximeter is not the same as the palpated pulse or the heart rate displayed by ECG monitor, the oxygen saturation reading is not reliable. If a digital display of the pulse waveform is present, it typically has an inconsistent or poor waveform in this setting. When the pulse oximeter does not detect a consistent pulse, suspect that the child has poor distal perfusion.

For a complete discussion see "Pulse Oximetry" in Respiratory Management Resources on the student CD.

Circulation

Circulation Assessment

Assessment of circulation includes evaluation of both cardiovascular function and end-organ function.

Cardiovascular function is assessed by the evaluation of

- skin color and temperature
- heart rate
- heart rhythm
- blood pressure
- pulses (both peripheral and central)
- capillary refill time

End-organ function is assessed by the evaluation of

- brain perfusion (mental status)
- skin perfusion
- renal perfusion (urine output)

Cardiovascular Function

Skin Color and Temperature

Normal skin color and temperature should be consistent over the trunk and extremities. Mucous membranes, nail beds, palms of the hands, and soles of the feet should be pink.

When perfusion deteriorates, the hands and feet are typically affected first. They may become cool, pale, dusky, or mottled. If the condition worsens, the skin over the trunk and extremities may undergo similar changes.

Consider the temperature of the child's environment when evaluating skin color and temperature. If the environment is cool, peripheral vasoconstriction may produce mottling or pallor with cool skin and delayed capillary refill, particularly in the extremities, despite normal cardiovascular function.[5]

To assess skin temperature, use the back of your hand. The back of the hand is more sensitive to temperature changes than the palm, which has thicker skin. Slide the back of your hand up the extremity to determine if there is a point where the skin changes from cool to warm. Monitor this area of demarcation between warm and cool skin over time to determine the child's response to therapy. The line should move distally as the child improves.

Heart Rate: Normal

Heart rate should be appropriate for the child's age, level of activity, and clinical condition (Table 2). Note that there is a wide range for normal heart rate and that it may vary in a sleeping or athletic child.

Table 2. Normal Heart Rates (per Minute) by Age

Age	Awake Rate	Mean	Sleeping Rate
Newborn to 3 months	85 to 205	140	80 to160
3 months to 2 years	100 to 190	130	75 to 160
2 years to 10 years	60 to 140	80	60 to 90
>10 years	60 to 100	75	50 to 90

Modified from: Hazinski[3] and Gillette[6]

To determine heart rate, check the pulse rate, listen to the chest, or view a monitor (ECG monitor or pulse oximeter). Attach a 3-lead ECG monitoring system when practical.

Heart Rate: Abnormal

An abnormal heart rate is defined as either tachycardia or bradycardia. See Chapter 6: Recognition and Management of Bradyarrhythmias and Tachyarrhythmias for a detailed discussion.

Tachycardia

Tachycardia is a heart rate faster than the normal range for a child's age measured when the child is at rest. Tachycardia is a common, nonspecific response to a variety of underlying conditions. Tachycardia is often appropriate when the child is seriously ill or injured. To determine if the tachycardia is a sinus tachycardia or represents a primary cardiac rhythm disturbance, evaluate the child's history, clinical condition, and ECG.

Bradycardia

Bradycardia is a heart rate lower than normal for a child's age. Bradycardia may be normal in athletic children, but it can be a worrisome sign and may indicate that cardiac arrest is imminent. Hypoxia is the most common cause of bradycardia in a child. If the child with bradycardia has decreased responsiveness or other signs of poor perfusion, immediately support ventilation and provide oxygen. If the child with bradycardia is alert and responsive, consider other causes of a slow heart rate, such as heart block or drug overdose.

Heart Rhythm

The normal heart rhythm is regular with only small fluctuations in rate. When checking the heart rate, assess for abnormalities in the pattern. Like bradycardia and tachycardia, an abnormal pattern of the heartbeat can be classified as an arrhythmia.

In healthy children the heart rate may fluctuate with the respiratory cycle, increasing with inspiration and slowing down with expiration. This condition is called a sinus arrhythmia. You should note if the child has an irregular rhythm with no relationship to breathing. An irregular rhythm may indicate an underlying rhythm disturbance, such as premature ventricular or atrial beats or variable heart block.

Blood Pressure

Accurate blood pressure measurement requires use of a properly sized cuff. Current recommendations require the use of a cuff bladder that covers about 40% of the mid-upper arm circumference.[7] The blood pressure cuff should extend at least 50% to 75% of the length of the upper arm (from the axilla to the antecubital fossa).

Normal Blood Pressures

Table 3 lists normal blood pressure values by age. This table summarizes the range from the 33rd to 67th percentile in the first year of life and from the 5th to 95th percentile for systolic and diastolic blood pressure according to age and gender and assuming the 50th percentile for height for children 1 year of age and older. Like heart rate, there is a wide range of values within the normal range.

Table 3. Normal Blood Pressures in Children by Age

Age	Systolic BP (mm Hg)		Diastolic BP (mm Hg)	
	Female	Male	Female	Male
Neonate (1st day)	60 to 76	60 to 74	31 to 45	30 to 44
Neonate (4th day)	67 to 83	68 to 84	37 to 53	35 to 53
Infant (1 mo)	73 to 91	74 to 94	36 to 56	37 to 55
Infant (3 mo)	78 to 100	81 to 103	44 to 64	45 to 65
Infant (6 mo)	82 to 102	87 to 105	46 to 66	48 to 68
Infant (1 y)	68 to 104	67 to 103	22 to 60	20 to 58
Child (2 y)	71 to 105	70 to 106	27 to 65	25 to 63
Child (7 y)	79 to 113	79 to 115	39 to 77	38 to 78
Adolescent (15 y)	93 to 127	95 to 131	47 to 85	45 to 85

Blood pressure ranges taken from the following sources: Neonate, Infant (1 to 6 mo)[8]; Infant (1 y), Child, Adolescent[9]

Hypotension

Hypotension is defined by the following thresholds of systolic blood pressure.

Table 4. Definition of Hypotension by Systolic Blood Pressure and Age

Age	Systolic Blood Pressure (mm Hg)
Term neonates (0 to 28 days)	<60
Infants (1 to 12 months)	<70
Children 1 to 10 years 5th BP percentile	<70 + (age in years × 2)
Children >10 years	<90

Note that these blood pressure thresholds approximate the 5th percentile systolic blood pressures for age, so will overlap with normal blood pressure values for 5% of healthy children. An observed fall of 10 mm Hg in systolic blood pressure from baseline should prompt serial evaluations for additional signs of shock. In addition, remember that these threshold values are in normal, resting children. Children with injury and stress will typically have increased blood pressure. A blood pressure in the low normal range may be inappropriate in a seriously ill child.

Hypotension in the child represents a state of shock in which physiologic compensatory mechanisms (eg, tachycardia and vasoconstriction) have failed. Hypotension with hemorrhage is thought to be consistent with an acute loss of 20% to 25% of circulating blood volume. Hypotension may be a sign of septic shock, in which there is inappropriate vasodilation rather than loss of intravascular volume. The hypotensive, tachycardic patient who further deteriorates may develop bradycardia, which is an ominous sign. Aggressive fluid resuscitation, along with management of airway and breathing, are needed to prevent cardiac arrest.

Pulses

Evaluation of pulses is critical to the assessment of systemic perfusion in an ill or injured child. Palpate both the central and peripheral pulses. Central pulses are ordinarily stronger than peripheral pulses because they are larger in caliber and located closer to the heart. Exaggeration of the difference in quality between central and peripheral pulse occurs with vasoconstriction associated with shock. In healthy infants and children (unless the child is obese or ambient temperature is cold), you should easily palpate the following pulses:

Central Pulses

- Femoral
- Carotid (in older children)
- Axillary

Peripheral Pulses

- Brachial
- Radial
- Dorsalis pedis
- Posterior tibial

When cardiac output decreases in shock, systemic perfusion decreases incrementally. The decrease in perfusion starts in the extremities with loss of peripheral pulses. It then extends toward the trunk with eventual weakening of central pulses. A cold environment can cause vasoconstriction and a discrepancy between peripheral and central pulses. Central pulses, however, should remain strong.

Weakening of central pulses is a worrisome sign requiring very rapid intervention to prevent cardiac arrest.

Beat-to-beat fluctuation in pulse volume may occur in children with arrhythmias (eg, premature atrial or ventricular beats). Fluctuation in pulse volume with the respiratory cycle (pulsus paradoxus) can occur in children with severe asthma and pericardial tamponade.

In the intubated patient receiving positive-pressure ventilatory support, a reduction in pulse volume with each positive-pressure breath may indicate hypovolemia.

Capillary Refill Time

Capillary refill reflects skin perfusion and may indicate abnormalities in cardiac output. Capillary refill time is the time it takes for blood to return to tissue blanched with pressure. Normal capillary refill time is less than 2 seconds.

To evaluate capillary refill, lift the extremity slightly above the level of the heart. This action facilitates assessment of arteriolar capillary refill. It is best to evaluate capillary refill in a neutral thermal environment (ie, room temperature).

Frequent causes of sluggish, delayed, or prolonged capillary refill (a refill time >2 seconds) include dehydration, shock, and hypothermia.

Shock can be present despite a normal capillary refill time. Children in "warm" septic shock may have excellent (ie, <2 seconds) capillary refill time.

End-Organ Perfusion

Brain

Clinical signs of brain perfusion are important indicators of circulatory function in the ill or injured pediatric patient. These signs include level of consciousness, muscle tone, and pupillary responses. Signs of inadequate oxygen delivery to the brain correlate with both the severity and duration of cerebral hypoxia.

Sudden and severe cerebral hypoxia may present with the following neurologic signs:

- Loss of muscular tone
- Generalized seizures
- Pupillary dilation
- Unconsciousness

You may observe other neurologic signs when cerebral hypoxia develops gradually. These signs can be subtle and are best detected with repeated measurements over time:

- Altered consciousness with confusion
- Irritability
- Lethargy
- Agitation alternating with lethargy

Alterations in neurologic signs may be caused by conditions other than cerebral hypoxia. Some drugs and metabolic conditions (eg, increased ammonia) or increased intracranial pressure may produce neurologic signs and symptoms.

The child's neurologic condition may be characterized using the Alert–Voice–Painful–Unresponsive (AVPU) scale and a description of pupillary responses. The AVPU Pediatric Response Scale and pupillary responses are reviewed in the section on disability assessment.

Skin

Skin color (as well as skin temperature and capillary refill time) can reflect either peripheral (end-organ) perfusion or central (cardiovascular) function. Monitor changes in skin color, temperature, and capillary refill over time to assess a child's response to therapy.

Look for the presence and progression of petechiae and purpura, nonblanching purple discolorations in the skin caused by bleeding from capillaries and small vessels. Petechiae appear as tiny dots and suggest a low platelet count. Purpura appear as larger spots and may represent septic shock.

Carefully evaluate *pallor, mottling,* and *cyanosis*, which may indicate inadequate oxygen delivery to the tissues.

Pallor

Pallor, or paleness, is a lack of normal skin or mucous membrane color. Causes of pallor include one or more of the following:

- Decreased blood supply to the skin (cold, stress, hypovolemic shock)
- Decreased number of red blood cells (anemia)
- Decreased skin pigmentation

Pallor does not necessarily indicate disease; it can result from lack of sunlight or inherited paleness. Pallor is more likely to be clinically significant if the child has pale mucous membranes (lips, lining of the mouth, tongue, lining of the eyes) or pale palms and soles. Pallor is often difficult to detect in a child with dark skin. Thick skin and variations in the vascularity of subcutaneous tissue also can make detection difficult. Family members often can tell you if a child's color is abnormal. Central pallor (ie, lips and mucus membranes) strongly suggests anemia or poor perfusion.

Mottling

Mottling, or mottled skin, is an irregular or patchy discoloration of the skin. Mottling may occur because of variations in the amount of melanin in the skin. But it also can be caused by hypoxemia, hypovolemia, or shock. These conditions can cause intense vasoconstriction, resulting in an irregular supply of oxygenated blood to the skin and even cyanosis in some areas.

Cyanosis

Cyanosis is a blue discoloration of the skin and mucous membranes. Blood saturated with oxygen is bright red whereas blood that has lost its oxygen is dark bluish-red. The location of cyanosis (peripheral or central) is important.

Peripheral cyanosis (ie, affecting the hands and feet) can be caused by diminished oxygen delivery to the tissues. It may be seen in conditions such as shock, congestive heart failure, or peripheral vascular disease, or in conditions causing venous stasis.

Central cyanosis is a blue color of the lips and other mucous membranes. Typically cyanosis is not apparent until at least 5 g/dL of hemoglobin are desaturated (not bound to oxygen). The oxygen saturation at which a child will appear cyanotic depends on the patient's hemoglobin concentration. For instance, in the child with a hemoglobin concentration of 16 g/dL, cyanosis will appear at an oxygen saturation of approximately 70% (ie, 30% of the hemoglobin, or 4.8 g/dL, is desaturated). If the hemoglobin concentration is low (eg, 8 g/dL), a very low arterial oxygen saturation (eg, less than 40%) is required to produce cyanosis. Thus, cyanosis may be apparent with milder degrees of hypoxemia in the child with cyanotic heart disease and polycythemia but may not be apparent despite significant hypoxemia if the child is anemic.

Causes of central cyanosis include all mechanisms of hypoxemia:

- Low ambient oxygen tension (eg, high altitude)
- Alveolar hypoventilation (eg, traumatic brain injury, drug overdose)
- Diffusion defect (eg, pneumonia)
- Ventilation/perfusion imbalance (eg, asthma, bronchiolitis, acute respiratory distress syndrome)
- Intracardiac shunt (eg, cyanotic congenital heart disease)

Cyanosis may be more obvious in the mucous membranes and nail beds, particularly in children with darker skin. It can also appear on the feet, nose, and ears. Because the level of hemoglobin can vary widely (eg, anemia, polycythemia), children with different hemoglobin levels will be cyanotic at different levels of oxygen saturation.

The development of central cyanosis typically indicates the need for emergency intervention, such as oxygen administration and ventilatory support.

Acrocyanosis is a bluish discoloration of the hands and feet. It is commonly seen in healthy newborns. Unlike central cyanosis, acrocyanosis in young infants usually is not associated with hypoxemia.

Renal Perfusion

Adequate urine output usually indicates adequate renal perfusion. Normal urinary output varies with age.

Normal urine output in well-hydrated infants, young children, older children, and adolescents is as follows:

Age	Normal Urine Output
Infants and young children	1.5 to 2 mL/kg per hour
Older children and adolescents	1 mL/kg per hour

Initial urine output on placement of a catheter represents the amount of urine currently held in the bladder. Subsequent measurements over time reflect ongoing urine production. Decreased urine output in the absence of known renal disease is typically a sign of hypovolemia. If urine output is low because of hypovolemic shock, it should improve with adequate fluid resuscitation.

High glucose acts like an osmotic diuretic, resulting in increased urine output and glucosuria. The blood glucose concentration is easy to detect using a bedside glucose test.

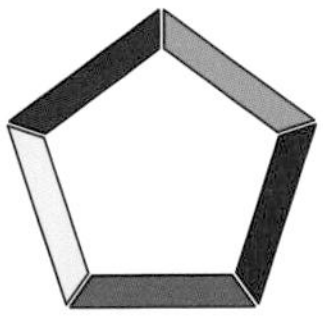

D

Disability

Disability Assessment

The disability assessment is a quick evaluation of 2 main components of the central nervous system: the cerebral cortex and the brainstem. Perform this evaluation at the end of the primary assessment, and repeat it during the secondary assessment to monitor for changes in the child's neurologic status. The disability assessment establishes the child's level of consciousness. Standard evaluations include

- AVPU Pediatric Response Scale
- Glasgow Coma Scale (GCS)
- pupillary response to light

AVPU

To rapidly evaluate cerebral cortex function, use the AVPU Pediatric Response Scale.[10] This scale is a system for rating a child's level of consciousness, an indicator of cerebral cortex function. The scale consists of 4 ratings:

A	Alert	The child is awake, active, and appropriately responsive to parents and external stimuli. "Appropriate response" is assessed in terms of the anticipated response based on the child's age and the setting or situation.
V	Voice	The child responds only when the parents or you call the child's name or speak loudly.
P	Painful	The child responds only to a painful stimulus, such as pinching the nail bed.
U	Unresponsive	The child does not respond to any stimulus.

Causes of a decreased level of consciousness in children include

- poor cerebral perfusion, such as from increased ICP
- traumatic brain injury
- encephalitis, meningitis
- hypoglycemia
- drugs
- hypoxemia
- hypercarbia

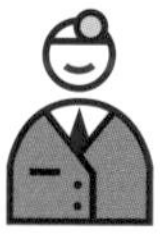

If an ill or injured child has an altered level of consciousness, immediately assess oxygenation, ventilation, and perfusion.

GCS Overview

The Glasgow Coma Scale (GCS) is the most widely used method of defining a child's level of consciousness and neurologic status. The child's *best* eye opening (E), verbal (V), and motor (M) responses are individually scored. The individual scores are then added together to produce the GCS score.

For example: A child who has spontaneous eye opening (E = 4), who is fully oriented (V = 5), and who is able to follow commands (M = 6) is assigned a GCS score of 15, the highest possible score. A child with no eye opening (E = 1), no verbal response (V = 1), and no motor response (M = 1) to a painful stimulus is assigned a GCS score of 3, the lowest possible score.

Head injury severity is categorized into 3 levels based on GCS score after initial resuscitation:

- Mild head injury: GCS 13 to 15
- Moderate head injury: GCS 9 to 12
- Severe head injury: GCS 3 to 8

GSC Scoring

The GCS has been modified for preverbal or nonverbal children (Table 5: Modified Coma Scale for Infants). Scores for eye opening are essentially the same as for the standard GCS. The best motor response score (of a possible 6) requires that a child follow commands, so this section was adapted to accommodate the preverbal or nonverbal child. The verbal score was also adapted to assess age-appropriate responses.

Important: When using the Glasgow Coma Scale or its pediatric modification, record the individual components of the score.

Table 5. Glasgow Coma Scale[11] for Adults and Modified Glasgow Coma Scale for Infants and Children*

Response	Adult	Child	Infant	Coded Value
Eye opening	Spontaneous	Spontaneous	Spontaneous	4
	To speech	To speech	To speech	3
	To pain	To pain	To pain	2
	None	None	None	1
Best verbal response	Oriented	Oriented, appropriate	Coos and babbles	5
	Confused	Confused	Irritable, cries	4
	Inappropriate words	Inappropriate words	Cries in response to pain	3
	Incomprehen-sible sounds	Incomprehensible words or nonspecific sounds	Moans in response to pain	2
	None	None	None	1
Best motor response†	Obeys	Obeys commands	Moves spontaneously and purposely	6
	Localizes	Localizes painful stimulus	Withdraws in response to touch	5
	Withdraws	Withdraws in response to pain	Withdraws in response to pain	4
	Abnormal flexion	Flexion in response to pain	Decorticate posturing (abnormal flexion) in response to pain	3
	Extensor response	Extension in response to pain	Decerebrate posturing (abnormal extension) in response to pain	2
	None	None	None	1
Total score				**3-15**

*Modified from Davis RJ, et al. Head and spinal cord injury. In: Rogers MC, ed. *Textbook of Pediatric Intensive Care.* Baltimore, Md: Williams & Wilkins; 1987. James H, Anas N, Perkin RM. *Brain Insults in Infants and Children.* New York, NY: Grune & Stratton; 1985. Morray JP, et al. Coma scale for use in brain-injured children. *Crit Care Med.* 1984;12:1018. Reproduced with permission from Hazinski MF. Neurologic disorders. In: Hazinski MF, ed. *Nursing Care of the Critically Ill Child.* 2nd ed. St Louis, Mo: Mosby Year Book; 1992.

†If the patient is intubated, unconscious, or preverbal, the most important part of this scale is motor response. Providers should carefully evaluate this component.

GCS Advantages and Disadvantages

The advantage of the GCS is its objectivity, reproducibility and simplicity. A change of at least 2 points in the GCS score from one assessment to the next indicates a clinically important change in neurologic status. The GCS also has predictive value in head-injured children with regard to ultimate neurologic outcome.

The GCS score has some potential disadvantages. It was validated in adults, and the pediatric modification was validated only in children with traumatic brain injury.[12] It is widely used, however, in children with nontraumatic causes of coma, such as metabolic, toxic or infectious causes. The implications of a low GCS in a drug overdose, for example, are clearly different than a low GCS in a child following a traumatic brain injury.

Pupillary Response to Light

Pupil response to light is a useful indicator of brainstem function. Normally pupils constrict in response to light and dilate in a dark environment. If the pupils fail to constrict in response to direct light stimulus (eg, flashlight directed at the eyes), you should suspect that brainstem injury is present. The pupils are generally equal in size, but slight variations are normal. Irregularities in pupil size or response to light may occur as a result of ocular trauma or other conditions, such as increased intracranial pressure.

During the disability assessment, assess and record the following for each eye:

- Diameter of pupils (in millimeters)
- Equality of pupil size
- Constriction of pupils to light (ie, the magnitude and rapidity of the response of the pupils to light)

The acronym PERRL (**P**upils **E**qual **R**ound **R**eactive to **L**ight) describes the normal pupillary responses to light.

E

Exposure

Exposure Assessment

Exposure is the final component of the primary assessment. You should undress the seriously ill or injured child as appropriate to facilitate a focused physical examination. Remove clothing as necessary an area at a time to carefully observe the child's face, trunk (front and back), extremities, and skin. Institute warming measures as indicated if significant hypothermia is detected. Use blankets and heat lamps if available to ensure that the child does not develop hypothermia.

During this part of the exam, look for evidence of trauma, such as bleeding, burns, or unusual markings suggestive of abuse. Palpate the extremities and note the child's response. If there is obvious tenderness on palpation, you should suspect injury to that area, and you may need to immobilize the extremity. Be sure to include an assessment of core temperature.

Note: Be careful to maintain spine precautions when turning any patient with suspected spine injury.

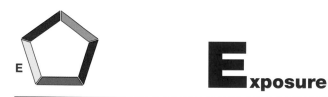

Life-threatening Conditions

Signs of a Life-threatening Condition

Signs of a life-threatening condition include the following:

Airway	Complete or severe airway obstruction
Breathing	Apnea, significant work of breathing, bradypnea
Circulation	Absence of detectable pulses, poor perfusion, hypotension, bradycardia
Disability	Unresponsiveness, depressed consciousness
Exposure	Significant hypothermia, significant bleeding, petechiae/purpura consistent with septic shock, abdominal distention consistent with an acute abdomen

Actions

Start life-saving interventions immediately and activate the ERS in the following circumstances:

- If the patient has a life-threatening condition
- If you are uncertain or "something feels wrong"

If the child does not have a life-threatening condition, initiate the secondary and tertiary assessments.

Secondary Assessment

Introduction

After you complete the primary assessment and appropriate interventions to stabilize the child, your next priority is the secondary assessment.

Components of Secondary Assessment

The components of the secondary assessment are

- focused history
- focused physical exam

SAMPLE

Use the SAMPLE mnemonic to identify important aspects of the child's history and presenting complaint. *Try to gain information that might help explain impaired respiratory, cardiovasular, or neurologic function.*

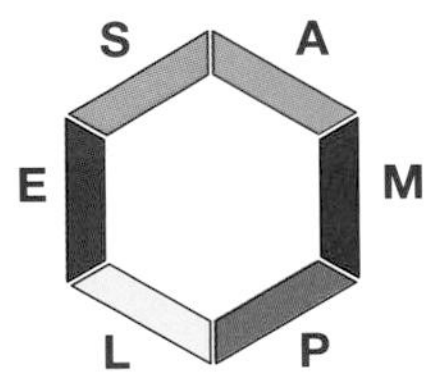

Signs and Symptoms	Signs and symptoms at onset of illness, such as • Breathing difficulty (eg, cough, rapid breathing, increased respiratory effort, breathlessness, abnormal breathing pattern, chest pain on deep inhalation) • Altered level of consciousness • Agitation, anxiety • Fever • Decreased oral intake • Diarrhea, vomiting • Bleeding • Fatigue • Time course of symptoms
Allergies	Medications, foods, latex, etc
Medications	• Medications • Last dose and time of recent medications
Past medical history	• Health history (eg, premature birth) • Significant underlying medical problems (eg, asthma, chronic lung disease, congenital heart disease, arrhythmia, congenital airway abnormality, seizures, head injury, brain tumor, diabetes, hydrocephalus, neuromuscular disease) • Past surgeries • Immunization status
Last meal	• Time and nature of last liquid or food (including breast or bottle feeding in infants)
Events	• Events leading to current illness or injury (eg, onset sudden or gradual, type of injury) • Hazards at scene • Treatment during interval from onset of disease or injury until your evaluation • Estimated time of arrival (if out-of-hospital onset)

Detailed Physical Examination

Next, perform a thorough head-to-toe physical exam. The severity of the child's illness or injury should determine the extent of the physical exam.

Tertiary Assessment

Overview

The tertiary assessment consists of ancillary studies to detect and identify the presence and severity of *respiratory* and *circulatory abnormalities*. Note that some of these tertiary assessments (such as rapid bedside glucose or point of care laboratory testing) may occur early in your evaluation. The term *tertiary* does not mean these are performed third. The timing of tertiary tests is dictated by the clinical situation.

Assessment of Respiratory Abnormalities

Introduction

Several ancillary studies help assess respiratory abnormalities:

Laboratory (blood) studies

- Arterial blood gas (ABG)
- Venous blood gas (VBG)
- Hemoglobin concentration

Nonlaboratory studies

- Pulse oximetry (oxyhemoglobin saturation)
- Exhaled CO_2 monitoring
- Capnography
- Chest x-ray
- Peak expiratory flow rate

Arterial Blood Gas

An arterial blood gas (ABG) analysis measures the partial pressure of arterial oxygen ($Pa{O_2}$) and carbon dioxide ($Pa{CO_2}$) dissolved in the blood plasma (ie, the liquid component of blood).

Measurement	Indicates
$Pa{O_2}$	Adequacy of oxygenation* of arterial blood (but not the oxygen content)
$Pa{CO_2}$	Adequacy of ventilation

*The adequacy of arterial oxygenation can also be derived from pulse oximetry.

Note that a normal $Pa{O_2}$ does not confirm adequate oxygen content of the blood because it reflects only the oxygen dissolved in the blood plasma. If the child's hemoglobin is only 3 g/dL, the $Pa{O_2}$ may be normal or high, but the oxygen delivery to the tissues may be inadequate.

The arterial oxygen saturation can be calculated using the $Pa{O_2}$ and pH, or it may be directly measured using a co-oximeter. Obtain co-oximeter measurement if there is uncertainty about the calculated oxygen saturation and to rule out the presence of carbon monoxide intoxication or methemoglobinemia.

Respiratory failure is traditionally diagnosed on the basis of inadequate oxygenation (hypoxemia) or inadequate ventilation (hypercarbia) as defined by ABG results[13]:

Diagnosis	ABG Result
Hypoxemia	Low $Pa{O_2}$
Hypercarbia	High $Pa{CO_2}$
Acidosis	pH <7.35

This approach is problematic for the following reasons:

- An ABG analysis may not be available (eg, during transport), thereby delaying initiation of therapy.
- A single ABG analysis will not provide information about trends in the patient's condition. Clinical response to therapy is often more valuable.
- Interpretation of ABG results requires consideration of the child's clinical appearance and condition.

For example, an infant with bronchopulmonary dysplasia (a form of chronic lung disease) is likely to have chronic hypoxemia and hypercarbia. Diagnosis of acute respiratory failure in this infant relies heavily on clinical examination and evaluation of arterial pH. The infant will compensate for chronic hypercarbia, and arterial pH will be normal or nearly normal at baseline. Uncompensated worsening hypercarbia leading to measured acidosis will be apparent if the child's respiratory status is significantly worse than the baseline status.

ABG analysis may be used to confirm your clinical impression or to evaluate the child's response to therapy, but it is not required to identify respiratory failure.

Venous Blood Gas

A pH obtained by venous blood gas (VBG) analysis typically correlates with the pH obtained with ABG analysis. But a VBG test is not as useful for monitoring blood gas status (PaO_2 and $PaCO_2$) in acutely ill children. If the child is well perfused, the venous PCO_2 is typically within 4 to 6 mm Hg of the arterial PCO_2. If the child is poorly perfused, however, the gradient between arterial and venous PCO_2 increases. In general, venous PCO_2 is not useful in the assessment of arterial oxygenation.

When interpreting the VBG results you should consider the source of the venous specimen. A peripheral specimen that is free flowing may be close to the ABG, but if a tourniquet is used and the specimen is from a poorly perfused extremity, it will often show a much higher PCO_2 and lower pH than an arterial specimen. A central venous specimen is preferable to a peripheral venous specimen for this reason.

Hemoglobin Concentration

Hemoglobin concentration helps determine adequacy of oxygen-carrying capacity if oxygen saturation is low. Oxygen content is the total amount of oxygen bound to hemoglobin plus unbound (dissolved) oxygen in arterial blood. At normal levels of hemoglobin, the oxygen bound to hemoglobin is the most significant component of total oxygen content in the blood. In other words, oxygen content is determined largely by the hemoglobin concentration (g/dL) and its saturation with oxygen (SaO_2) rather than by the partial pressure of arterial O_2 (PaO_2), which determines the amount of oxygen dissolved in the liquid phase of blood.

$$O_2 \text{ Content} = \text{Oxygen bound to Hemoglobin ([Hb concentration} \times \text{\% saturation)} + \text{Dissolved } O_2 \text{ (}PaO_2 \times 0.003 \text{ mL/mm Hg)}$$

Pulse Oximetry

Pulse oximetry provides a noninvasive estimate (SpO_2) of the arterial oxyhemoglobin saturation (SaO_2). Pulse oximetry can be used to monitor

- adequacy of oxygenation of the blood
- increase in oxygenation in response to treatment

Pulse oximetry should be used during stabilization of a child in respiratory distress or failure. It also should be used during transport for definitive care, including intra-hospital transport.

Pulse oximetry monitors only the oxyhemoglobin saturation. It does not evaluate oxygen content or delivery to the tissues or the effectiveness of ventilation (elimination of CO_2).

Exhaled CO_2 Monitoring

Evaluation of exhaled carbon dioxide can be used to estimate arterial carbon dioxide tension and to confirm ET tube placement. It is particularly accurate (both sensitive and specific) to confirm ET tube placement when the child >2 kg body weight has a perfusing rhythm. Exhaled CO_2 is typically monitored by attaching a carbon dioxide detector to an ET tube to quantify the amount of carbon dioxide present in exhaled gas. Exhaled CO_2 can be monitored by a specially designed nasal cannula.

Capnography

In the intubated patient capnography provides a continuous quantitative measure of end-tidal CO_2 concentration that is displayed as a waveform. In patients with adequate cardiac output and without lower airway obstruction, P_{ETCO_2} (partial pressure of end-tidal CO_2) measured by capnography is a good estimate of Pa_{CO_2}. For some patients this means that repeat assessments of Pa_{CO_2} by ABG analysis can be avoided. For more information about capnography, see Respiratory Management Resources on the student CD.

Chest X-ray

A chest x-ray is useful in respiratory illness to assist in the diagnosis of the following conditions:

- Airway obstruction (upper airway or lower airway)
- Lung tissue disease
- Barotrauma
- Pleural disease (pleural effusion/pneumothorax)

A chest x-ray also can be used to evaluate the depth of ET tube placement, but an anterior-posterior (or posterior-anterior) x-ray will *not* help to determine tracheal versus esophageal placement.

Peak Expiratory Flow Rate

The peak expiratory flow rate (PEFR) represents the maximum flow rate generated during forced expiration. Measurement of the PEFR requires cooperation, so it must be used in children who are alert, can follow directions, and can provide a maximum effort. The PEFR decreases in the presence of airway obstruction, such as asthma. You evaluate the child's PEFR by comparing measurements with the child's personal best and also with normal values predicted from the child's height and gender. The PEFR measurement should improve in response to therapy. An asthmatic patient in severe distress may not be able to cooperate with PEFR measurements. This in itself suggests that the child has very significant respiratory distress.

Assessment of Circulatory Abnormalities

Introduction

Ancillary studies may be performed to assess circulatory abnormalities. Such studies include

Laboratory Studies

- Arterial blood gas
- Venous blood gas
- Central venous oxygen saturation (Sv_{O_2})
- Total serum CO_2
- Arterial lactate
- Hemoglobin concentration

Nonlaboratory Studies

- Invasive arterial pressure monitoring
- Central venous pressure monitoring
- Chest x-ray
- Echocardiography

Arterial Blood Gas

The arterial pH and bicarbonate (HCO_3^-) concentrations obtained with ABG analysis may be useful in the diagnosis of acid-base imbalances. Arterial blood gas values do not reliably indicate the severity of tissue hypoxia, hypercarbia, or acidosis but are useful to follow over time as an index of improving or worsening tissue oxygenation, as reflected by an increasing base deficit.

Venous Blood Gas

VBG may be used if an arterial sample is unavailable. There is generally adequate correlation with ABG samples to make venous pH useful in the diagnosis of acid-base imbalance.

Central Venous Oxygen Saturation

Venous blood gases may provide a useful monitor of changes in the child's tissue oxygen delivery. Normal venous oxygen saturation (Svo_2) is approximately 70% to 75% assuming arterial oxygen saturation is 100%. Measurement of Svo_2 may be used as a surrogate to help evaluate the adequacy of tissue oxygen delivery (ie, the product of cardiac output and arterial oxygen content). Alternatively, Svo_2 may be interpreted by knowing that there should be a 25% to 30% absolute difference between the arterial and central venous oxygen saturation. For example, if the child has cyanotic heart disease and the arterial oxygen saturation is 80%, then the Svo_2 should be approximately 55%. If the flow to the tissues is low, more oxygen is consumed and the Svo_2 is lower. For more information about Svo_2, see the Management of Shock chapter.

Total Serum CO_2

The total serum CO_2 is the total amount of carbon dioxide in the blood. It is present in 3 forms:

- Bicarbonate (HCO_3^-)
- Carbonic acid (H_2CO_3)
- Dissolved CO_2

The total serum CO_2 predominantly reflects the serum bicarbonate concentration. On an electrolyte panel it is often called the bicarbonate concentration, although this is technically incorrect. Total CO_2 can be used to evaluate the severity of an acid-base imbalance and determine whether the etiology is primarily metabolic (due to increased or decreased levels of bicarbonate). It is an important element of the anion gap equation, helping to identify if an acidosis is due to the presence of unmeasured anions.

Arterial Lactate

The arterial concentration of lactate reflects the balance between lactate production and use. In seriously ill or injured patients, the arterial lactate can rise as the result of increased production of lactate (metabolic acidosis) associated with tissue hypoxia and anaerobic metabolism. Arterial lactate is easy to measure, is a good prognostic indicator, and can be followed sequentially to assess the child's response to therapy.

Lactate concentration may also be elevated in conditions associated with increased glucose production, such as stress hyperglycemia. It does not always represent tissue ischemia when the concentration is increased, especially when there is no accompanying metabolic acidosis. In general, following lactate concentrations over time is useful because the failure of the lactate concentration to fall in response to therapy is more predictive of outcome than the initial lactate concentration.

Central venous lactate concentration can be followed if arterial concentrations are not readily available. Again, the trend in the concentrations over time is more predictive than the initial concentration.

Hemoglobin Concentration

Since hemoglobin (Hgb) is the major substance that transports oxygen in the blood, the hemoglobin concentration indicates the oxygen-carrying capacity of the blood. You can use the total hemoglobin concentration (Hgb) to calculate the total amount of oxygen bound to hemoglobin (mL oxygen/dL blood).

Invasive Arterial Pressure Monitoring

Invasive arterial pressure monitoring enables continuous evaluation and display of the systolic and diastolic blood pressure. The arterial waveform pattern may provide information about systemic vascular resistance and visual indications of a compromise in cardiac output (eg, pulsus paradoxus or alternating strength of pulse waveform with positive-pressure ventilation). Invasive arterial pressure monitoring requires an arterial cannula, a monitoring line, a transducer, and a monitoring system.

Central Venous Pressure Monitoring

Central venous pressure can be monitored through a central venous catheter. Measurement of central venous pressure may provide helpful information to guide fluid and vasoactive therapy.

The triad of low arterial blood pressure, high central venous pressure, and tachycardia is consistent with poor myocardial contractility, extrinsic cardiac compression (eg, tension pneumothorax, cardiac tamponade, or excessive positive end-expiratory pressure), or obstruction of pulmonary arterial flow (severe pulmonary hypertension or massive pulmonary embolus).

Chest X-Ray

The chest x-ray can be used in assessment of circulatory abnormalities to assess heart size and the presence or absence of congestive heart failure (pulmonary edema). A small heart implies that preload is reduced; a large heart suggests normal or increased preload or pericardial effusion.

Echocardiography

Echocardiography is a valuable noninvasive tool for imaging

- cardiac chamber size
- wall thickness
- wall motion (contractility)
- valve configuration and motion
- pericardial space
- estimated ventricular pressures
- interventricular septal position
- congenital anomalies

It can be useful in the diagnosis and evaluation of cardiac disease. Technical expertise in performing and interpreting the echocardiogram is essential.

References

1. Nadkarni VM, Larkin GL, Peberdy MA, et al. First documented rhythm and clinical outcome from in-hospital cardiac arrest among children and adults. *Jama*. Jan 4 2006;295(1):50-57.

2. Dieckmann R, Gausche-Hill M, Brownstein D, eds. *Pediatric Education for Prehospital Professionals*. Sudbury, Mass: Jones and Barlett Publishers, American Academy of Pediatrics; 2000.

3. Hazinski M. Children are different. In: Hazinski M, ed. *Manual of Pediatric Critical Care*. St. Louis, Mo: Mosby-Year Book; 1999.

4. Singer JI, Losek JD. Grunting respirations: chest or abdominal pathology? *Pediatr Emerg Care*. Dec 1992;8(6):354-358.

5. Gorelick MH, Shaw KN, Baker MD. Effect of ambient temperature on capillary refill in healthy children. *Pediatrics*. 1993 Nov 1993;92(5):699-702.

6. Gillette PC, Garson A, Jr., Porter CJ, et al. Dysrhythmias. In: Adams FH, Emmanouildies GC, Riemenschneider TA, eds. *Moss' Heart Disease in Infants, Children and Adolescents*. 4th ed. Baltimore, MD: Williams & Wilkins; 1989:725-741.

7. National High Blood Pressure Education Program Working Group on High Blood Pressure in Children and Adolescents. The fourth report on the diagnosis, evaluation, and treatment of high blood pressure in children and adolescents. *Pediatrics*. 2004;114(Suppl 2):1-22.

8. Gemelli M, Manganaro R, Mami C, et al. Longitudinal study of blood pressure during the 1st year of life. *Eur J Pediatr.* Feb 1990;149(5):318-320.

9. *Fourth Report on the Diagnosis, Evaluation, and Treatment of High Blood Pressure in Children and Adolescents:* NHLBI; May 2004.

10. Hannan EL, Farrell LS, Meaker PS, et al. Predicting inpatient mortality for pediatric trauma patients with blunt injuries: a better alternative. *J Pediatr Surg.* Feb 2000;35(2):155-159.

11. Teasdale G, Jennett B. Assessment of coma and impaired consciousness: a practical scale. *Lancet*. 1974 Jul 13 1974;2(7872):81-84.

12. Holmes JF, Palchak MJ, MacFarlane T, et al. Performance of the pediatric Glagow Coma Scale in children with blunt head trauma. *Acad Emerg Med.* 2005;12:814-819.

13. Downes JJ, Fulgencio T, Raphaely RC. Acute respiratory failure in infants and children. *Pediatr Clin North Am.* 1972;19:423-445.

Chapter 2

Recognition of Respiratory Distress and Failure

Overview

Introduction

It is not difficult to distinguish a child who is breathing from one who is not. But it can be difficult to distinguish on clinical grounds a child who is merely working hard to breathe (in respiratory distress) from one who is deteriorating toward full respiratory arrest (in respiratory failure). You must be alert to respiratory conditions that are treatable with simple measures (eg, administration of oxygen or nebulized albuterol). It may be even more important to identify respiratory conditions that are subtly yet rapidly progressing toward cardiopulmonary failure. These conditions require timely intervention with more advanced airway techniques (eg, assisted bag-mask ventilation).

Respiratory failure in infants and children can quickly progress to respiratory arrest and then to cardiac arrest. Good outcome (ie, neurologically intact survival to hospital discharge) is more likely following respiratory arrest than following cardiac arrest. Once the child is in cardiac arrest, the outcome is generally poor. You can greatly improve outcome by early recognition and treatment of respiratory distress and respiratory failure (and even respiratory arrest) before deterioration to cardiac arrest.

The earlier you detect respiratory distress or respiratory failure and start appropriate therapy, the better chance the child has for a good outcome.

Learning Objectives

After completing this section, you should be able to

- recognize the signs of inadequate oxygenation and inadequate ventilation
- define respiratory distress and respiratory failure
- recognize signs that a child is in respiratory distress or respiratory failure
- recall the categories of respiratory problems (type and severity)

Fundamental Factors Associated With Respiratory Problems

Treatment of the seriously ill or injured child with respiratory distress or failure requires an understanding of fundamental factors associated with abnormal breathing in respiratory illness. The next two sections discuss

- impairment of oxygenation and ventilation in respiratory illness
- physiology of breathing in respiratory illness

Impairment of Oxygenation and Ventilation in Respiratory Problems

Physiologic Role of the Respiratory System

The main role of the respiratory system is to exchange gases. Oxygen is taken into the lungs through inspiration and diffuses across the alveoli into the blood to dissolve in the plasma and attach to hemoglobin (oxygenation). Carbon dioxide (CO_2) diffuses from the blood across the capillaries into the alveoli, where it is excreted through expiration (ventilation). Acute respiratory problems can result from any airway, pulmonary, or neuromuscular disease that impairs oxygenation or ventilation.

The pediatric patient has a high metabolic rate, so oxygen demand is high per kilogram of body weight. Oxygen consumption in infants is 6 to 8 mL/kg per minute, compared with 3 to 4 mL/kg per minute in adults.[1] For this reason, in the presence of apnea or inadequate alveolar ventilation, hypoxemia and potential tissue hypoxia can develop more rapidly in the child than in the adult.

The presence and severity of respiratory problems may result in

- hypoxemia—inadequate arterial blood oxygenation
- hypercarbia—inadequate ventilation
- both hypoxemia and hypercarbia

Hypoxemia (Inadequate Oxygenation)

Inadequate oxygenation of blood results in hypoxemia, a decreased oxyhemoglobin saturation in the blood. Pulse oximetry gives a noninvasive estimate of arterial oxygen saturation ($Sa{O_2}$) by calculating the saturation of oxyhemoglobin ($Sp{O_2}$). A room air $Sp{O_2}$ <94% in a normal child indicates hypoxemia.

Tissue hypoxia is present when tissue oxygenation is inadequate. The child may initially compensate by increasing respiratory rate and effort to increase arterial oxygenation. In addition, the child will often have tachycardia to increase cardiac output and help compensate for lower oxygen content by increasing blood flow to maintain oxygen delivery. As tissue hypoxia increases, the clinical signs of cardiorespiratory distress become more severe.

Signs of tissue hypoxia include

- tachypnea
- pallor
- nasal flaring, retractions
- agitation, anxiousness
- cyanosis (late)
- altered mental status
- fatigue
- bradypnea, apnea (late)
- tachycardia (early)
- bradycardia (late)

It is important to distinguish between *tissue hypoxia* and *hypoxemia*. When tissue hypoxia is present, oxygen delivery to the tissues is inadequate. Hypoxemia is a low arterial oxygen saturation defined by consensus as an arterial oxygen saturation <94%. Note that hypoxemia does not always lead to tissue hypoxia. Compensatory mechanisms may increase blood flow and oxygen-carrying capacity (ie, hemoglobin concentration) to maintain tissue oxygenation despite hypoxemia. Conversely, arterial oxygen tension and oxyhemoglobin saturation may be adequate, but arterial oxygen content and oxygen delivery to the tissues may be inadequate.

Additional terms are sometimes used to describe the etiology of tissue hypoxia:

- Hypoxemic hypoxia—arterial oxygen saturation is reduced
- Anemic hypoxia—arterial oxygen saturation is normal, but total oxygen content of the blood is reduced by a low hemoglobin concentration. This state leads to inadequate oxygen-carrying capacity.
- Ischemic hypoxia—blood flow to the tissues is too low. Both hemoglobin concentration and oxygen saturation may be normal, but intense vasoconstriction, poor cardiac pumping function, hypovolemia, or other conditions lead to low tissue blood flow.
- Histotoxic (cytotoxic) hypoxia—the quantity of oxygen reaching the tissue is normal, but the tissue is unable to use the oxygen (eg, with cyanide or carbon monoxide poisoning).

Oxygenation of the tissues is determined by several factors, such as hemoglobin concentration. Arterial oxygen content is the quantity of oxygen bound to hemoglobin plus unbound (dissolved) oxygen in arterial blood. It is determined largely by the hemoglobin (Hgb) concentration (g/dL) and its saturation with oxygen (Sa_{O_2}). Use the following equation to calculate arterial oxygen content:

$$\text{Arterial Oxygen Content} = [1.36 \times \text{Hgb concentration} \times Sa_{O_2}] + (0.003 \times Pa_{O_2})$$

Under normal conditions the dissolved oxygen term ($0.003 \times Pa_{O_2}$) is an inconsequential portion of total arterial oxygen content. But an increase in dissolved oxygen can substantially increase arterial oxygen content in a child with severe anemia.

Precipitating factors leading to respiratory distress and failure may cause hypoxemia by several mechanisms (Table).

Table. Mechanisms of Hypoxemia

Factor	Mechanism	Treatment	Causes
Low ambient Po_2	Decreased Pao_2	Supplementary oxygen	Increase in altitude (decreased barometric pressure)
Alveolar hypoventilation	Increased arterial carbon dioxide tension ($Paco_2$ or hypercarbia) displaces alveolar O_2, resulting in decreased alveolar and arterial oxygen tension (Pao_2 or hypoxemia)	Restore normal ventilation; supplementary oxygen	• CNS infection • Traumatic brain injury • Drug overdose
Diffusion defect	Impaired movement of O_2 and CO_2 across the alveolar/capillary membrane, resulting in decreased Pao_2 and if severe, an increased $Paco_2$ (hypercarbia)	Supplementary oxygen with continuous positive airway pressure (CPAP) or advanced airway with ventilation and positive end-expiratory pressure (PEEP)	• Alveolar proteinosis • Interstitial pneumonia
Ventilation/perfusion (V/Q) imbalance	Mismatch of ventilation and perfusion allowing inadequately oxygenated blood to pass through the lung, resulting in decreased Pao_2 and to a lesser extent increased $Paco_2$ (hypercarbia)	PEEP to increase the mean airway pressure*; supplementary oxygen; ventilatory support	• Pneumonia • Acute respiratory distress syndrome (ARDS) • Asthma • Bronchiolitis • Aspiration pneumonia
Shunt	Absolute/fixed shunting or perfusion of nonventilated areas of the lung, resulting in decreased Pao_2 and eventual increase in $Paco_2$	Correction of defect (supplementary oxygen alone is insufficient)	• Intracardiac (cyanotic congenital heart disease) • Extracardiac (pulmonary) • Same causes listed for V/Q imbalance†

*The use of PEEP in children with asthma should be carefully titrated with expert consultation.

†With pneumonia, ARDS, and other lung tissue diseases, the pathophysiology is often characterized by a mix of V/Q mismatch and absolute shunting of blood through completely nonventilated lung units.

Hypercarbia (Inadequate Ventilation)

Inadequate alveolar ventilation results in hypercarbia, ie, increased CO_2 tension ($Paco_2$) in the blood.

CO_2 is a byproduct of tissue metabolism. It normally is eliminated by the lungs to maintain acid-base homeostasis. When ventilation is inadequate, CO_2 elimination decreases and the $Paco_2$ rises, producing a respiratory acidosis. Inadequate ventilation may be due to decreased respiratory effort (central hypoventilation). It can also result from airway disease or lung tissue disease.

> *Hypoxemia is readily detected noninvasively with pulse oximetry monitoring. Hypercarbia, however, is more difficult to detect because of overlap of clinical signs with hypoxemia and requires invasive measurement to confirm.*

A child with inadequate ventilation typically presents with tachypnea (an attempt to eliminate excess CO_2). An exception is the child with impaired respiratory drive induced by drugs or the central nervous system and resulting in hypercarbia without a compensatory increase in respiratory rate. Detection of the child with inadequate respiratory drive requires careful observation and assessment. Consequences of inadequate ventilation become more severe as the partial pressure of CO_2 in the blood rises and respiratory acidosis worsens.

Signs of inadequate ventilation are somewhat nonspecific and include one or more of the following:

- Tachypnea or inadequate respiratory rate for age and clinical condition
- Nasal flaring, retractions
- Agitation, anxiety
- Altered mental status

It is extremely important that you monitor for evidence of inadequate ventilation. The clinical signs of inadequate ventilation and hypoxemia may be identical. When a child presents with evidence of hypoxemia, administer oxygen to increase oxygen saturation in the blood. You can detect hypercarbia with an arterial blood gas test (if readily available).

One critical indicator of inadequate ventilation is *altered mental status*. If hypoxemia is being treated with supplementary oxygen but CO_2 concentration is increasing, the child's clinical condition will progress from agitation and anxiety to decreased responsiveness.

Note that even if the pulse oximeter indicates adequate oxyhemoglobin saturation, ventilation can still be impaired. If the child demonstrates decreased level of consciousness despite adequate oxygenation, you should suspect that ventilation is inadequate and that hypercarbia and respiratory acidosis may be present.

Physiology of Breathing in Respiratory Problems

Introduction

Normal spontaneous breathing is accomplished with minimal work. Breathing is quiet with easy inspiration and passive expiration. In children with respiratory disease, the "work of breathing" increases with increased use of respiratory muscles. Factors that contribute to increased work of breathing are increased airway resistance (upper or lower) and decreased lung compliance. The effectiveness of respiration is also affected by muscle tone, strength, and coordination and by central nervous system control of breathing.

Important components of the mechanism of breathing include

- airway resistance (upper and lower)
- lung compliance
- muscles of respiration
- central nervous system control of breathing

Airway Resistance

Airway resistance is the impedance to airflow caused by forces of friction. Resistance is primarily increased by reduction in the size of the conducting airways (either by airway constriction or inflammation).

Larger airways have lower resistance to airflow. Airway resistance decreases as lung volume increases because of the airway dilation that accompanies lung inflation. Airway resistance is also affected by the number of parallel airways present: the large and medium-sized airways provide greater resistance to airflow than do the more numerous small airways because the cumulative cross-sectional area of the larger airways is smaller than the cumulative small airway area.

Increased airway resistances may be caused by turbulent airflow, such as during crying, and decreased airway size. Decreased airway size may result from edema, bronchoconstriction, secretions, mucus, or a mediastinal mass impinging on large airways. Resistance in the upper airway, particularly in the nasal or nasopharyngeal passages in infants, may also significantly contribute to airway resistance.

Work of breathing increases in an attempt to maintain airflow despite an increase in airway resistance.

Airway Resistance in Laminar Airflow

During normal breathing, airflow is laminar with relatively low resistance. That is, only a small driving pressure (difference in pressure between the pleural space and the atmosphere) is needed to produce adequate airflow. When airflow is laminar (quiet), resistance to airflow is inversely proportional to the *fourth* power of the airway radius. Any reduction in airway diameter results in an exponential increase in airway resistance and work of breathing (see the Figure).

Airway Resistance in Turbulent Airflow

Resistance is higher when airflow is turbulent. In turbulent airflow, resistance is inversely proportional to the *fifth* power of the radius of the airway lumen. In this state a larger driving pressure is required to produce the same rate of airflow. Therefore, patient agitation with rapid, turbulent airflow results in a much greater increase in airway resistance and work of breathing than that seen with laminar flow. To prevent generation of turbulent airflow (eg, during crying), try to keep a child with airway obstruction as calm as possible.

Figure. Effects of edema on airway resistance in the infant versus the adult. Normal airways are shown on the left; edematous airways (with 1 mm of circumferential edema) are on the right. Resistance to flow is inversely proportional to the *fourth* power of the radius of the airway lumen for laminar flow and to the *fifth* power for turbulent flow. The net result is a 75% decrease in cross-sectional area and a 16-fold increase in airway resistance in the infant versus a 44% decrease in cross-sectional area and a 3-fold increase in airway resistance in the adult during quiet breathing. Turbulent flow in the infant (eg, crying) increases airway resistance and thus the work of breathing from 16- to 32-fold. Modified with permission from Coté and Todres.[2]

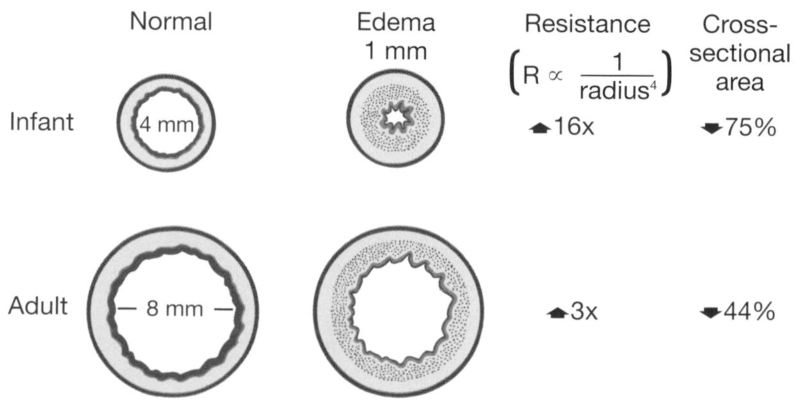

Lung Compliance

Compliance refers to the distensibility (stiffness) of the lung, chest wall, or both. Lung compliance is defined as the change in lung volume produced by a change in driving pressure across the lung. In a child with low lung compliance, the lungs are stiffer, and more effort (ie, driving pressure) is required to inflate the alveoli. In the spontaneously breathing child, increased inspiratory effort reduces the pressure in the pleural space to a level well less than atmospheric pressure to create airflow into the lung. During mechanical ventilation, increased positive airway pressure is needed to achieve adequate ventilation when lung compliance is decreased.

> *Work of breathing increases in an attempt to maintain airflow despite decreased lung compliance.*

Compliance varies within the lung according to the degree of lung inflation. Extrapulmonary conditions that cause decreased compliance are pneumothorax and pleural effusion. Intrapulmonary conditions that cause decreased compliance are pneumonia and inflammatory lung tissue disease (eg, ARDS, fibrosis). These conditions are associated with an increase in the water content in the interstitial space and alveoli. The impact of this increase in water content on lung compliance is similar to the expansion properties of a wet sponge versus a normal sponge. A normal sponge reexpands quickly when it is compressed. A wet sponge is harder to compress and reexpands more slowly because its normal elasticity is opposed by the extra weight of the fluid.

The chest wall of infants and young children is compliant. This means that relatively small pressure changes can move the chest wall. During normal breathing diaphragm contraction in infants pulls the lower ribs in slightly but does not result in sinking in of the chest. Conversely, forceful contraction of the diaphragm results in a greater drop in the pressure within the chest compared with atmospheric pressure, pulling the chest inward during normal breathing. When lung compliance is reduced, maximum inspiratory effort may not produce adequate tidal volume because marked inspiratory retractions of the chest wall limit lung expansion during inspiration. Similarly, children with neuromuscular disorders have a weak chest wall and weak respiratory muscles that make breathing and coughing ineffective and result in the characteristic seesaw breathing seen with neuromuscular weakness.

Muscles of Respiration

During spontaneous breathing the inspiratory muscles (chiefly the diaphragm) increase intrathoracic volume, which results in a fall in intrathoracic pressure. When intrathoracic pressure is less than atmospheric pressure, air flows into the lungs (inspiration). The inspiratory muscles include

- diaphragm (main muscle)
- intercostals
- accessory muscles

Normally the intercostal muscles stiffen the chest wall as the diaphragm contracts. Diaphragm contraction creates a sufficient fall in intrathoracic pressure to produce airflow into the lungs. The accessory muscles of respiration are not typically needed during normal ventilation. In respiratory disorders that increase airway resistance or reduce lung compliance, accessory muscles may be needed to help create the fall in intrathoracic pressure and maintain adequate chest wall stiffness to produce inspiratory flow.

During spontaneous breathing *expiratory flow* is primarily a passive process. Expiratory flow results from relaxation of the inspiratory muscles and elastic recoil of the lung and chest wall. These changes increase intrathoracic pressure to a level that is higher than atmospheric pressure. Expiration may become an active process in the presence of increased lower airway resistance. It also may involve muscles of the abdominal wall and the intercostals.

The normal diaphragm is dome-shaped, and it contracts most forcefully when in this shape. When the diaphragm is flattened, as occurs with lung hyperinflation (eg, as in acute asthma), contraction is less forceful and ventilation is less efficient. If movement of the diaphragm is impeded by abdominal distention and high intra-abdominal pressure (eg, gastric inflation) or by air trapping due to airway obstruction, respiration will be compromised. During infancy and early childhood, the intercostal muscles cannot effectively lift the chest wall to increase intrathoracic volume and compensate for the loss of diaphragm motion.

Central Nervous System Control of Breathing

Breathing is controlled by complex mechanisms involving

- brainstem respiratory centers
- central and peripheral chemoreceptors
- voluntary control

Spontaneous breathing is controlled by a group of respiratory centers located in the brainstem. It is regulated mainly by input from central and peripheral chemoreceptors. Central chemoreceptors respond to changes in the hydrogen ion concentration of cerebrospinal fluid, which is largely determined by the level of arterial CO_2 ($Paco_2$). Peripheral chemoreceptors (carotid body) respond primarily to a fall in arterial O_2 (Pao_2), but some receptors also respond to a rise in $Paco_2$.

Breathing can be overridden by voluntary control from the cerebral cortex. Examples of voluntary control include breathholding, panting, and sighing. Conditions such as infection of the central nervous system, traumatic brain injury, and drug overdose can impair respiratory drive, resulting in hypoventilation or apnea.

Categorization of Respiratory Problems by Severity

Respiratory Distress

Respiratory distress is a clinical state characterized by increased respiratory rate (tachypnea) and increased respiratory effort (resulting in nasal flaring, retractions, and use of accessory muscles). Respiratory distress can be associated with changes in airway sounds, skin color, and mental status.

Respiratory distress can range from mild to severe. For example, a child with mild tachypnea and a mild increase in respiratory effort with changes in airway sounds is in *mild* respiratory distress. But a child with marked tachypnea, significantly increased respiratory effort, and changes in airway sounds and deterioration in skin color and mental status is in *severe* respiratory distress. Severe respiratory distress can be an indication of respiratory failure.

Clinical signs of respiratory distress typically include some or all of the following:

- Tachypnea
- Tachycardia
- Increased respiratory effort (nasal flaring, retractions)
- Abnormal airway sounds (eg, stridor, wheezing, grunting)
- Pale, cool skin
- Changes in mental status

These indicators may vary in severity.

Respiratory distress is apparent when a child tries to maintain adequate gas exchange despite airway obstruction, reduced lung compliance, or lung tissue disease. As the child tires or as respiratory function or effort deteriorate, adequate gas exchange cannot be maintained. When this happens, clinical signs of respiratory failure develop.

Respiratory Failure

Respiratory failure is a clinical state of inadequate oxygenation, ventilation, or both.

Respiratory failure is often the end stage of respiratory distress. But the child with respiratory failure may have little or no respiratory effort if there is abnormal central nervous system control of breathing. The diagnosis of probable respiratory failure may be made based on clinical findings. But confirmation of respiratory failure may require an arterial blood gas (ABG) analysis, which may not be readily available.

Probable respiratory failure may be recognized clinically by some of the following indicators:

- Marked tachypnea (early)
- Bradypnea, apnea (late)
- Tachycardia (early)
- Bradycardia (late)
- Increased, decreased, or no respiratory effort
- Cyanosis
- Poor to absent distal air movement
- Stupor, coma

Respiratory failure may be caused by upper or lower airway obstruction, lung tissue disease, and disordered control of breathing (eg, apnea or shallow, slow respirations). *When respiratory effort is inadequate, respiratory failure may occur without typical signs of respiratory distress.*

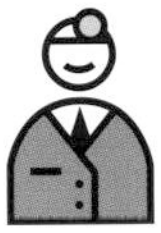

It is difficult to define strict criteria for respiratory failure because the baseline (ie, when not ill) respiratory function of an individual infant or child may be abnormal. For example, an infant with cyanotic congenital heart disease and a baseline arterial oxygen saturation (SaO_2) of 75% is not in respiratory failure based on his oxygen saturation. But that degree of hypoxemia would be a sign of respiratory failure in a child with normal baseline cardiopulmonary physiology.

Respiratory failure may be functionally characterized as a clinical state that *requires intervention* to prevent respiratory arrest and ultimately cardiac arrest.

Classification of Respiratory Problems by Type

Introduction

Respiratory distress or failure can be classified into one or more of the following types:

- Upper airway obstruction
- Lower airway obstruction
- Lung tissue (parenchymal) disease
- Disordered control of breathing

Respiratory problems do not always occur in isolation. A child may demonstrate one or more types of respiratory distress or failure. For example, a child may have disordered control of breathing due to a head injury and then develop pneumonia (lung tissue disease).

Upper Airway Obstruction

Obstruction of the upper airways (ie, the airways outside the thorax) may occur in the nose, pharynx, or larynx. Obstructions can range from mild to severe. Common causes of upper airway obstruction are foreign-body aspiration (eg, aspiration of food or a small object) and swelling of the tissues lining the upper airway (eg, anaphylaxis, tonsillar hypertrophy, croup, or epiglottitis). A mass that compromises the airway lumen (eg, pharyngeal or peritonsillar abscess or tumor) can also cause upper airway obstruction. Thick secretions obstructing the nasal passages or a congenital airway abnormality resulting in narrowing (eg, congenital complete tracheal rings) are other causes. Upper airway obstruction also may be iatrogenic. For example, subglottic stenosis may develop secondary to trauma induced by endotracheal intubation.

Clinical signs of upper airway obstruction include general signs of increased respiratory rate and effort. Typical signs are observed predominantly during *inspiration* and may include

- tachypnea
- increased inspiratory respiratory effort (inspiratory retractions, nasal flaring)
- change in voice (eg, hoarseness), cry, or presence of a seal-like cough
- stridor (usually inspiratory but may be biphasic)
- poor chest rise
- poor air entry on auscultation

Other signs, such as cyanosis, drooling, cough, or seesaw breathing, may be present. Respiratory rate is often only mildly elevated because rapid rates create turbulent flow and further increase the resistance to airflow.

Lower Airway Obstruction

Obstruction of the lower airways (ie, the airways within the thorax) may occur in the lower trachea, the bronchi, or the bronchioles. Asthma and bronchiolitis are common causes of lower airway obstruction.

Clinical signs of lower airway obstruction include general signs of increased rate and effort. Typical signs occur during *expiration* and include

- tachypnea
- wheezing (expiratory—most common; also inspiratory or biphasic)
- increased respiratory effort (retractions, nasal flaring, and prolonged expiration)
- prolonged expiratory phase associated with increased expiratory effort (ie, expiration is an active rather than a passive process)
- cough

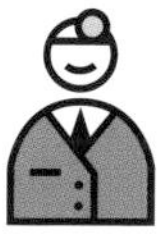

In children with acute lower airway obstruction (eg, status asthmaticus), the increase in intrapleural pressure produced by forced expiration compresses airways proximal to the alveoli. This airway compression leads to further expiratory obstruction with no increase in expiratory flow. If this small airway collapse is severe, it leads to air trapping and lung hyperinflation. With acute severe asthma in the child, the respiratory rate may slow and the child may attempt to increase tidal volume. These responses minimize frictional forces and the work of breathing. In comparison, when lower airway obstruction is present in infants, the respiratory rate tends to be high. The infant has a compliant chest wall. If the infant attempts to breathe more deeply, the greater subatmospheric intrapleural pressure may result in greater chest wall collapse. It is more efficient for the infant to breathe at a fast rate with small tidal volumes to maintain minute ventilation, keeping a relatively larger volume of gas in the lungs when there is significant lower airway obstruction.

Lung Tissue Disease

Lung tissue (parenchymal) disease is a term given to a heterogeneous group of clinical conditions that affect the substance of the lung. Lung tissue disease generally affects the lung at the level of the alveolar-capillary unit and is often characterized by alveolar and small airway collapse or fluid-filled alveoli. For this reason abnormalities in oxygenation and, with severe disease, ventilation are typical. Lung compliance is typically reduced and pulmonary infiltrates are present on chest x-ray.

Lung tissue disease has many causes. Pneumonia from any cause (eg, bacterial, viral, chemical), pulmonary edema (eg, associated with congestive heart failure or capillary leak, such as sepsis), and acute respiratory distress syndrome (ARDS) can cause lung tissue disease. Pulmonary contusion (trauma) is another possible cause. Other potential causes of lung tissue disease include allergic reaction, toxins, vasculitis, and infiltrative disease.

Clinical signs of lung tissue disease are

- tachypnea (often marked)
- tachycardia
- increased respiratory effort
- grunting
- hypoxemia (may be refractory to supplementary oxygen)
- crackles (rales)
- diminished breath sounds

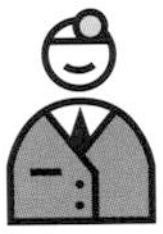

In children with lung tissue disease, ventilation (ie, carbon dioxide elimination) can often be maintained with a relatively small number of functional alveoli whereas oxygenation cannot be maintained. Compromised ventilation, indicated by hypercarbia, is typically a late manifestation of the disease process.

Grunting produces early glottic closure during expiration in an effort to maintain positive airway and prevent collapse in the alveoli and small airways.

Disordered Control of Breathing

Disordered control of breathing is an abnormal breathing pattern that produces symptoms of inadequate respiratory rate, effort, or both. Often the parent will say the child is "breathing funny." Common causes are neurologic disorders (eg, seizures, CNS infections, head injury, brain tumor, hydrocephalus, neuromuscular disease). Because disordered control of breathing is typically associated with conditions that impair neurologic function, these children often have a depressed level of consciousness.

Clinical signs of disordered control of breathing are

- variable or irregular respiratory rate (tachypnea alternating with bradypnea)
- variable respiratory effort
- shallow breathing (frequently resulting in hypoxemia and hypercarbia)
- central apnea (ie, apnea without any respiratory effort)

References

1. Baraff LJ. Capillary refill: is it a useful clinical sign? *Pediatrics*. 1993;92:723-724.

2. Coté CJ, Ryan JF, Todres ID, Groudsouzian NG, eds. *A Practice of Anesthesia for Infants and Children.* 2nd ed. Philadelphia, Pa: WB Saunders; 1993.

Chapter 3

Management of Respiratory Distress and Failure

Overview

Introduction

Respiratory problems are the major cause of cardiac arrest in children. Progressive respiratory insufficiency is the root problem in the majority of infants and children who require CPR, whether in hospital or out of hospital.

There are often no clear clinical indicators that demarcate respiratory distress from respiratory failure. Failure can occur even with few or no signs of distress. Children have unique anatomic and physiologic features of the respiratory system. In children clinical deterioration in respiratory function may progress rapidly. Thus, there is little time to waste debating initial or subsequent steps in management.

Prompt recognition and effective management of respiratory problems are fundamental to pediatric advanced life support.

To optimize patient outcome, PALS providers must intervene quickly to restore respiratory function. If respiratory insufficiency is treated promptly, neurologically intact survival is likely. Once respiratory arrest progresses to cardiac arrest, outcome is generally poor.

Learning Objectives

After completing this chapter, you should be able to

- describe appropriate actions to manage respiratory distress and respiratory failure
- discuss specific actions for management of upper airway obstruction, lower airway obstruction, lung tissue disease, and disordered control of breathing
- explain the use of pulse oximetry and describe its limitations

Initial Management of Respiratory Distress and Failure

Introduction

The primary goal of initial treatment for respiratory distress or failure is to support or restore adequate oxygenation and ventilation. To achieve this goal, you should anticipate and recognize respiratory distress or failure and begin treatment as soon as possible. Since respiratory conditions are the major cause of cardiac arrest, the first priority in the management of any seriously ill or injured child is evaluation of airway and breathing.

Initial intervention for a child in respiratory distress or failure is based on a rapid, focused assessment to categorize the type and severity of respiratory compromise. You should prioritize the initial steps of management based on the type and severity of the child's respiratory compromise rather than the precise etiology of the respiratory problem. Once oxygenation and ventilation are established, identification of the cause of respiratory dysfunction will facilitate targeted interventions. You will need to reassess the child frequently to evaluate response to therapy and prioritize further treatment.

Management of Respiratory Distress and Failure

Initial stabilization and management of a child in respiratory distress or respiratory failure may include the following actions (Table 1):

Table 1. Initial Management of Respiratory Distress or Failure

Assess	Action (as indicated)
Airway	• Support the airway (allow child to assume position of comfort) or open airway (perform manual airway maneuvers). — If a cervical spine injury is suspected, open the airway using a jaw thrust without head extension. If this maneuver does not open the airway, use a head tilt–chin lift or jaw thrust with gentle head extension because opening the airway is a priority. • Clear the airway (suction the nose and mouth as indicated, remove visualized foreign body). • Insert an oropharyngeal airway (OPA) or nasopharyngeal airway (NPA) as indicated.
Breathing	• Assist ventilation (eg, bag-mask ventilation) if needed. • Provide oxygen (humidified if available). Use a high concentration for severe respiratory distress or respiratory failure; use a nonrebreathing system if available. • Continuously monitor oxygen saturation by pulse oximetry. • Prepare for endotracheal intubation as indicated. • Administer medication as needed (eg, albuterol, epinephrine).
Circulation	• Monitor heart rate and rhythm. • Establish vascular access as indicated (for fluid therapy and medications).

Targeted Management Principles

Once oxygenation and ventilation are stabilized, identify the cause of respiratory dysfunction to help determine the best treatment. This chapter discusses targeted management principles for the following 4 types of respiratory illness:

- Upper airway obstruction
- Lower airway obstruction
- Lung tissue (parenchymal) disease
- Disordered control of breathing

Management of Upper Airway Obstruction

Introduction

Upper airway obstruction is a block in the extrathoracic, large airways that may range from mild to severe. Common causes are an aspirated foreign body, tissue edema (above, at, or below the vocal cords), and decreased consciousness resulting in obstruction by the tongue's falling into the posterior pharynx.

Several factors can contribute to airway compromise in infants and children. The tongue is a common cause of upper airway obstruction because it is large in proportion to the oropharyngeal cavity. If the infant with decreased level of consciousness is supine, the large occiput can cause flexion of the neck that can lead to upper airway obstruction. In young infants nasal obstruction may impair ventilation. Secretions, blood, and debris in the nose, pharynx, and larynx from infection, inflammation, or trauma can also obstruct the airway.

General Management of Upper Airway Obstruction

General management recommendations for treatment of upper airway obstruction include the initial actions listed in Table 1. Additional measures focus on relieving the obstruction. These measures may include opening the airway by

- removing an obstructive object
- suctioning the nose or mouth
- reducing airway swelling
- allowing the child to assume a position of comfort
- avoiding unnecessary agitation, which often worsens upper airway obstruction
- deciding if an airway adjunct or advanced airway is needed
- deciding early if a surgical airway (tracheostomy) is needed

Suctioning is helpful if secretions, blood, or debris is present. *But use caution if the cause of upper airway swelling is edema caused by an infection (eg, croup). In many of these patients blind suctioning is relatively contraindicated.* The increased agitation produced by suctioning increases respiratory distress. Instead allow the infant or child to assume a position of comfort, and give a nebulizer treatment of epinephrine or racemic epinephrine if there is swelling of the airway below the tongue. Corticosteroids (inhaled, intravenous, oral, or intramuscular) may also be helpful in this situation.

When upper airway obstruction is severe, *call early* for advanced help. The provider with the greatest skill and experience in airway management is most likely to successfully establish an airway. Failure to treat an acute upper airway obstruction aggressively may lead to complete airway obstruction and ultimately cardiac arrest.

In less severe cases of upper airway obstruction, infants and children may benefit from specific airway adjuncts. For example, an OPA or NPA can be helpful in a child with Pierre Robin Syndrome causing obstruction at the level of the tongue. An OPA should be used only in an unconscious patient because it will stimulate gagging and may cause vomiting in the conscious child. NPAs should be inserted carefully to avoid nasopharyngeal trauma and bleeding. In a child with swelling of the soft tissues of the upper airway due to infection or inflammation, application of continuous positive airway pressure (CPAP) using prongs can be beneficial.

Specific Management Recommendations for Upper Airway Obstruction by Etiology

Introduction

Specific causes of upper airway obstruction require specific treatments. This section gives specific recommendations for management of upper airway obstruction due to the following common causes:

- Croup
- Anaphylaxis
- Other obstruction (eg, foreign-body airway obstruction, retropharyngeal abscess)

Management of Croup Based on Severity

Croup is managed according to your assessment of the clinical severity. Croup severity is described as follows[1-7]:

- Mild croup: occasional barking cough, limited to no stridor at rest, few to no retractions
- Moderate croup: frequent barking cough, easily audible stridor at rest, retractions at rest, little to no agitation, and good distal air entry on auscultation
- Severe croup: frequent barking cough, prominent inspiratory and occasionally expiratory stridor, marked retractions, decreased air entry on auscultation, significant agitation
- Impending respiratory failure: barking cough (may not be prominent if child's respiratory effort is declining secondary to severe hypoxemia and hypercarbia), audible stridor at rest (can be difficult to hear with failing respiratory effort), retractions (may not be marked with failing respiratory effort), poor air movement on auscultation, lethargy or decreased level of consciousness, often dusky skin and mucous membrane color in the absence of supplementary oxygen

Pulse oxygen saturation may be mildly depressed with mild and moderate croup and is commonly suppressed with severe croup.

General management recommendations for treatment of upper airway obstruction include the initial actions described in Table 1. *Specific measures for the management of croup* may include the actions described below.[1-7]

Severity of Croup	Action
Mild	• Consider giving a single oral dose of dexamethasone. • Provide cool mist.
Moderate to severe	• Administer oxygen. • Provide cool mist. • Keep NPO. • Administer nebulized racemic epinephrine or L-epinephrine. • Administer single oral dose or IM dose of dexamethasone. • Observe for at least 2 hours after giving epinephrine for "rebound" (recurrence of stridor). • Consider use of heliox (helium-oxygen mixture).

Severity of Croup	Action
Impending respiratory failure	• Assist ventilation (ie, bag-mask ventilation) if necessary (eg, persistent hypoxemia, inadequate ventilation, or changes in mental status). • Administer a high concentration of oxygen; use a nonrebreathing mask if available. • Perform endotracheal intubation if indicated; to avoid further injury to the subglottic area, use a size of ET tube that is smaller than the size calculated based on age. • Prepare for surgical airway if needed. *Note: If you anticipate rapid sequence intubation using neuromuscular blockade in a child with severe subglottic edema, be sure that you can adequately visualize the airway. If you cannot visualize the airway adequately, it is best to avoid using neuromuscular blockade.* • Administer dexamethasone IV.

Management of Anaphylaxis

In addition to initial management described in Table 1, specific measures for the *management of anaphylaxis* may include the actions described below.[8-10]

Action
Administer IM epinephrine by autoinjector or draw up appropriate dose and give IM or IV depending on severity of symptoms.
Prepare for endotracheal intubation if indicated.
• If bronchospasm (wheezing) is present, administer albuterol by metered-dose inhaler (MDI) or nebulizer solution. • Give continuous nebulization if indicated (ie, severe bronchospasm).
• Administer diphenhydramine and H_2 blocker.
If hypotension is present: • Place in Trendelenburg position as tolerated. • Administer epinephrine by small boluses or infusion titrated to achieve adequate blood pressure for age. • Administer isotonic crystalloid (eg, normal saline [NS] or lactated Ringer's [LR]) 20 mL/kg IV bolus (repeat PRN).
Administer methylprednisolone or equivalent corticosteroid.

Management of Other Obstructions

In addition to the general management recommendations for the treatment of upper airway obstruction, specific measures for the *management of other obstructions* (eg, foreign-body airway obstruction, retropharyngeal abscess) may include the actions described below.

Action
Provide initial support. *In cases of mild to moderate upper airway obstruction* where the child is still breathing effectively: • Allow the child to assume a position of comfort (mild to moderate upper airway obstruction, conscious child)

(continued)

Action
• Administer oxygen in high concentration as tolerated; use a nonrebreathing mask if available *If the child has more severe symptoms:* • Perform jaw thrust or head tilt–chin lift (severe or complete upper airway obstruction, unconscious child) • Proceed immediately for definitive treatment by an appropriately skilled provider (eg, anesthesiologist or otolaryngologist) *If you suspect a foreign body,* try to remove the foreign body as indicated (complete or severe upper airway obstruction where the child is unable to breathe adequately): • For a conscious infant or child, use manual techniques appropriate for age: — <1 year: back slaps and chest thrusts — ≥1 year: abdominal thrusts • If the child becomes unconscious, look in the mouth and remove any visible object. Try to provide bag-mask ventilation. If you cannot provide effective ventilation despite several attempts, proceed to cycles of compressions and attempted ventilation (even if a palpable pulse is present) until specialty assistance is available. Before you give each breath, look in the mouth and remove any visible object. Chest compressions may help displace the object. Note: The *blind finger* sweep is not recommended to relieve an upper airway obstruction. This technique may displace the foreign body further into the airway or cause trauma and bleeding.
Attempt ventilation (ie, bag-mask ventilation) as indicated; may require high inflating pressures—if so, disable pop-off valve if present; consider using a 2-person bag-mask ventilation technique.
Attempt endotracheal intubation as indicated.
Obtain specialty consultation.
Administer nebulized racemic epinephrine or L-epinephrine as indicated (eg, stridor).
Consider chest imaging studies as indicated.
Refer for definitive treatment (eg, bronchoscopy).

Management of Lower Airway Obstruction

Introduction

Lower airway obstruction involves the intrathoracic, smaller airways (eg, bronchi and bronchioles). Common causes are bronchiolitis and asthma.

General Management of Lower Airway Obstruction

General management of lower airway obstruction includes the initial actions described in Table 1.

In infants and children with lower airway obstruction, be careful to provide assisted ventilation at a relatively slow respiratory rate with adequate expiratory time (see below).

In infants or children with respiratory failure or severe respiratory distress, the priority is restoration of adequate oxygenation. Correction of hypercarbia is not as important because children typically tolerate hypercarbia without adverse effects.

> If assisted ventilation is required for lower airway obstruction, perform *bag-mask ventilation at a relatively slow respiratory rate.*

Providing ventilation at a slow rate allows more time for expiration and reduces the risk of air trapping. With a slow rate you can also lengthen the inspiratory time to prevent high airway pressure and its complications. High airway pressure results in gastric distension (air preferentially enters the stomach), which increases the risk of regurgitation and aspiration. High airway pressure also increases the risk of pneumothorax and may compromise venous return and cardiac output. Gastric distension can prevent normal movement of the diaphragm, limiting effective ventilation. Severe air trapping may cause severe hypoxia or significantly reduced cardiac output.

Specific Management Recommendations for Lower Airway Obstruction by Etiology

Introduction

Specific causes of lower airway obstruction require specific treatments. This section gives recommendations for management of lower airway obstruction due to the following common causes:

- Bronchiolitis
- Acute asthma

Note: Distinguishing between bronchiolitis and asthma in the wheezing infant can be difficult. A history of previous wheezing episodes suggests that the infant has reversible bronchospasm (ie, asthma). Consider a trial of bronchodilators if the diagnosis is unclear.

Management of Bronchiolitis

In addition to initial management described in Table 1, specific measures for the *management of bronchiolitis* may include the actions described below.

Action
Perform oral or nasal suctioning as needed.
Perform ancillary testing as indicated: viral studies, chest x-ray, arterial blood gas analysis (ABG).

Randomized controlled trials have shown mixed results following administration of bronchodilators or corticosteroids for bronchiolitis.[11-13] Results of additional trials are awaited. Some infants respond to nebulized epinephrine or albuterol. Nebulized epinephrine has been shown to improve symptoms better than albuterol.[14-16] Other infants may experience worsening of their symptoms with nebulizer therapy. Therefore, consider a trial of nebulized epinephrine or albuterol and discontinue the treatment if there is no benefit.

Management of Acute Asthma

In addition to initial management described in Table 1, specific measures for the *management of acute asthma* may include the actions described below.[17-22]

Asthma is managed according to your assessment of the clinical severity (Table 2).

Table 2. Asthma Severity Score: Classification of Mild, Moderate, and Severe Asthma*

Parameter†	Mild	Moderate	Severe	Respiratory Arrest Imminent
Breathless	Walking Can lie down	Talking (Infant will have softer, shorter cry; difficulty feeding) Prefers sitting	At rest (Infant will stop feeding) Hunched forward	
Talks in	Sentences	Phrases	Words	
Alertness	May be agitated	Usually agitated	Usually agitated	Drowsy or confused
Respiratory rate	Increased	Increased	Often >30/min	
	Age <2 months 2-12 months 1-5 years 6-8 years	**Normal rate** <60/min <50/min <40/min <30/min		
Accessory muscles and suprasternal retractions	Usually not	Usually	Usually	Paradoxical thoraco-abdominal movement
Wheeze	Moderate, often only end-expiration	Loud	Usually loud	Absence of wheeze
Pulse/minute	<100	100-120	>120	Bradycardia
	Guide to limits of normal pulse rate in children: **Age** Infants (2-12 months) Toddler (1-2 years) Preschool/school age (2-8 years)	 **Normal rate** <160/min <120/min <110/min		
Pulsus paradoxus	Absent <10 mm Hg	May be present 10-25 mm Hg	Often present >25 mm Hg (adult) 25-40 mm Hg (child)	Absence suggests respiratory muscle fatigue
PEF after initial bronchodilator % predicted or % personal best	>80%	Approximately 60%-80%	<60% predicted or personal best (<100 L/min adults) or response lasts <2 hours	
Pao_2 (on air)‡ **and/or** **$Paco_2$‡**	Normal, test usually not necessary <45 mm Hg§	>60 mm Hg <45 mm Hg§	<60 mm Hg Possible cyanosis >45 mm Hg; possible respiratory failure	
Sao_2 %	>95%	91%-95%	<90%	

*Reproduced from National Heart, Lung, and Blood Institute and World Health Organization: Global Strategy for Asthma Management and Prevention NHLBI/WHO Workshop Report, US Department of Health and Human Services, Revised September 1997. Publication no. 97-4051.

†The presence of several parameters, but not necessarily all, indicates the general classification of the attack.

‡Kilopescals are used internationally; conversion would be appropriate in this regard.

§Hypercapnia (hypoventilation) develops more readily in young children than in adults and adolescents.

Asthma Severity	Action
Mild to moderate	• Administer humidified oxygen in high concentration; titrate using pulse oximetry. • Administer albuterol by metered dose inhaler (MDI) or nebulizer solution. • Administer corticosteroids PO.
Moderate to severe	• Administer humidified oxygen in high concentrations to keep oxygen saturation >90%; use a nonrebreathing mask if needed. • Administer albuterol by MDI or nebulizer solution. • Administer ipratropium bromide by nebulizer solution. (Note: Albuterol and ipratropium can be mixed together for nebulization made up to a volume of 3 mL with saline.) • Consider establishing vascular access for administration of fluids or medications. • Administer corticosteroids PO/IV. • Consider magnesium sulfate by slow (15 to 20 minutes) IV bolus infusion while monitoring heart rate and blood pressure. • Perform ancillary testing as indicated (eg, ABG, chest x-ray).
Impending respiratory failure	• Administer oxygen in high concentrations; use a nonrebreathing mask if available. • Administer albuterol by continuous nebulizer or by MDI if child is intubated. • Administer ipratropium bromide by nebulizer solution or by MDI if child is intubated. • Assist ventilation (ie, bag-mask ventilation) as indicated. • Consider bilevel positive airway pressure (BiPAP) noninvasive positive-pressure assistance, especially in cooperative children. • Establish vascular access for administration of fluids and medications. • Administer IV methylprednisolone or an equivalent corticosteroid. • Administer terbutaline SQ or IV, titrate to effect while monitoring for toxicity (or use IV salbutamol if available). (Note: You may administer SQ L-epinephrine as an alternative.) • Consider magnesium sulfate IV—watch for hypotension and bradycardia. • Perform endotracheal intubation as needed (preferably performed in-hospital using rapid sequence intubation by airway expert because there is high potential for respiratory and circulatory complications). Consider use of a cuffed ET tube. • Perform ancillary testing as indicated (eg, ABG, chest x-ray).

Management of Lung Tissue Disease

Introduction

Lung tissue disease (also called parenchymal lung disease) refers to a heterogeneous group of clinical conditions. Common causes of lung tissue disease include pneumonia (eg, infectious, chemical, aspiration) and cardiogenic pulmonary edema. Acute respiratory distress syndrome (ARDS) and trauma resulting in pulmonary contusion are other common causes. Lung tissue disease can also result from allergic, vascular, infiltrative, environmental, and other factors.

General Management of Lung Tissue Disease

General management of lung tissue disease includes the initial actions described in Table 1. In children with hypoxemia that is refractory to high concentrations of oxygen alone, specific management of lung tissue disease consists of the use of positive expiratory pressure (CPAP, BiPAP, or mechanical ventilation with PEEP). Treatment may also include administration of bronchodilators if wheezing is present or if there is evidence of airway obstruction. Monitor clinical signs of cardiac output and tissue perfusion and support as necessary.

Specific Management Recommendations for Lung Tissue Disease by Etiology

Introduction

Specific causes of lung tissue disease require specific recommendations. This section gives recommendations for management of lung tissue disease from the following causes:

- Infectious pneumonia
- Chemical pneumonitis
- Aspiration pneumonitis
- Cardiogenic pulmonary edema
- Noncardiogenic pulmonary edema (ARDS)

Management of Infectious Pneumonia

Infectious pneumonia results from inflammation of the alveolar space caused by invasion by bacteria, viruses, or fungi.[23]

A recent study showed that the most common type of bacteria in children with acute community-acquired pneumonia was *Streptococcus pneumoniae. Mycoplasma pneumoniae* and *Chlamydia pneumoniae were less common.*[23] In hospitalized children methicillin-resistant *Staphylococcus aureus* is increasingly common and often causes an empyema.[24]

In addition to initial management described in Table 1, specific measures for the *management of acute infectious pneumonia* may include the actions described below.

Action
Perform ancillary testing as indicated (eg, ABG, chest x-ray, viral studies, complete blood count, blood culture, sputum gram stain and culture).
Administer antimicrobial therapy to treat potential gram-positive organisms such as pneumococcus and methicillin-resistant *Staphylococcus aureus* and consider coverage for mycoplasma or chlamydia with a macrolide antibiotic.
Administer albuterol by MDI or nebulizer solution if wheezing is present.
Consider use of CPAP or BiPAP to reduce the need for mechanical ventilation.
If febrile, reduce temperature, which reduces metabolic demand and thus the need to provide as much minute ventilation.

Management of Chemical Pneumonitis

Chemical pneumonitis is characterized by inflammation of the lung tissue that is caused by inhalation or aspiration of toxic substances. Toxic substances may be liquids, gases, or particulate matter such as dust or fumes. Chemical pneumonitis may also be caused by aspiration of hydrocarbons or inhalation of irritant gases (eg, chlorine). For example, aspiration of hydrocarbons or inhalation of irritant gases (eg, chlorine) can produce noncardiogenic pulmonary edema. This condition is characterized by pulmonary edema resulting from increased capillary permeability.

In addition to initial management described in Table 1, specific measures for the *management of chemical pneumonitis* may include the actions described below.

Action
Administer nebulized bronchodilator if wheezing is present.
Consider use of CPAP or BiPAP to reduce the need for mechanical ventilation.
In children with rapidly progressive symptoms, obtain early consultation and referral to a specialized center because advanced technologies (such as high frequency oscillation or extracorporeal membrane oxygenation (ECMO) may be required.

Management of Aspiration Pneumonitis

Aspiration pneumonitis is a form of chemical pneumonitis. In this condition lung tissue inflammation results from the toxic effects of stomach acid and enzymes along with a reaction to the particulate material and other contents in the stomach.

General management of lung tissue disease includes the initial actions described in Table 1. Specific measures for the *management of aspiration pneumonitis* may include the additional actions described below.

Action
Consider use of CPAP or BiPAP to reduce the need for mechanical ventilation.
Consider administration of antibiotics if an infiltrate is present on the chest x-ray and a fever is present.

Prophylactic antimicrobial therapy is not indicated in aspiration pneumonitis.

Management of Cardiogenic Pulmonary Edema

Cardiogenic pulmonary edema represents the accumulation of fluid in the lung interstitium and alveoli due to elevated pulmonary capillary pressure. Increased capillary pressure can be caused by conditions such as obstruction of pulmonary venous return or blood flow through the left heart or by impaired left ventricular function. The most common cause of acute cardiogenic pulmonary edema is congestive heart failure. Another important cause is acute myocardial dysfunction. Cardiac-depressant drugs (eg, β-adrenergic blockers, tricyclic antidepressants, and verapamil) may also cause this condition. Myocardial infarction is an uncommon cause in children with the exception of a cocaine-induced MI in an adolescent or a congenital anomalous coronary artery in an infant.

In addition to initial management described in Table 1, specific measures for the *management of cardiogenic pulmonary edema* may include the actions described below.

Action
Provide ventilatory support as indicated (ie, noninvasive positive-pressure ventilation or mechanical ventilation with PEEP).
Administer medical therapy to support cardiovascular function as indicated. Consider expert consultation. The advanced provider will reduce left atrial pressure, reduce left ventricular afterload, and provide inotropic or inodilator therapy.
Reduce metabolic demand by reducing temperature and the work of breathing.

Indications for endotracheal intubation and mechanical ventilation in children with cardiogenic pulmonary edema include

- persistent hypoxemia despite maximal noninvasive supplementary oxygen administration
- impending respiratory failure
- hemodynamic compromise (eg, hypotension, severe tachycardia)
- failure of noninvasive ventilation

If mechanical ventilation is needed, PEEP is added to help reduce the need for high oxygen concentrations. It is usually started at 6 to 10 cm H_2O and adjusted until oxyhemoglobin saturation is improved. Too much PEEP may impede venous return and thus cardiac output and oxygen delivery.

In general the goals of medical therapy in cardiogenic pulmonary edema are

- reduction of pulmonary venous return (preload reduction)
- reduction of systemic vascular resistance (afterload reduction)
- reduction of myocardial metabolic demand

Management of Noncardiogenic Pulmonary Edema (ARDS)

Acute respiratory distress syndrome (ARDS) may follow a pulmonary (eg, pneumonia or aspiration) or systemic (eg, sepsis, pancreatitis) insult that injures the alveolar-capillary unit and triggers release of inflammatory mediators. Early recognition and treatment of bacteremia, shock, and respiratory failure may effectively minimize the process that precipitates ARDS.

ARDS is defined by the following:

- Acute onset
- PaO_2/FiO_2 <300 (regardless of PEEP)
- Bilateral infiltrates on chest x-ray
- No evidence for a cardiogenic cause of pulmonary edema

In addition to initial management described in Table 1, specific measures for the *management of ARDS* may include the actions described below.

Action
Initiate monitoring (eg, cardiac, pulse oximetry, end-tidal CO_2).
Obtain laboratory studies such as arterial blood gas, central venous blood gas, and complete blood count.
Provide ventilatory support as indicated (ie, noninvasive pressure support ventilation or mechanical ventilation with PEEP).

The general indication for noninvasive pressure support ventilation or endotracheal intubation with mechanical ventilation in children with ARDS is worsening clinical and radiographic lung disease with hypoxemia that is refractory to high inspired oxygen concentrations. The most important respiratory parameter that needs to be addressed is correction of hypoxemia. "Permissive" hypercarbia is a treatment approach that recognizes that correction of increased $PaCO_2$ is less important. Indeed, keeping the peak inspiratory pressure less than approximately 35 cm H_2O is more important than correcting the $PaCO_2$.

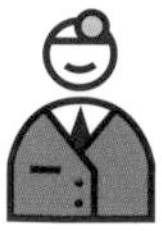

When endotracheal intubation is anticipated in children with lung tissue disease, one should anticipate the need to use PEEP and higher airway pressures. To ensure that both can be provided effectively, a cuffed ET tube may be helpful to prevent glottic air leak. When using a cuffed tube, carefully monitor cuff inflation pressure and maintain less than 20 cm H_2O.[25]

Management of Disordered Control of Breathing

Introduction

Disordered control of breathing results in an abnormal respiratory pattern producing inadequate minute ventilation. Causes include increased intracranial pressure (ICP) and other conditions that depress the level of consciousness (eg, from central nervous system infection, seizures, metabolic disorders such as hyperammonemia, and poisoning or drug overdose). Neuromuscular disease (ie, weakness) can also cause disordered control of breathing.

General management recommendations for treatment of disordered control of breathing include the initial actions described in Table 1.

Specific causes of *disordered control of breathing* require specific treatments. This section provides specific recommendations for management of disordered control of breathing caused by the following common problems:

- Increased intracranial pressure (ICP)
- Poisoning or drug overdose
- Neuromuscular disease

Management of Respiratory Distress/Failure With Increased ICP

Increased ICP can complicate a variety of disorders, including meningitis, encephalitis, intracranial abscess, subarachnoid hemorrhage, subdural or epidural hematoma, traumatic brain injury, hydrocephalus, and central nervous system tumor.

An irregular respiratory pattern can be a sign of increased ICP. The combination of irregular breathing or apnea, a rise in mean arterial pressure, and bradycardia is called "Cushing's triad." It suggests a marked increase in ICP. Cushing's triad typically signals impending brain herniation. Children with increased ICP often present with tachycardia, hypertension, and irregular breathing rather than with bradycardia.

In addition to the general management recommendations described in Table 1, *management of disordered control of breathing due to increased ICP* may include the following actions.

Action
When opening the airway, use a jaw thrust maneuver and manually stabilize the cervical spine if trauma is suspected; keep the head in midline.
Verify patent airway, adequate oxygenation, and adequate ventilation. A brief period of hyperventilation may be used as a temporizing rescue therapy in response to signs of impending brain herniation (eg, irregular respirations, dilated pupil[s] not responsive to light, bradycardia, hypertension, and decerebrate or decorticate posturing).
If the child has poor perfusion or inadequate cerebral perfusion pressure, administer 20 mL/kg IV isotonic crystalloid (NS or LR).
Administer pharmacologic therapy such as hypertonic saline for management of increased ICP.
Treat agitation and pain aggressively once the airway is secured and adequate ventilation is ensured.
Avoid hyperthermia.

Management of Respiratory Distress/Failure in Poisoning or Drug Overdose

One of the most common causes of respiratory distress or failure following a poisoning or drug overdose is depression of central respiratory drive. A less common cause is weakness or paralysis of respiratory muscles.

Frequent complications of disordered breathing in this setting are upper airway obstruction, poor respiratory effort and rate, hypoxemia, aspiration, and respiratory failure. Complications from a depressed level of consciousness such as aspiration pneumonitis and noncardiogenic pulmonary edema may also result in respiratory failure. If poisoning is suspected, contact your local poison control center. For more information on toxicology, see Part 10.2 of the *2005 AHA Guidelines for CPR and ECC*.

Support of airway and ventilation is the main therapeutic intervention in this setting. In addition, *management of disordered control of breathing due to poisoning or drug overdose* may include the following actions.[26]

Action
Administer antidote as indicated.
Contact poison control.
Be prepared to suction the airway if vomiting occurs.
Perform ancillary testing as indicated (eg, ABG, ECG, chest x-ray, electrolytes, glucose, serum osmolality, and drug screen).

Management in Neuromuscular Disease

Chronic neuromuscular disease affects the muscles of respiration in various degrees. Eventually children with these diseases have an ineffective cough and develop complications such as atelectasis, restrictive lung disease, pneumonia, chronic respiratory insufficiency, and respiratory failure. Consider the general management recommendations described in Table 1 for disordered control of breathing due to neuromuscular disease. For children with advanced restrictive lung disease, noninvasive positive pressure ventilation (NPPV) may improve ventilation and comfort, improve sleep-related respiratory parameters, and decrease hospitalizations.

Recall that these children may have severe reactions to the use of succinylcholine for rapid sequence intubation. Several commonly used drugs, such as aminoglycosides, can worsen respiratory muscle weakness due to the intrinsic neuromuscular blocking activity of this class of agents.

References

1. Croup Working Committee. Guideline for the diagnosis and management of croup. Alberta Medical Association Clinical Practise Guidelines (Canada). Available at: http://www.albertadoctors.org/bcm/ama/amawebsite.nsf/AllDocSearch/87256DB000705C3F.
2. Geelhoed GC, Turner J, Macdonald WB. Efficacy of a small single dose of oral dexamethasone for outpatient croup: a double blind placebo controlled clinical trial. *BMJ*. 1996;313:140-142.
3. Westley CR, Cotton EK, Brooks JG. Nebulized racemic epinephrine by IPPB for the treatment of croup: a double-blind study. *Am J Dis Child.* 1978;132:484-487.
4. Kristjansson S, Berg-Kelly K, Winso E. Inhalation of racemic adrenaline in the treatment of mild and moderately severe croup: clinical symptom score and oxygen saturation measurements for evaluation of treatment effects. *Acta Paediatr*. 1994;83:1156-1160.
5. Taussig LM, Castro O, Beaudry PH, et al. Treatment of laryngotracheobronchitis (croup): use of intermittent positive-pressure breathing and racemic epinephrine. *Am J Dis Child*. 1975;129:790-793.

6. Luria JW, Gonzalez-del-Rey JA, DiGiulio GA, et al. Effectiveness of oral or nebulized dexamethasone for children with mild croup. *Arch Pediatr Adolesc Med.* 2001;155:1340-1345.
7. Kairys SW, Olmstead EM, O'Connor GT. Steroid treatment of laryngotracheitis: a meta-analysis of the evidence from randomized trials. *Pediatrics.* 1989;83:683-693.
8. Gold MS, Sainsbury R. First aid anaphylaxis management in children who were prescribed an epinephrine autoinjector device (EpiPen). *J Allergy Clin Immunol.* 2000;106:171-176.
9. Dibs SD, Baker MD. Anaphylaxis in children: a 5-year experience. *Pediatrics*. 1997;99(1):E7.
10. Sampson HA, Mendelson L, Rosen JP. Fatal and near-fatal anaphylactic reactions to food in children and adolescents. *N Engl J Med.* 1992;327:380-384.
11. Ralston S, Hartenberger C, Anaya T, et al. Randomized, placebo-controlled trial of albuterol and epinephrine at equipotent beta-2 agonist doses in acute bronchiolitis. *Pediatr Pulmonol.* 2005;40(4):292-299.
12. Patel H, Platt R, Lozano JM, et al. Glucocorticoids for acute viral bronchiolitis in infants and young children. *Cochrane Database Syst Rev.* 2004(3):CD004878.
13. Schuh S, Coates AL, Binnie R, et al. Efficacy of oral dexamethasone in outpatients with acute bronchiolitis. *J Pediatr.* 2002;140(1):27-32.
14. Langley JM, Smith MB, LeBlanc JC, et al. Racemic epinephrine compared to salbutamol in hospitalized young children with bronchiolitis; a randomized controlled clinical trial [ISRCTN46561076]. *BMC Pediatr.* 2005;5(1):7.
15. Ray MS, Singh V. Comparison of nebulized adrenaline versus salbutamol in wheeze associated respiratory tract infection in infants. *Indian Pediatr.* 2002;39(1):12-22.
16. Bertrand P, Aranibar H, Castro E, et al. Efficacy of nebulized epinephrine versus salbutamol in hospitalized infants with bronchiolitis. *Pediatr Pulmonol.* 2001;31(4):284-288.
17. Ciarallo L, Sauer AH, Shannon MW. Intravenous magnesium therapy for moderate to severe pediatric asthma: results of a randomized, placebo-controlled trial. *J Pediatr.* 1996;129:809-814.
18. Khine H, Fuchs SM, Saville AL. Continuous vs. intermittent nebulized albuterol for emergency management of asthma. *Acad Emerg Med.* 1996;3:1019-1024.
19. Stephanopoulos DE, Monge R, Schell KH, et al. Continuous intravenous terbutaline for pediatric status asthmaticus. *Crit Care Med.* 1998;26:1744-1748.
20. Ciarallo L, Brousseau D, Reinert S. Higher-dose intravenous magnesium therapy for children with moderate to severe acute asthma. *Arch Pediatr Adolesc Med.* 2000;154:979-983.
21. Plotnick LH, Ducharme FM. Combined inhaled anticholinergics and b2 agonists in the initial management of acute paediatric asthma. *The Cochrane Library.* Chichester, UK: John Wiley & Sons; 2003.
22. Smith M, Iqbal S, Elliott TM, et al. Corticosteroids for hospitalized children with acute asthma (Cochrane Review). *The Cochrane Library.* Chichester, UK: John Wiley & Sons; 2003.
23. Michelow IC, Olsen K, Lozano J, et al. Epidemiology and clinical characteristics of community-acquired pneumonia in hospitalized children. *Pediatrics.* 2004;113:701-707.
24. Fridkin SK, Hageman JC, Morrison M, et al. Methicillin-resistant *Staphylococcus aureus* disease in three communities. *N Engl J Med.* 2005;352(14):1436-1444.
25. Parwani V, Hahn IH, Hsu B, et al. Experienced emergency physicians cannot safely or accurately inflate endotracheal tube cuffs or estimate endotracheal tube cuff pressure using standard technique. *Acad Emerg Med.* 2004;11(5):490-491.
26. Olson KR. Emergency evaluation and treatment. In: Olson KR, ed. *Poisoning & Drug Overdose.* 4th ed. New York, NY: Lange Medical Books/McGraw-Hill; 2004.

Chapter 4

Recognition of Shock

Overview

Introduction

Outcomes in critically ill or injured children can be greatly improved with *early recognition and treatment of shock.* If left untreated, shock can quickly progress to cardiopulmonary failure and then cardiac arrest. If the child in shock develops cardiac arrest, the outcome is poor.

This chapter discusses the following topics:

- Physiology of shock
- Effect of different types of shock on blood pressure
- Use of systolic blood pressure to categorize the severity of shock (ie, compensated versus hypotensive shock)
- Causes (etiology) and signs of the 4 common types of shock
- Systematic approach to assessment of the cardiovascular system

Once you *categorize* the child's shock based on type and severity, then you *decide* which life-saving actions to begin. These *actions* are discussed in Chapter 5: Management of Shock.

The earlier you can recognize shock, establish priorities, and start therapy, the better the child's chance for a good outcome.

Learning Objectives

After completing this chapter you should be able to

- explain the basic pathophysiology of shock
- describe how to evaluate clinical signs of systemic perfusion
- differentiate between compensated shock and hypotensive shock
- recall the types of shock (hypovolemic, distributive, cardiogenic, and obstructive)
- recognize clinical signs and symptoms of shock
- explain the elements and interpretation of the systematic assessment evaluating cardiovascular performance

Definition of Shock

Shock is a critical condition that results from inadequate delivery of oxygen and nutrients to the tissues relative to tissue metabolic demand. It is often, but not always, characterized by inadequate perfusion. The definition of shock does not depend on blood pressure; shock may occur with a normal, increased, or decreased systemic arterial pressure. In children most shock is characterized by low cardiac output, but some forms of shock may have a high cardiac output, such as in sepsis or in the child with severe anemia. All forms of shock can result in impaired function of vital organs, such as the brain (depressed mental status) and kidneys (low urine output, ineffective filtering).

Shock can result from

- inadequate blood volume or inadequate oxygen-carrying capacity (hypovolemic shock, including hemorrhagic shock)
- inappropriately distributed blood volume (distributive shock)
- impairment of heart contractility (cardiogenic shock)
- obstructed blood flow (obstructive shock)

Conditions such as fever, infection, injury, respiratory distress, and pain may contribute to shock by increasing tissue demand for oxygen and nutrients. Whether due to inadequate supply of oxygen to the tissues or increased demand of the tissues for oxygen, *tissue perfusion in shock is inadequate relative to metabolic needs.*

Inadequate tissue perfusion can lead to tissue hypoxia, anaerobic metabolism, accumulation of lactic acid and carbon dioxide, and irreversible cell and organ damage. Death may then rapidly result from cardiovascular collapse or later from multiple organ failure.

The treatment goal for shock is to prevent end-organ injury and halt the progression to cardiopulmonary failure and cardiac arrest.

Definition of Tissue Hypoxia

Tissue hypoxia is a pathologic condition in which a region of the body or an organ is deprived of adequate oxygen supply. Low oxygen saturation in the blood (hypoxemia) does not necessarily result in tissue hypoxia. In many hypoxemic children acute compensatory increases in blood flow or chronic increases in hemoglobin concentration (polycythemia) maintain systemic (tissue) oxygen delivery. Tissue oxygenation (oxygen delivery) depends on the amount of blood pumped per minute (cardiac output) and the arterial oxygen content of that blood. The causes of tissue hypoxia fall into the following 4 categories:

- Hypoxemic hypoxia
- Anemic hypoxia
- Ischemic hypoxia
- Histotoxic hypoxia

Hypoxemic Hypoxia

Hypoxemic hypoxia results from reduced arterial oxygen content. It is caused by

- inadequate partial pressure of oxygen in the inspired air (such as at high altitude)
- airway obstruction (upper or lower) that is usually severe
- inadequate alveolar-capillary transfer (eg, lung disease resulting in ventilation/perfusion [V/Q] mismatch or intrapulmonary shunt) often due to lung tissue disease
- intracardiac shunt (eg, congenital heart disease)

Administration of oxygen may be helpful, but oxygen alone may not correct hypoxemic hypoxia. Correction often depends on addressing the underlying cause of low arterial oxygen saturation.

Anemic Hypoxia

Anemic hypoxia is caused by an abnormality in the oxygen-carrying capacity of the blood, specifically a low hemoglobin concentration. These abnormalities include

- excessive blood loss (hemorrhage)
- excessive red blood cell destruction (hemolysis)
- deficient red blood cell production (aplastic anemia or cancer)

Administration of oxygen may not correct anemic hypoxia. It may, however, improve symptoms by increasing the concentration of oxygen dissolved in the blood. The normal compensatory mechanism to maintain oxygen delivery is an increase in cardiac output. The treatment of anemic hypoxia is to restore the hemoglobin concentration (eg, blood transfusion) and manage the underlying problem.

Ischemic Hypoxia

Ischemic hypoxia results from inadequate delivery of oxygen to the tissues because blood flow is insufficient. Hemoglobin concentration and oxygen saturation can be normal. Causes include any condition characterized by a low cardiac output, such as

- hypovolemia
- intense vasoconstriction
- poor heart function
- severe obstruction to blood flow (eg, pulmonary embolus, coarctation of the aorta)

Treatment of the underlying problem is crucial. Oxygen administration is helpful to maximize oxygen content, but it will not correct ischemic hypoxia. Instead, focus efforts on increasing cardiac output and improving tissue perfusion.

Histotoxic Hypoxia

Histotoxic hypoxia (also called cytotoxic hypoxia) results from impaired cellular metabolic (mitochondrial) oxygen use despite normal or even increased oxygen delivery. Causes include

- cyanide poisoning, which inhibits a critical mitochondrial enzyme (cytochrome oxidase)
- carbon monoxide poisoning
- methemoglobinemia

Septic shock is also characterized by disordered mitochondrial function and thus has elements of cytotoxic hypoxia in addition to ischemic hypoxia. Treatment of the cause of cellular poisoning is indicated.

Physiology of Shock

Introduction

The fundamental goal of the cardiorespiratory system is to maintain delivery of oxygen to body tissues and remove the metabolic byproducts of cellular metabolism. When oxygen delivery is inadequate to meet tissue demand, there is high extraction of oxygen from the blood, resulting in low central venous oxygen saturation. As tissue hypoxia worsens, the cells use anaerobic metabolism to produce energy and generate lactic acid as a byproduct of this process. Anaerobic metabolism can only maintain limited cell function. Hypoxic cells become dysfunctional or die, leading to organ dysfunction or failure.

Components of Tissue Oxygen Delivery

Adequate delivery of oxygen to tissues (Figure 1) depends on

- sufficient oxygen content in the blood
- adequate flow of blood to tissues (cardiac output)
- adequate matching of blood flow to local tissue metabolic demand

Oxygen content of the blood is determined by the concentration of hemoglobin and percent of hemoglobin that is saturated with oxygen (SaO_2).

Adequate flow of blood to tissues is determined by both cardiac output and local regulation of blood flow to tissues based on their metabolic demand. Cardiac output is the volume of blood that flows through the tissues in 1 minute. Cardiac output is determined by stroke volume (the volume of blood ejected with each cardiac contraction) and heart rate (the number of cardiac contractions each minute).

$$\text{Cardiac Output} = \text{Stroke Volume} \times \text{Heart Rate}$$

In children low cardiac output is most often the result of low stroke volume rather than low heart rate. In infants, however, stroke volume is relatively fixed, and cardiac output depends more on heart rate. Conversely, with certain toxic ingestions or in children with supraventricular tachycardia, the heart rate may be too fast to permit adequate stroke volume because there is inadequate time to fill the heart (ie, the diastolic phase is too short).

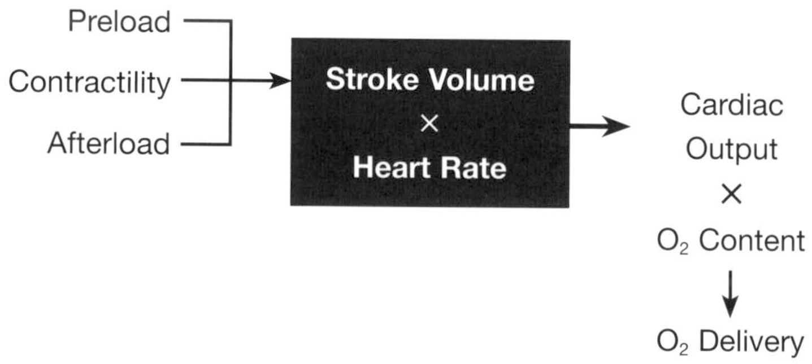

Figure 1. Factors influencing oxygen delivery.

Stroke Volume

Stroke volume is the amount of blood ejected by the heart with each beat. Stroke volume is determined by 3 factors:

Factor	Definition
Preload	Volume of blood present in the ventricle before contraction
Contractility	Strength of contraction
Afterload	Resistance against which the ventricle is contracting

Inadequate preload is the most common cause of low stroke volume and therefore low cardiac output. Inadequate preload may be caused by a number of factors (eg, hemorrhage, severe dehydration, or vasodilation). It results in hypovolemic shock.

Preload is often estimated by the central venous pressure (CVP), but the relationship between this pressure and the volume of blood in the heart is complex. In general, as CVP increases, the amount of blood in the heart at the end of diastole (end-diastolic volume) increases. An increase in the CVP, however, does not always ensure a higher end-diastolic volume. Similarly, a fall in CVP does not always mean that the end-diastolic volume is lower.

Preload is not the same as total blood volume. At steady state, most of the blood (about 70%) is in the veins. If the veins are dilated, the total blood volume may be increased, but an inadequate amount of blood may be returning to the heart. This is part of the problem with sepsis: there is an inappropriate venodilation and maldistribution of blood flow and blood volume.

Poor contractility (myocardial dysfunction) impairs stroke volume and cardiac output and may lead to cardiogenic shock. Poor contractility may be due to an intrinsic problem with pump function or to an acquired abnormality, such as an inflamed heart muscle during myocarditis. Poor contractility may also occur from metabolic problems, such as hypoglycemia or carbon monoxide intoxication.

Increased afterload is an uncommon primary cause of low stroke volume and impaired cardiac output in children, but it commonly affects stroke volume in children with poor contractility. When the heart pumping function is reduced, an increased afterload further compromises stroke volume. An essential component of the treatment of cardiogenic shock is afterload reduction.

Compensatory Mechanisms

To maintain oxygen delivery to the tissues, compensatory mechanisms are activated. Several common compensatory mechanisms are

- Tachycardia
- Increased systemic vascular resistance
- Increased strength of cardiac contraction (contractility)
- Increased venous tone

The body's first line of defense in maintaining cardiac output is to compensate for low stroke volume by increasing heart rate (tachycardia). Tachycardia will increase cardiac output to a point. However, if tachycardia is excessive, ventricular filling time is so abbreviated that stroke volume and cardiac output fall. Assuming that oxygen content remains the same, this reduces oxygen delivery to the tissues.

When decreased cardiac output results in decreased tissue oxygen delivery, the body's second line of defense is to redirect or shunt blood from nonvital to vital organs. This redirection occurs through an increase in systemic vascular resistance (vasoconstriction), which preferentially sends blood to vital organs while reducing flow to nonvital areas, such as the skin, skeletal muscles, gut, and kidneys. Clinically the result is reduced peripheral perfusion (ie, delayed capillary refill, cool extremities, and decreased peripheral pulses).

Another mechanism to maintain stroke volume is to increase the strength of cardiac contraction, resulting in more complete emptying of the ventricle.

The stroke volume may also be maintained by increasing venous smooth muscle tone, resulting in more blood moving from the high capacity venous system to the heart.

Effect on Blood Pressure

An increase in systemic vascular resistance may maintain perfusion pressure to vital organs despite decreased blood flow. As a result the child's systolic blood pressure may be normal or slightly elevated. Pulse pressure is often narrowed. Pulse pressure is the difference between the systolic and diastolic blood pressure. When systemic vascular resistance is increased, the diastolic blood pressure increases. Similarly, if systemic vascular resistance is low (as in sepsis), the diastolic blood pressure decreases, widening the pulse pressure.

Blood pressure is determined by the cardiac output and systemic vascular resistance. If cardiac output continues to fall, the blood pressure will begin to fall when the systemic vascular resistance cannot increase further. Similarly, delivery of oxygen to vital organs will be compromised despite elevated systemic vascular resistance. Clinically end-organ dysfunction occurs, such as impaired mental status and decreased urine output. Ultimately oxygen delivery to the myocardium will become inadequate, causing myocardial dysfunction, decreased stroke volume, and hypotension. This can rapidly lead to cardiovascular collapse, cardiac arrest, and irreversible end-organ injury.

Categorization of Shock by Severity (Effect on Blood Pressure)

Introduction

The severity of shock is frequently characterized by its effect on systolic blood pressure. Shock is described as *compensated* as long as compensatory mechanisms are able to maintain a systolic blood pressure within a normal range (ie, defined as greater than the fifth percentile systolic blood pressure for age). When compensatory mechanisms fail and systolic blood pressure drops, shock is then classified as *hypotensive* (previously referred to as *decompensated* shock).

Hypotensive shock is an easy diagnosis to make when blood pressure measurement is readily available; recognition of compensated shock is more difficult. Shock may range from mild to moderate to severe. The signs and symptoms of shock are affected by the type of shock and the child's compensatory responses. *Severe shock may occur with normal or low blood pressure.* In some cases children will present with low systolic blood pressure but will still maintain adequate blood flow to meet tissue metabolic demand; in these cases metabolic acidosis, decreased central venous oxygen saturation, and elevation of lactate may be mild.

Since blood pressure is an important method of categorizing the severity of shock, it is important to recognize that automated blood pressure devices are accurate only when there is adequate distal perfusion. If you cannot palpate distal pulses and the extremities are cool and poorly perfused, automated blood pressure readings are not always reliable. You should treat the patient based on your entire clinical examination. Likewise, if blood pressure measurement is unavailable, then treatment is guided by your clinical examination of the adequacy of tissue perfusion.

Compensated Shock

If the systolic blood pressure is within the normal range but signs of inadequate tissue perfusion are present, the child is in compensated shock. In this stage of shock the body is able to maintain blood pressure despite impaired delivery of oxygen and nutrients to the vital organs.

Note that the term *compensated shock* refers to the child with signs of poor perfusion but a normal systolic blood pressure (ie, with blood pressure compensation). In the absence of established normative data about mean arterial blood pressure in infants and children, by convention and consensus the systolic blood pressure is used to determine the presence or absence of hypotension with shock. Infants and children with compensated shock may be critically ill with severe shock despite a "normal" systolic blood pressure. Furthermore, automated blood pressure devices can provide normal blood pressure readings (ie, falsely high blood pressure results) in children with severe shock and hypotension. In general, if you cannot palpate the radial or brachial pulses and the central (eg, femoral) pulses are weak or absent, assume that the child is hypotensive. Do not rely on an automated blood pressure device in the child with clinical signs of shock.

Although by definition the systolic pressure is normal in compensated shock, the diastolic pressure may not be normal. For example, in compensated hypovolemic shock, diastolic pressure is increased (due to increased systemic vascular resistance), producing a narrowed pulse pressure.

When oxygen delivery is limited, compensatory mechanisms try to maintain normal blood flow to the brain and heart. These compensatory mechanisms are clues to the presence of shock and vary according to the type of shock. Table 1 lists common compensatory mechanisms in shock and their associated cardiovascular signs.

Table 1. Common Signs of Shock Resulting From Cardiovascular Compensatory Mechanisms

Compensatory Mechanism	Area	Sign
Increased heart rate	Heart	Tachycardia
Increased systemic vascular resistance	Skin	Cold, pale, diaphoretic
	Circulation	Delayed capillary refill
	Pulses	Weak peripheral pulses and narrow pulse pressure (raised diastolic blood pressure)
Increased splanchnic vascular resistance	Kidney Intestine	Oliguria (decreased urine output), vomiting, ileus

Signs specific to shock type are discussed later in this chapter.

Hypotensive Shock

If systolic hypotension and signs of inadequate tissue perfusion are present, the child is in hypotensive shock. Hypotension develops when physiologic attempts to maintain systolic blood pressure and perfusion are no longer effective. One key clinical sign that a child's condition is deteriorating is a change in mental status as brain perfusion declines. Hypotension itself is a late finding in most types of shock and may signal irreversible organ injury or impending cardiac arrest.

Hypotension may be present early in septic shock because of the effects of sepsis on reducing systemic vascular resistance. In this setting the hypotensive child may initially appear alert and responsive. In sepsis the hypotension is caused by release or activation of inflammatory mediators that produce vasodilation and increased capillary permeability. In this case hypotension is an early rather than a late sign of shock.

Hypotension Formula

In children 1 to 10 years of age, hypotension is defined as a systolic blood pressure reading as follows:

$$<70 \text{ mm Hg} + [\text{child's age in years} \times 2] \text{ mm Hg}$$

See Table 4: Definition of Hypotension by Systolic Blood Pressure and Age in Chapter 1.

Physiologic Continuum

You must be alert to the progression of clinical signs that may signal a worsening of the child's condition along the physiologic continuum from compensated shock to hypotensive shock and ultimately to cardiac arrest. Warning signs include loss of peripheral pulses and deterioration in mental status. Bradycardia and weak-to-absent central pulses in a child who is still responsive are ominous signs of impending cardiac arrest.

Accelerating Process

It may take hours for compensated shock to progress to hypotensive shock but only minutes for hypotensive shock to progress to cardiopulmonary failure and cardiac arrest. The progression from compensated shock to hypotensive shock and then to cardiac arrest is typically an *accelerating process.*

Compensated Shock

↓ Possibly hours

Hypotensive Shock

↓↓↓ Potentially minutes

Cardiac Arrest

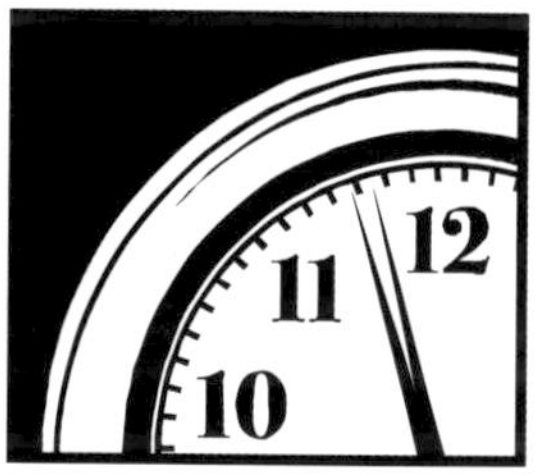

Early recognition and timely intervention are critical to halting the progression from compensated shock to hypotensive shock to cardiopulmonary failure and arrest.

These and other clinical manifestations are discussed in greater detail later in this chapter.

Categorization of Shock by Type

Types of Shock

Shock can be categorized into 4 basic types:

- Hypovolemic
- Distributive
- Cardiogenic
- Obstructive

Hypovolemic Shock

Introduction

Hypovolemia is the most common cause of shock in children worldwide. Fluid loss due to diarrhea is the leading cause of hypovolemic shock. In fact, diarrhea and associated dehydration and electrolyte abnormalities are a major worldwide cause of infant mortality. Causes of volume loss that can lead to hypovolemic shock include

- diarrhea
- hemorrhage (internal and external)
- vomiting
- inadequate fluid intake
- osmotic diuresis (eg, diabetic ketoacidosis)
- third-space losses (fluid leak into tissues)
- burns

Hypovolemic shock is the result of an absolute deficiency of intravascular blood volume. However, it typically represents depletion of both intravascular and extravascular fluid volume. Adequate fluid resuscitation often requires IV infusions that exceed estimated intravascular volume loss in order to restore and maintain intravascular and extravascular fluid volumes.

Tachypnea is often observed in hypovolemic shock. It represents a respiratory compensation to maintain acid-base homeostasis (balance). The respiratory alkalosis from hyperventilation partially compensates for the metabolic acidosis (lactic acidosis) that accompanies shock.

Physiology of Hypovolemic Shock

Hypovolemic shock is characterized by decreased preload leading to reduced stroke volume and low cardiac output. Compensatory mechanisms are tachycardia, increased contractility, and increased systemic vascular resistance.

Hypovolemic Shock	Preload	Contractility	Afterload
	Decreased	Normal or increased	Increased

Signs of Hypovolemic Shock

Table 2 outlines typical signs of hypovolemic shock that might be detected when evaluating the child during the general and primary assessments.

Although septic, anaphylactic, neurogenic, and other distributive forms of shock are not typically classified as hypovolemic shock, all are characterized in large part by *relative* hypovolemia that results from arterial and venous vasodilation, increased capillary permeability, and plasma loss into the interstitium ("third spacing" or capillary leak).

Table 2. Findings Consistent With Hypovolemic Shock

Primary Assessment	Finding
A	
B	• Tachypnea without increased effort (quiet tachypnea)
C **Assessment of Cardiovascular Function**	• Tachycardia • Normal blood pressure or hypotension with a narrow pulse pressure • Weak or absent peripheral pulses • Normal or weak central pulses • Delayed capillary refill
Assessment of End-Organ Function	• Cool to cold, pale, diaphoretic skin • Changes in mental status • Oliguria
D	• Changes in mental status
E	

Distributive Shock

Introduction

Distributive shock is characterized by inappropriate distribution of blood volume with inadequate organ and tissue perfusion (especially the splanchnic vascular bed).

The most common forms of distributive shock are

- septic shock
- anaphylactic shock
- neurogenic shock (eg, head injury, spinal injury)

Distributive shock caused by sepsis can be characterized by an abnormal reduction in systemic vascular resistance resulting in abnormal distribution of blood flow. This inappropriate vasodilation combined with venodilation causes pooling of blood in the venous capacitance system and a relative hypovolemia. Septic shock also causes increased capillary permeability, so there is loss of plasma from the vascular space, increasing the severity of the hypovolemia.

In anaphylactic shock, venodilation, systemic vasodilation, and increased capillary permeability combine with pulmonary vasoconstriction to reduce cardiac output due to relative hypovolemia and increased right ventricular afterload.

Neurogenic shock is characterized by generalized loss of vascular tone, most often following a high cervical spine injury.

Physiology of Distributive Shock

In distributive shock cardiac output may be increased, normal, or decreased. Although myocardial dysfunction is typically present, stroke volume may be adequate, particularly if aggressive volume resuscitation is provided. Tachycardia and an increase in the end-diastolic volume of the heart help maintain the cardiac output. Tissue perfusion is compromised by maldistribution of blood flow. Some tissue beds may be inadequately perfused (eg, the splanchnic circulation), whereas others (eg, skeletal muscle and skin) may receive blood flow that exceeds metabolic demand. Children may present with

- low systemic vascular resistance and increased blood flow to the skin producing warm extremities and bounding peripheral pulses (warm shock)
- high systemic vascular resistance resulting in decreased blood flow to the skin, cold extremities, and weak pulses (cold shock)

As distributive shock progresses, concomitant hypovolemia or myocardial dysfunction produces a fall in cardiac output. Tissues without adequate oxygen delivery generate lactic acid, leading to metabolic acidosis. Unlike hypovolemic and cardiogenic shock, however, central venous oxygen saturation may be normal or even increased in sepsis because of the inappropriate blood flow to organ beds that far exceeds their metabolic demand so that there is little oxygen extraction.

Distributive Shock	Preload	Contractility	Afterload
	Normal or decreased	Normal or decreased	Variable

Distributive shock can be characterized by high, normal, or low cardiac output but is most often characterized by multiple derangements, including

- low systemic vascular resistance, which causes the wide pulse pressure characteristic of distributive shock and contributes to early hypotension
- increased flow to peripheral tissue beds
- inadequate perfusion of the splanchnic vascular bed
- release of inflammatory mediators and vasoactive substances, complement cascade activation, and microcirculatory thrombosis
- volume depletion caused by capillary leak
- accumulation of lactic acid in poorly perfused tissue beds

Although most forms of distributive shock are not typically classified as hypovolemic shock, all are characterized by relative hypovolemia prior to fluid resuscitation.

Signs of Distributive Shock

Table 3 outlines typical signs of distributive shock that might be detected during the general and primary assessments of the child. The **boldface** text denotes type-specific signs that distinguish distributive shock from other forms of shock.

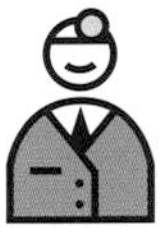

The high cardiac output and low systemic vascular resistance often observed in distributive shock are the opposite of the low cardiac output and high systemic vascular resistance seen in hypovolemic, cardiogenic, and obstructive shock.

A wide pulse pressure due to low systemic vascular resistance may be characterized by a diastolic blood pressure that is equal to or less than half of the systolic blood pressure.

Table 3. Findings Consistent With Distributive Shock

Primary Assessment	Finding
A	Usually patent unless level of consciousness is significantly impaired
B	• Tachypnea, usually without increased work of breathing ("comfortable tachypnea") unless the patient has pneumonia or is developing ARDS or cardiogenic pulmonary edema
C **Assessment of Cardiovascular Function**	• Tachycardia • **Hypotension with a wide pulse pressure (warm shock) or narrow pulse pressure (cold shock)** or normotension • **Bounding peripheral pulses** • **Brisk or delayed capillary refill** • **Warm, flushed skin (extremities) or pale skin with vasoconstriction**
Assessment of End-Organ Function	• Changes in mental status • Oliguria
D	• Changes in mental status
E	• Variable temperature • Petechial or purpuric rash (septic shock)

Septic Shock

Introduction

Septic shock is the most common form of distributive shock. It is caused by infectious organisms or their byproducts (eg, endotoxin) that stimulate the immune system and trigger release or activation of inflammatory mediators.

Septic shock in children typically evolves along a continuum from a systemic inflammatory response in the early stages to septic shock in the late stages. This continuum may evolve over days or hours with wide variability in clinical presentation and progression. The pathophysiology of the septic cascade includes the following:

- The infectious organism or its byproducts (eg, endotoxin) activate the immune system, including neutrophils, monocytes, and macrophages.
- These cells, or their interaction with the infecting organism, stimulate release or activation of inflammatory mediators, called cytokines.
- Cytokines produce vasodilation and increased capillary permeability.

Uncontrolled activation of inflammatory mediators can lead to organ failure, particularly cardiovascular and respiratory failure, systemic thrombosis, and adrenal dysfunction.[1]

Vasodilation and increased capillary permeability can produce maldistribution of blood flow, hypovolemia, and hypotension. Cardiac output may be normal or increased as a result of tachycardia and low afterload. In some patients specific inflammatory mediators produce myocardial dysfunction that combined with vasodilation and capillary leak can cause low cardiac output with inadequate systemic perfusion and oxygen delivery.

Septic Shock	Preload	Contractility	Afterload
	Decreased	Normal to decreased	Variable

Absolute or relative adrenal insufficiency is often present and will contribute to cardiovascular dysfunction.

Consensus Definitions and Clinical Characteristics of Pediatric Sepsis

In 2005 an international panel of experts developed the following consensus definitions and clinical characteristics of pediatric sepsis and its consequences[2]:

- Systemic Inflammatory Response Syndrome (SIRS)
- Sepsis
- Severe sepsis
- Septic shock

Systemic Inflammatory Response Syndrome (SIRS)

Systemic Inflammatory Response Syndrome (SIRS) is defined by the presence of at least 2 of the following 4 criteria, one of which must be abnormal temperature or leukocyte count:

- Core temperature of >38.5°C or <36°C.
- Tachycardia (mean HR >2 standard deviations above normal for age) in the absence of external stimulus, chronic drugs or pain, or otherwise unexplained persistent elevation over a ½-hour to 4-hour time period

  or

  For children <1 year old, bradycardia (mean HR <10th percentile for age in absence of external vagal stimulus, β-adrenergic blocker drugs, or congenital heart disease) or otherwise unexplained persistent depression over a ½-hour time period
- Mean respiratory rate >2 standard deviations above normal for age or mechanical ventilation for an acute process not related to underlying neuromuscular disease or general anesthesia
- Leukocyte count elevated or depressed for age (not leukopenia induced by chemotherapy) or >10% immature neutrophils

Sepsis

Sepsis is defined as SIRS in the presence of, or as a result of, suspected or proven infection.

Severe Sepsis

Severe sepsis is defined as

- Sepsis *plus* either cardiovascular dysfunction or acute respiratory distress syndrome

  or

- Sepsis *plus* 2 or more other organ failures

Respiratory failure as a sign of organ dysfunction in sepsis is characterized by any of the following:

- PaO_2/FiO_2 <300 in absence of cyanotic heart disease or preexisting lung disease
- $PaCO_2$ >65 mm Hg or 20 mm Hg above baseline
- Proven need for inspired O_2 concentration >50% to maintain oxyhemoglobin saturation ≥92%
- Need for nonelective mechanical ventilation (invasive or noninvasive)

Pulmonary edema and resultant hypoxemia and respiratory distress may develop, particularly during aggressive fluid resuscitation.

Septic Shock

Septic shock is defined as

- Sepsis (SIRS in the presence of, or as a result of, suspected or proven infection)

  and

- Cardiovascular dysfunction* despite administration of isotonic intravenous fluid boluses ≥40 mL/kg in 1 hour

*Cardiovascular dysfunction is characterized by the following:

- Hypotension (SBP <5th percentile for age or SBP <2 standard deviations below normal for age)

  or

- Need for vasoactive drug to maintain BP in normal range

  or

- Two of the following characteristics of inadequate organ perfusion:
  - Unexplained metabolic acidosis: base deficit >5 mEq/L
  - Increased arterial lactate greater than twice the upper limit of normal
  - Oliguria: urine output <0.5 mL/kg per hour
  - Prolonged capillary refill: >5 seconds
  - Core to peripheral temperature gap >3°C

Signs of Septic Shock

In its early stages septic shock is often subtle and may be difficult to recognize because peripheral perfusion may appear to be good. Because septic shock is triggered by an infection or its byproducts, the child may also demonstrate fever or hypothermia and an elevated or decreased white blood cell count.

In addition to the findings listed in Table 3, the child with septic shock may demonstrate petechiae or purpura. Other findings of septic shock (eg, metabolic acidosis, respiratory alkalosis, and leukocytosis, leukopenia, or increased bands [immature white blood cells]) are identified in the tertiary assessment.

Treatment Considerations

Because capillary permeability is increased, providers should anticipate the development of pulmonary edema during volume resuscitation. The risk of pulmonary edema should not prevent adequate volume resuscitation to restore vital organ perfusion even if mechanical ventilatory support is needed. Vasoactive therapy is often needed to control the vasodilation and restore an adequate blood pressure. Myocardial dysfunction may develop and is an indication for inotropic support. If adrenal dysfunction is present or suspected, cortisol therapy is indicated.

Early recognition and treatment of septic shock are critically important determinants of outcome. You should evaluate systemic perfusion and clinical signs of end-organ function to identify sepsis before hypotensive shock develops. Once sepsis is identified, aggressively search for and treat the causative organism. See the Management of Shock chapter for details on the treatment of septic shock.

Goal-directed therapy to maintain oxygen delivery can reduce morbidity and mortality from pediatric septic shock.

Anaphylactic Shock

Introduction

Anaphylactic shock results from a severe reaction to a drug, vaccine, food, toxin, plant, venom, or other antigen. This acute multisystem allergic response often occurs in seconds to minutes after exposure. It is characterized by venodilation, systemic vasodilation, and increased capillary permeability combined with pulmonary vasoconstriction. The vasoconstriction acutely increases right heart work and may add to the hypotension by reducing the delivery of blood from the right ventricle to the left ventricle. Death may occur immediately, or the child may develop acute-phase symptoms, which typically begin 5 to 10 minutes after exposure.

Signs and Symptoms of Anaphylactic Shock

Signs and symptoms may include

- anxiety or agitation
- nausea and vomiting
- urticaria (hives)
- angioedema (swelling of the face, lips, and tongue)
- respiratory distress with stridor or wheezing
- hypotension
- tachycardia

Angioedema may result in complete upper airway obstruction. Hypotension is caused by vasodilation; hypovolemia is caused by capillary leak and intravascular volume loss.

Neurogenic Shock

Introduction

Neurogenic shock, including spinal shock, results from an injury to the head or spine that disrupts the sympathetic nervous system innervation of blood vessels and the heart. The cause of neurogenic shock is usually a cervical spine (neck) injury, but neurogenic shock may also result from head injury or injury to the thoracic spine above the sixth thoracic (T6) spinal level.

Physiology of Neurogenic Shock

The sudden loss of sympathetic nervous system signals to the smooth muscle in the vessel walls results in uncontrolled vasodilation.

Signs of Neurogenic Shock

Primary signs of neurogenic shock are

- hypotension with a wide pulse pressure
- normal heart rate or bradycardia

Other signs may include increased respiratory rate, diaphragmatic breathing (use of muscles in the diaphragm rather than the chest wall), and other evidence of a high thoracic or cervical spine injury.

Neurogenic shock must be differentiated from hypovolemic shock. Hypovolemic shock is typically associated with hypotension, a narrow pulse pressure from compensatory vasoconstriction, and compensatory tachycardia. In neurogenic shock, hypotension occurs without compensatory tachycardia or peripheral vasoconstriction because sympathetic innervation of the heart is also disrupted, reducing the expected compensatory tachycardia.

Cardiogenic Shock

Introduction

Cardiogenic shock is a condition of inadequate tissue perfusion resulting from myocardial dysfunction. This dysfunction can be caused by pump failure (poor contractility), congenital heart disease, or rhythm abnormalities (eg, supraventricular tachycardia or ventricular tachycardia).

Common causes of cardiogenic shock are

- congenital heart disease
- myocarditis (inflammation of the heart muscle)
- cardiomyopathy (an inherited or acquired abnormality of pumping function)
- arrhythmias
- sepsis
- poisoning or drug toxicity
- myocardial injury (eg, trauma)

Physiology of Cardiogenic Shock

Cardiogenic shock is characterized by decreased cardiac output, marked tachycardia, and high systemic vascular resistance. The work of breathing may be increased secondary to pulmonary edema. Typically intravascular volume is normal or increased unless a concurrent illness causes hypovolemia (eg, in a child who has a viral myocarditis with recent vomiting and fever).

Cardiogenic Shock	Preload	Contractility	Afterload
	Variable	Decreased	Increased

Cardiogenic shock is often characterized by sequential compensatory and pathologic mechanisms, including

- compensatory increase in systemic vascular resistance to redirect blood flow from peripheral and splanchnic tissues to the heart and brain
- increase in heart rate and left ventricular afterload, which increases left ventricular work and myocardial oxygen consumption
- as afterload increases, stroke volume decreases when pumping function of the heart is poor
- increased venous tone, which increases central venous (right atrial) and pulmonary capillary (left atrial) pressures
- renal fluid retention
- pulmonary edema resulting in part from the last two mechanisms noted above

The compensatory mechanisms that maintain perfusion to the brain and heart during hypovolemic shock are often harmful during cardiogenic shock. For example, compensatory peripheral vasoconstriction can maintain adequate blood pressure during hypovolemic shock but may have detrimental effects in children with cardiogenic shock because the vasoconstriction increases left ventricular afterload (increased resistance to left ventricular ejection). See Figure 2.

Because the heart is also an end organ (ie, the heart muscle needs adequate oxygen delivery), almost any child with severe or sustained shock may experience inadequate delivery of oxygen to the myocardium relative to its increased metabolic demand. Therefore, severe or sustained shock of any type typically leads to impaired myocardial function (ie, these children then develop cardiogenic shock in addition to the primary cause of shock). Once a child begins to develop poor myocardial function, clinical status usually declines rapidly.

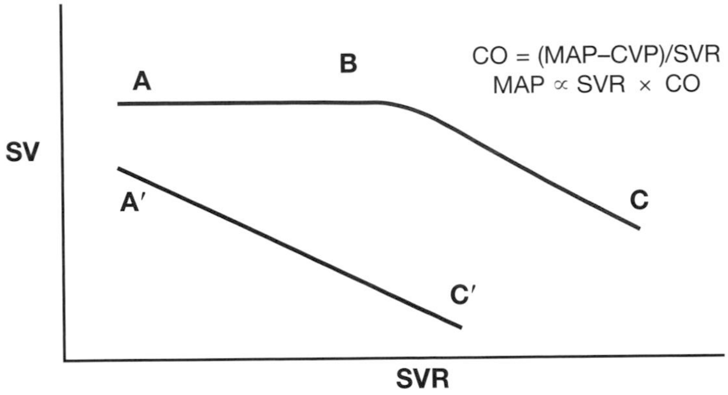

Figure 2. The relationship between stroke volume (SV) and systemic vascular resistance (SVR). The upper curve shows changes in SV in a patient with normal ventricular contractility and function. As SVR increases from point A to B, blood pressure (MAP) increases because the healthy ventricle maintains SV (and thus CO) constant. Further increases in SVR eventually depress SV, moving the patient to point C. The lower curve illustrates the relation between SVR and SV in a patient with poor ventricular function. As SVR increases, SV falls proportionately. Note that the reciprocal changes between SV and SVR may cause little to no change in MAP as the patient moves from point A′ to C′. Conversely, note that reducing SVR (moving from C′ to A′ by using a vasodilator) may improve SV with no change in MAP.

Signs of Cardiogenic Shock

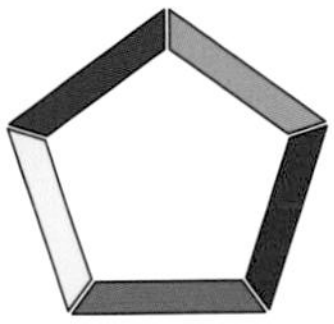

Table 4 outlines typical signs of cardiogenic shock that might be detected during the general and primary assessments of the child. The **boldface** text denotes type-specific signs that distinguish cardiogenic shock from other forms of shock.

Table 4. Findings Consistent With Cardiogenic Shock

Primary Assessment	Finding
A	
B	• Tachypnea • **Increased respiratory effort (retractions, nasal flaring) resulting from pulmonary edema**
C Assessment of Cardiovascular Function	• Tachycardia • Normal or low blood pressure with a narrow pulse pressure • Weak or absent peripheral pulses • Normal and then weak central pulses • Delayed capillary refill with cool extremities • **Signs of congestive heart failure (eg, pulmonary edema, hepatomegaly, jugular venous distention)**
Assessment of End-Organ Function	• **Cyanosis (caused by cyanotic congenital heart disease or pulmonary edema)** • Cold, pale, diaphoretic skin • Changes in mental status • Oliguria
D	• Changes in mental status
E	• Variable temperature

For cardiogenic shock the pulse oximetry may be low if there is pulmonary edema (lung tissue disease).

> *Increased respiratory effort* often distinguishes cardiogenic shock from hypovolemic shock. Hypovolemic shock is characterized by *quiet tachypnea*.

If a child has *cardiogenic* shock caused by poor myocardial function, rapid volume resuscitation could aggravate pulmonary edema and myocardial function, further compromising respiratory function and cardiac output. Volume resuscitation should be more gradual, with smaller (5 to 10 mL/kg) isotonic fluid boluses delivered over longer periods of time with careful monitoring during fluid infusion. Infants and children with cardiogenic shock often require drug therapy to increase and redistribute cardiac output to improve myocardial function and reduce systemic vascular resistance. In addition, treatment should include methods of decreasing metabolic demand, such as reducing the work of breathing or controlling fever. This will allow limited cardiac output to better meet tissue metabolic demand.

Obstructive Shock

Introduction

Obstructive shock is a condition of impaired cardiac output caused by physical obstruction of blood flow. Types of obstructive shock include

- cardiac tamponade
- tension pneumothorax
- ductal-dependent congenital heart lesions
- massive pulmonary embolism

The physical obstruction to blood flow results in low cardiac output, inadequate tissue perfusion, and a compensatory increase in systemic vascular resistance. The early clinical presentation of obstructive shock can be indistinguishable from severe hypovolemic shock, although careful clinical examination may reveal signs of systemic or pulmonary venous congestion that would not be consistent with simple hypovolemia. As the condition progresses, increased respiratory effort, cyanosis, and signs of vascular congestion become more apparent.

Physiology and Clinical Signs

Physiology and clinical signs vary according to the cause of obstructive shock. The 4 primary causes of obstructive shock and major distinguishing signs of each are briefly described in this chapter.

Cardiac Tamponade

Cardiac tamponade is caused by an accumulation of fluid, blood, or air in the pericardial space. Increased intrapericardial pressure and compression of the heart impede systemic venous and pulmonary venous return, reduce ventricular filling, and cause a fall in cardiac output. If untreated, cardiac tamponade will result in cardiac arrest characterized by pulseless electrical activity.

In children cardiac tamponade most often occurs after penetrating trauma or cardiac surgery, although it may develop with pericardial effusion complicating an inflammatory disorder. Distinguishing signs are

- muffled or diminished heart sounds
- pulsus paradoxus (decrease in systolic blood pressure by more than 10 mm Hg during inspiration)
- distended neck veins (may be difficult to see in infants if hypotension is severe)

Note that in children following cardiovascular surgery, signs of tamponade may be indistinguishable from those of cardiogenic shock. Favorable outcome depends on urgent diagnosis and immediate treatment. The diagnosis can be made with echocardiography. The electrocardiogram typically shows small QRS complexes with a large pericardial effusion.

Tension Pneumothorax

Tension pneumothorax is caused by the entry of air into the pleural space. This air can enter from injured lung tissue, which may occur from an internal tear or following a penetrating chest injury. A simple pneumothorax occurs when air leaks into the space and then stops. When air continues to leak into and accumulates in the pleural space, it generates positive intrathoracic pressure. This ongoing leak is often due to the use of positive-pressure ventilation that forces air out of the injured lung and into the pleural space. As the pleural pressure rises, it compresses the lung and pushes the mediastinum to the opposite side. Compression of the lung rapidly causes respiratory failure, whereas the high pleural pressure and direct pressure on mediastinal structures (heart and great vessels) impair venous return. This leads to a rapid fall in cardiac output. Untreated tension pneumothorax will lead to cardiac arrest characterized by pulseless electrical activity.

You should suspect tension pneumothorax in the victim of chest trauma or in any intubated child who deteriorates suddenly during positive-pressure ventilation (including overzealous bag-mask ventilation). Distinguishing signs are

- hyperresonance on the affected side
- diminished breath sounds on the affected side
- distended neck veins (may be difficult to appreciate in infants or if hypotension is severe)
- tracheal deviation toward contralateral side (may be difficult to appreciate in infants and young children)
- rapid deterioration in perfusion and often rapid evolution from tachycardia to bradycardia as the cardiac output falls

Favorable outcome depends on immediate diagnosis and treatment.

Ductal-Dependent Lesions

Ductal-dependent lesions are congenital cardiac abnormalities that generally present in the first weeks of life. Ductal-dependent lesions include

- forms of cyanotic congenital heart disease (ductal dependent for pulmonary blood flow)
- left ventricular outflow tract obstructive lesions (ductal dependent for systemic blood flow)

The ductal-dependent pulmonary blood flow lesions usually present with cyanosis and not shock. The left ventricular outflow tract obstructive lesions often present in obstructive shock in the first 2 weeks of life when the patent ductus arteriosus closes. These left-sided lesions include coarctation of the aorta, interrupted aortic arch, critical aortic stenosis, and hypoplastic left heart syndrome. Maintaining patency of the ductus arteriosus as a conduit for blood flow bypassing the left-sided obstruction is crucial to survival.

Distinguishing signs of left ventricular outflow tract obstructive lesions include

- rapidly progressive deterioration in systemic perfusion
- congestive heart failure
- preductal versus postductal differential blood pressure (coarctation or interrupted aortic arch)
- preductal versus postductal differential cyanosis (coarctation or interrupted aortic arch)
- absence of femoral pulses (coarctation or interrupted aortic arch)
- rapid deterioration in mental status
- respiratory failure with signs of pulmonary edema or inadequate respiratory effort

You should rapidly recognize ductal-dependent lesions and initiate specific therapy to maintain patency of the ductus arteriosus.

Massive Pulmonary Embolism

Pulmonary embolism is a total or partial obstruction of the pulmonary artery or its branches by a clot or by fat, air, amniotic fluid, catheter fragment, or injected matter. A pulmonary embolus is most commonly a thrombus that migrates to the pulmonary circulation. Pulmonary embolism may lead to pulmonary infarction.

Pulmonary embolism is relatively rare in children but may develop when an underlying condition predisposes the child to embolic phenomena. Examples of these conditions and other predisposing factors are indwelling central venous catheters, sickle cell disease, malignancy, connective tissue disorders, and inherited disorders of coagulation (eg, antithrombin, protein S, and protein C deficiencies).

Pulmonary embolism results in a vicious cycle of events, including

- ventilation/perfusion mismatch (proportional to the size of pulmonary infarction)
- systemic hypoxemia
- increased pulmonary vascular resistance leading to right heart failure and a fall in cardiac output
- leftward shift of the intraventricular septum leading to impaired left ventricular filling and further reduction in cardiac output
- rapid fall in end-tidal CO_2 if this is being monitored

This condition may be difficult to diagnose because signs are subtle and providers may not suspect it. The presentation is more general and includes cyanosis, tachycardia, and hypotension. The signs of congestion and right heart failure, however, distinguish it from hypovolemic shock.

Summary

Treatment of obstructive shock is cause-specific. Immediate recognition and correction of the underlying cause of the obstruction can be life-saving. Therefore, the most critical tasks for PALS providers are prompt recognition, diagnosis, and treatment of obstructive shock.

Without immediate treatment, patients with obstructive shock often progress rapidly to cardiopulmonary failure and cardiac arrest.

References

1. Carcillo JA. Pediatric septic shock and multiple organ failure. *Crit Care Clin.* 2003;19:413-440, viii.
2. Goldstein B, Giroir B, Randolph A. International pediatric sepsis consensus conference: definitions for sepsis and organ dysfunction in pediatrics. *Pediatr Crit Care Med.* 2005;6:2-8.

Chapter 5

Management of Shock

Overview

Introduction

Once shock is recognized in the seriously ill or injured child, early treatment can greatly improve outcome.

This chapter discusses goals and priorities in shock management, fundamentals of treatment, general and advanced management of shock, and specific management according to etiology.

After completing this chapter you should be able to

- describe the general goals of shock management
- summarize initial treatment priorities, monitoring, and ongoing management
- describe effective fluid resuscitation principles
- explain how effective shock therapy depends on targeting the etiology and degree of shock
- summarize principles of acute management of hypovolemic, distributive, cardiogenic, and obstructive shock

Goals of Shock Management

Introduction

The goals in treatment of shock are to reverse perfusion abnormalities, improve the balance between perfusion and tissue metabolic demand, restore organ function, and prevent cardiac arrest. The speed of intervention is crucial: having the knowledge and skills to respond to a seriously ill or injured child at the moment of presentation may be life-saving. The longer the interval between the precipitating event and the start of resuscitation, the poorer the outcome. Once a child is in cardiac arrest, the prognosis is poor.

Warning Signs

You must be alert to signs that compensatory mechanisms are failing in a seriously ill or injured child; you and the other members of the resuscitation team must act decisively with effective resuscitative therapy. Warning signs that indicate progression from compensated to hypotensive shock include

- marked tachycardia
- absent peripheral pulses
- weakening central pulses
- cold distal extremities with very prolonged capillary refill
- narrowing pulse pressure
- altered mental status
- hypotension (late finding)

Once hypotension is present, organ perfusion is typically severely compromised and organ dysfunction may occur even if the child does not progress to cardiac arrest.

Early recognition of compensated shock is critical to effective treatment and good outcome.

Fundamentals of Shock Management

Introduction

Shock treatment focuses on restoring oxygen delivery to the tissues and improving the balance between tissue perfusion and metabolic demand. Treatment consists of

- optimizing oxygen content of the blood
- improving volume and distribution of cardiac output
- reducing oxygen demand
- correcting metabolic derangements

Restoring effective oxygen delivery to the tissues may also require correction of metabolic derangements such as hypoglycemia or profound metabolic acidosis as well as focusing therapy on reversing the underlying cause of shock.

Optimizing Oxygen Content of the Blood

Optimizing oxygen content of the blood involves ensuring that 100% of the available hemoglobin is saturated with oxygen. This is accomplished by

- administration of a high concentration of oxygen
- transfusion in circumstances in which hemoglobin is low because of blood loss or other processes
- using CPAP, PEEP, or other airway interventions to correct V/Q abnormalities or other respiratory disorders affecting oxygenation

Improving Volume and Distribution of Cardiac Output

Measures to improve the volume and distribution of cardiac output are based on the type of shock:

- Hypovolemic shock
- Distributive shock
- Cardiogenic shock
- Obstructive

Hypovolemic Shock

Rapid administration of fluids is indicated for most children who present with signs and symptoms of hypovolemic shock. Reassess the child's response to each fluid bolus and look for ongoing evidence of hypovolemia or fluid loss to determine the need for additional fluids.

Distributive Shock

Suspect distributive shock when there is evidence of a low systemic vascular resistance (wide pulse pressure) and maldistribution of blood flow (eg, vasodilation and warm skin in the presence of altered mental status and lactic acidosis). Although the end result is inadequate oxygen delivery to some organ systems, the primary abnormality is low systemic vascular resistance caused by the host response to invading organisms (eg, sepsis) or loss of vasomotor tone (eg, anaphylaxis or spinal cord injury) and increased capillary permeability.

In the presence of low systemic vascular resistance, the body normally attempts to maintain blood pressure by increasing cardiac output (ie, stroke volume and heart rate). Clinically the child has signs of hyperdynamic cardiovascular function with bounding pulses. Often the child has a flushed appearance to the skin caused by vasodilation. Impaired oxygen delivery results from inadequate blood flow to some tissues. Despite the fact that cardiac output is increased, blood flow is "maldistributed": there is excessive blood flow to some tissues (such as the skin and skeletal muscles) and inadequate blood flow to other tissues. The resulting end-organ dysfunction is similar to that of other forms of shock.

Management of distributive shock is aimed at rapidly restoring intravascular volume to better fill the vasodilated vascular space. Administration of vasoconstrictors may be needed to combat the primary problem of low systemic vascular resistance. Inotropic agents are sometimes needed to help improve contractility.

Cardiogenic Shock

Suspect cardiogenic shock when there are signs of pulmonary or systemic venous congestion (eg, increased work of breathing, grunting respirations, distended neck veins, or hepatomegaly). When these signs are not present, consider cardiogenic shock when there is clinical deterioration in perfusion and respiratory function in response to fluid resuscitation.

If you identify cardiogenic shock, focus treatment on improving cardiac output while reducing metabolic demand when possible. Specific treatments may include use of BiPAP or mechanical ventilation to reduce the work of breathing and improve oxygenation. You may consider a cautious trial of fluid administration using 5 to 10 mL/kg infused slowly under careful observation. Selection of inotropic and vasodilator therapy is determined by the need to maintain adequate blood pressure, restore tissue perfusion, and minimize the adverse effects of inotropes on myocardial oxygen demand.

Early consultation with experts in the management of these children is recommended. Selection of the best vasoactive drug may depend on information obtained by echocardiogram or other invasive studies. Often vasodilator therapy is indicated even when blood pressure is low. This is because the primary end point of therapy is to increase blood flow and not to correct blood pressure.

Obstructive Shock

Suspect obstructive shock when there are signs of elevated CVP and venous congestion with poor perfusion. The key to management of obstructive shock is to identify and treat the cause. You will need to support cardiovascular function (eg, with volume administration and possible vasoactive agents) while performing appropriate assessment and diagnostic studies. Expert consultation is often necessary. Rapid diagnosis and treatment of the obstruction is essential.

Reducing Oxygen Demand

For all forms of shock the imbalance between oxygen consumption and supply can be improved by measures to reduce oxygen demand. The most common factors that contribute to increased oxygen demand include

- increased work of breathing
- fever
- pain and anxiety

Controlling these factors reduces metabolic demands and thereby reduces oxygen consumption. Control increased work of breathing with assisted ventilation and endotracheal intubation. To achieve intubation and mechanical ventilation, you may need to administer sedatives or analgesics and paralytics; use sedative and analgesic agents cautiously because they suppress the patient's endogenous stress hormone response, which may be critically important to maintain compensation. Control fever by administering antipyretics and other cooling measures. Control pain and anxiety with analgesics and sedatives, but recall the caution noted above on the use of these agents.

Correcting Metabolic Derangements

Many conditions that lead to shock may result in or be complicated by metabolic derangements, including

- hypoglycemia
- hypocalcemia
- hyperkalemia
- metabolic acidosis

Hypoglycemia and hypocalcemia are frequently found in children with septic shock; both conditions can adversely affect cardiac contractility. Hyperkalemia may develop when renal insufficiency or cell death complicates severe shock or when severe metabolic acidosis is present. Metabolic acidosis is characteristic of all forms of shock.

Hypoglycemia is low serum glucose. Glucose is vital for proper cardiac function. Hypoglycemia can also cause brain injury.

Hypocalcemia is an abnormally low ionized plasma calcium concentration. Calcium is essential for effective cardiac function and vasomotor tone.

Hyperkalemia is higher-than-normal plasma or serum potassium concentration that may result from renal dysfunction, cell death, or acidosis.

Metabolic acidosis develops from production of acids such as lactic acid when there is inadequate tissue perfusion. Metabolic acidosis can be caused by renal or gastrointestinal dysfunction. Renal dysfunction can produce retention of organic acids or loss of bicarbonate ions. Gastrointestinal dysfunction, such as diarrhea, can result in loss of bicarbonate ions. Severe metabolic acidosis may depress myocardial contractility and impair the effect of vasopressors. Rather than directly correcting metabolic acidosis, it is initially treated with fluid resuscitation and inotropic therapy to restore tissue perfusion. If this therapy is effective, the patient will clear the metabolic acidosis.

On occasion, buffers (eg, sodium bicarbonate) may be needed to acutely correct profound acidosis. Sodium bicarbonate works by combining with hydrogen ions (acids) to produce carbon dioxide and water; carbon dioxide is then eliminated through increased alveolar ventilation. Support of ventilation may be required in the critically ill child if sodium bicarbonate is used to treat metabolic acidosis.

Correcting metabolic derangements may be essential to optimize organ function. In particular, you should measure and replenish the ionized calcium concentration (active form of calcium in the body) and glucose concentration if indicated. Consider administration of sodium bicarbonate or tromethamine to treat metabolic acidosis that is refractory to fluid resuscitation and other efforts to improve cardiac output.

Therapeutic End Points

No single resuscitation end point has been identified as a consistent marker of adequate tissue perfusion and cellular homeostasis.[1] Clinical improvement toward hemodynamic normality may be indicated by

- normal pulses (no differential between peripheral and central pulses)
- capillary refill less than 2 seconds
- warm extremities
- normal mental status
- normal blood pressure
- urine output greater than 1 mL/kg per hour
- decreased serum lactate
- reduced base deficit
- venous oxygen saturation (SvO_2) greater than 70%

Although blood pressure is an easily measured and traditional end point of resuscitation, it is important to assess all the signs of tissue perfusion. Blood pressure may be normal in children with severe shock, and blood pressure measurement may be inaccurate if perfusion is poor. These therapeutic end points can be combined with other appropriate treatment interventions designed to reverse or correct the underlying cause of the child's shock.

General Management of Shock

Components of General Management

General management of shock consists of the following (2 or more of these actions may be implemented by the team simultaneously):

- Positioning
- Oxygen administration
- Vascular access
- Fluid resuscitation
- Monitoring
- Frequent assessment
- Ancillary studies
- Pharmacologic support
- Subspecialty consultation

Positioning

Positioning of a critically ill or injured child in shock may be an important component of initial management. Place a hypotensive child in the Trendelenburg position (supine, head down at a 30° angle below the feet) as long as breathing is not compromised. Allow a stable child to remain in her most comfortable position (eg, in the arms of a caregiver, as appropriate for infants and young children) to decrease anxiety and activity during the general and primary assessments.

Oxygen Administration

High-flow oxygen is indicated in all children with shock. Usually this is delivered by a high-flow oxygen delivery system. Sometimes oxygen delivery needs to be combined with ventilatory support. This can range from the use of CPAP or BiPAP to mechanical ventilation following endotracheal intubation.

Vascular Access

Once airway and breathing are supported, the priority in shock treatment is gaining vascular access for fluid resuscitation and administration of medications. For compensated shock, initial attempts at peripheral venous cannulation are preferred. For hypotensive shock, emergent vascular access is critical, so early intraosseous access is encouraged. Depending on the provider's experience and expertise and the clinical circumstances, central venous access may be obtained. If peripheral vascular access cannot be readily achieved in children with compensated shock, then central venous or intraosseous access are appropriate alternatives.

Be prepared to establish intraosseous (IO) access as soon as possible if needed in compensated or hypotensive shock.

For a complete discussion of vascular procedures, see Vascular Access Procedures on the student CD.

Fluid Resuscitation

Once vascular access is established, start fluid resuscitation immediately.

Give isotonic crystalloid in a 20 mL/kg bolus over 5 to 20 minutes. Repeat 20 mL/kg boluses to restore blood pressure and tissue perfusion.

Repeat fluid bolus infusion based on clinical signs of end-organ perfusion, including heart rate, capillary refill, level of consciousness, and urine output. Remember that in cases of suspected cardiogenic shock, large fluid boluses are not recommended; monitor for development of pulmonary edema or worsening tissue perfusion during the infusion. Be prepared to support oxygenation and ventilation if necessary.

Monitoring

Assess the effectiveness of fluid resuscitation and pharmacologic support by frequent or continuous monitoring of the following:

- Oxyhemoglobin saturation with pulse oximetry (Spo_2)
- Heart rate
- Blood pressure and pulse pressure
- Mental status
- Temperature
- Urine output

Monitor Spo_2 and heart rate early; measure blood pressure as soon as practical. Assess neurologic function and temperature. Insert a urinary catheter for accurate measurement of urine output.

Start advanced monitoring as soon as possible, depending on the provider's experience in placement of advanced forms of vascular access (eg, arterial and central venous catheterization).

Frequent Assessment

Frequently reassess the child's respiratory, cardiovascular, and neurologic status to

- evaluate trends in the child's condition
- determine response to therapy
- plan the next treatment interventions

At any point the child's condition could deteriorate, requiring life-saving interventions such as endotracheal intubation or needle thoracostomy. Continue frequent reassessment until the child's condition is stable or the child is transferred to definitive care.

The condition of a child in shock is dynamic. Continuous monitoring and frequent reassessment are essential to evaluate trends in the child's condition and determine response to therapy.

Ancillary Studies

Ancillary laboratory and nonlaboratory studies provide important information to help you

- identify the etiology and severity of shock
- evaluate for organ dysfunction secondary to shock
- identify metabolic derangements
- evaluate the response to therapeutic interventions

Shock may effect end-organ function. Additional information regarding evaluation of end-organ function is provided in the Postresuscitation Management chapter. In addition, consider expert consultation regarding the diagnosis and management of end-organ failure.

Table 1 outlines some laboratory studies that might be used to better identify the etiology and severity of shock and to guide therapy.

Table 1. Laboratory Studies to Evaluate Shock and Guide Therapy

Ancillary Study	Finding	Possible Etiology	Action/ Intervention
CBC	Hgb/Hct decreased	• Hemorrhage • Fluid resuscitation • Hemolysis	• Administer 100% oxygen • Transfuse • Control bleeding • Titrate fluid administration
	WBC increased or decreased	• Sepsis	• Obtain appropriate cultures • Give antibiotics
	Platelets decreased	• Disseminated intravascular coagulation (DIC) • Decreased production	• Obtain prothrombin time (PT)/partial thromboplastin time (PTT), fibrinogen and D-dimers • Look for etiology of DIC • Transfuse platelets if patient has serious bleeding
Glucose	Increased or decreased	• Stress (usually increased) • Sepsis • Decreased production (eg, liver failure)	• Give dextrose bolus and start infusion of dextrose-containing solution for hypoglycemia

Ancillary Study	Finding	Possible Etiology	Action/ Intervention
Potassium	Increased or decreased	• Renal dysfunction • Acidosis (increases potassium concentration) • Diuresis	• Treat hyperkalemia or hypokalemia • Correct acidosis
Calcium	Decreased (measure ionized calcium concentration)	• Sepsis • Transfusion of blood products	• Give calcium
Lactate	Increased as product of anaerobic metabolism Increased as substrate for gluconeogenesis	• Tissue hypoxia • Increased glucose production (gluconeogenesis)	• Evaluate base deficit and glucose; gluconeogenesis causes increased lactate and glucose with normal base deficit • Correct acidosis as needed
ABG	pH decreased in lactic acidosis and other causes of metabolic acidosis; increased with alkalosis	• Lactic acid accumulation caused by tissue hypoperfusion • Renal failure • Inborn error of metabolism • DKA–diabetic ketoacidosis • Poisoning/overdose • Diarrhea or ileostomy losses	• Give fluid • Support ventilation • Consider buffer • Correct shock • Evaluate anion gap to determine if acidosis is from increased unmeasured ions (increased anion gap) or is more likely from loss of bicarbonate (normal anion gap)
Venous oxygen saturation (Svo_2)	Variable	• Low saturation—inadequate oxygen delivery or increased consumption • High saturation—maldistribution of blood flow or decreased oxygen consumption	• Attempt to maximize oxygen delivery and minimize oxygen demand

Pharmacologic Support

Vasoactive agents are used in the management of shock because they affect myocardial contractility, heart rate, vascular smooth muscle tone, or some combination of these actions. The choice of agents depends on the child's physiologic state.

Vasoactive agents are often indicated when shock persists after adequate volume resuscitation to optimize preload. For example, a child with septic shock who remains hypotensive and poorly perfused despite administration of fluids will likely benefit from an agent that increases systemic vascular resistance. In children with cardiogenic shock, early use of vasoactive agents is indicated because fluid resuscitation is usually unimportant. Most children with cardiogenic shock benefit from afterload reduction to improve cardiac output (provided that blood pressure is adequate).

Pharmacologic Agents

Common classes of pharmacologic agents used in shock are inotropes, phosphodiesterase inhibitors (so-called inodilators), vasodilators, and vasopressors. Table 2 lists drugs by class and pharmacologic effect.

Table 2. Pharmacologic Agents Used in the Treatment of Shock

Class	Drug	Effect
Inotropes	Dopamine Epinephrine Dobutamine	• Increase cardiac contractility • Increase heart rate • Produce variable effects on systemic vascular resistance (SVR) *Note:* Includes agents with both α-adrenergic and β-adrenergic effects
Phosphodiesterase inhibitors (inodilators)	Milrinone Inamrinone	• Reduce afterload • Improve coronary artery blood flow • Improve contractility
Vasodilators	Nitroglycerin Nitroprusside	• Reduce afterload • Reduce venous tone
Vasopressors (vasoconstrictors)	Epinephrine Norepinephrine Dopamine Vasopressin	• Increase systemic vascular resistance • Norepinephrine has inotropic effects whereas vasopressin is a pure vasoconstrictor

Please see the Pharmacology chapter for dosing information.

Subspecialty Consultation

For specific categories of shock, life-saving diagnostic and therapeutic interventions may be required that are beyond the scope of practice of many PALS providers. For example, a provider may not be trained to interpret an echocardiogram or may have never performed a thoracostomy or pericardiocentesis. You must recognize your own scope-of-practice limitations and the importance of calling for help when indicated. Early subspecialty consultation (eg, pediatric critical care, pediatric cardiology, pediatric surgery) is an essential component of shock management and may influence outcome.

Obtaining the appropriate level of care for a critically ill or injured child is a life-saving intervention.

Summary: General Management

Table 3 summarizes general management components discussed in this section.

Table 3. Fundamentals of Shock Management

Position the child • Stable—allow to remain with caregiver • Unstable—if hypotensive, place in Trendelenburg position unless breathing is compromised
Optimize arterial oxygen content • Administer a high concentration of oxygen • Provide transfusion in cases of blood loss • Consider use of CPAP, BiPAP, or mechanical ventilation with PEEP
Support ventilation as indicated (invasive or noninvasive)
Establish vascular access • Consider IO access early
Begin fluid resuscitation • Give an isotonic crystalloid 20 mL/kg bolus over 5 to 20 minutes. Repeat in 20 mL/kg boluses to restore blood pressure and tissue perfusion. For trauma and hemorrhage administer packed red blood cells as needed. • Modify volume and rate of bolus fluid therapy for cases of suspected cardiogenic shock or severe myocardial dysfunction.
Start monitoring • Spo_2 • Heart rate • Blood pressure • Neurologic function • Temperature • Urine output
Perform frequent reassessment • Evaluate trends • Determine response to therapy
Conduct ancillary studies • To identify shock etiology and severity • To evaluate for organ dysfunction secondary to shock • To identify metabolic derangements • To evaluate the response to therapeutic interventions
Administer pharmacologic support—see Table 2: Pharmacologic Agents Used in the Treatment of Shock • To improve or redistribute cardiac output (increase contractility, reduce or increase afterload, improve organ perfusion) • To correct metabolic derangements • To manage pain and anxiety
Obtain subspecialty consultation

Advanced Management of Shock

Introduction

As initial therapy is completed, further therapy can be guided by invasive hemodynamic monitoring to evaluate and adjust preload, systemic vascular resistance, cardiac output, and oxygen delivery. Invasive hemodynamic monitoring may include monitoring

- mean arterial pressure (MAP)
- central venous pressure (CVP)
- mixed venous oxygen saturation ($S_{MV}O_2$) or central venous oxygen saturation (SvO_2)

Mean Arterial Pressure

Continuous arterial blood pressure monitoring can be accomplished with placement of an arterial catheter. The child's physiology can be better understood by evaluating the arterial pressure tracing. For example:

- In cardiogenic shock, pulsus alternans (alternating height of pulse waveform) indicates low cardiac output and very poor myocardial function
- Provided there is not a mechanical obstruction in the pressure waveform, the initial upstroke of the arterial pressure wave is determined by the strength of contraction. A vertical upstroke is consistent with good contractility, whereas a sloped upstroke suggests decreased contractility

Central Venous Pressure (CVP)

Accurate evaluation of right ventricular end-diastolic pressure (preload) can be accomplished using a central venous catheter to measure CVP. Central venous catheters provide only an indirect measure of right ventricular preload. It is also important to recall that CVP is not the same as preload (end-diastolic volume). In general, as the CVP increases, the preload increases. As CVP decreases, the preload decreases.

The use of vasodilators and PEEP in addition to other interventions may change this relationship. It is also important to know that left ventricular pressure and preload may be the same, lower, or higher than right ventricular end-diastolic pressure.

Use of CVP monitoring varies according to the clinical setting, for example:

- In the setting of decreased contractility, the child with myocardial dysfunction may require a higher-than-normal filling pressure to maintain stroke volume.
- For the child with septic shock, measurement of CVP may distinguish between the need for additional volume administration versus titration of vasoactive agents in the hypotensive child. If the CVP is high and perfusion is poor, it is unlikely that additional fluid will be helpful, and vasoactive therapy is needed.
- CVP monitoring may also be helpful in the recognition of obstructive shock. In the presence of pericardial tamponade and tension pneumothorax, CVP is elevated because of increased pericardial pressure despite poor right atrial filling. Conversely, a large pulmonary embolus causes acute right heart failure due to the sudden increase in right ventricular afterload, which produces elevated right atrial pressure. The finding of elevated CVP in conjunction with evidence of venous congestion (eg, neck vein distention) and hypotension is pathognomonic of obstructive shock.

Mixed or Central Venous Oxygen Saturation

Monitoring of cardiac output usually requires placement of a pulmonary artery catheter. This procedure may be technically difficult in infants and young children, and it has a significant rate of complications. Although measurement of the oxygen saturation of a pulmonary artery blood sample is ideal for determination of total body oxygen consumption (mixed venous sample, SvO_2), a central venous sample may be used as a surrogate to help evaluate the adequacy of tissue oxygen delivery (ie, the product of cardiac output and arterial oxygen content). When the central venous O_2 is measured in lieu of the SvO_2 from a pulmonary artery catheter, it is important to note the position of the central venous catheter. In general, the venous oxygen saturation is higher in samples drawn from the inferior versus the superior vena cava since oxygen extraction is higher in blood draining from the brain compared with the lower body. If the catheter is in the right atrium, one should cautiously interpret the results since the sample may be contaminated by a high quantity of coronary sinus blood, which normally has a low (<60%) oxygen saturation.

Assuming that oxygen consumption and arterial oxygen content remain constant, SvO_2 will be inversely related to changes in cardiac output. In other words, the slower the flow of blood through tissues, the greater the percentage of oxygen extracted from arterial blood. This results in decreased oxygen saturation in venous blood.

But in septic shock, oxygen extraction by the tissues may be abnormal due to a combination of increased flow well beyond metabolic demand in some tissues and alterations in oxygen use due to mitochondrial dysfunction in some patients. SvO_2 is often high in sepsis, but lactic acidosis will also be present when there is tissue hypoxia, reflecting inadequate flow to some organs (eg, the splanchnic circulation) and cellular inability to use oxygen.

Fluid Therapy

Introduction

Intravenous (IV) fluid therapy is indicated for the treatment of shock. The primary objective of fluid resuscitation is to restore intravascular volume and thus tissue perfusion. Rapid and aggressive fluid resuscitation is required for hypovolemic shock and distributive shock. Cardiogenic shock and obstructive shock, as well as special shock conditions (eg, severe poisonings or diabetic ketoacidosis [DKA]) may dictate alternative fluid resuscitation therapies.

Fluid resuscitation may be achieved with either isotonic crystalloid solutions or colloid solution. Blood and blood products generally are not the first choice for immediate volume expansion in children with shock, but they are used for replacement of blood loss or correction of some coagulopathies.

Isotonic Crystalloid Solutions

Isotonic crystalloid solutions such as normal saline (NS) or lactated Ringer's (LR) are the preferred initial fluids for volume replacement in management of shock. They are inexpensive, readily available, and do not produce sensitivity reactions.

Isotonic crystalloids effectively expand the extravascular (interstitial) space and correct sodium deficits. But they do not efficiently expand the intravascular (circulating) space because only about ¼ of administered isotonic crystalloids remain in the vascular space. A large trial comparing isotonic saline to albumin found that about 1½ times more crystalloid was needed for volume resuscitation compared with albumin.[2]

Because isotonic crystalloids are distributed throughout the extracellular space, a large quantity of crystalloid solution may be needed to restore intravascular volume.

Rapid infusion of a large volume of fluid may be well tolerated by a healthy child but may cause pulmonary and peripheral edema in the critically ill child with underlying cardiac or renal disease.

Colloid Solutions

Colloid solutions contain relatively large molecules that remain in the intravascular compartment hours longer than isotonic crystalloids. As a result they are more efficient intravascular volume expanders than crystalloid solutions.[3] Colloid solutions include 5% albumin, fresh frozen plasma, and synthetic plasma expanders (eg, hetastarch, dextran 40, and dextran 60).

Blood-derived colloid solutions may cause sensitivity reactions, however. Synthetic colloids may cause coagulopathy; their use is usually limited to 20 to 40 mL/kg. As with crystalloids, excessive administration of colloids may lead to pulmonary edema, particularly in children with cardiac or pulmonary disease.

Crystalloid vs Colloid

Although there are decades of data analyzing the use of crystalloid versus colloid solutions in the patient with shock, the results and analysis of the trials yielded contradictory results. In general, the choice of resuscitation fluid is based on the patient's condition and response to initial isotonic crystalloid resuscitation.

For most children with shock, isotonic crystalloid solutions are equally effective compared with colloids for initial resuscitation.[2]

After administering 20 to 60 mL/kg of isotonic crystalloid, if additional fluid is indicated, consider administration of colloid. Colloids may also be indicated in children who have an underlying predisposition to decreased plasma oncotic pressure (eg, malnutrition, hypoproteinemia, nephrotic syndrome).

Rate and Volume of Fluid Administration

Start fluid resuscitation for shock with 20 mL/kg of isotonic crystalloid administered as a bolus over 5 to 20 minutes. Then administer repeat boluses of 20 mL/kg as needed to restore blood pressure and perfusion.

The amount of fluid needed is often difficult to predict based on history. Instead, it is most appropriate to use the patient's clinical examination and supporting laboratory studies to identify the needed volume.

Give fluid boluses more rapidly to correct hypotensive shock and septic shock. Resuscitation of most children in hypotensive or septic shock may require at least 40 to 80 mL/kg of isotonic crystalloid solution during the first hour(s) of therapy; as much as 240 mL/kg has been used in the first 8 hours of septic shock therapy.[4-6]

Give smaller volumes of fluid more slowly if myocardial dysfunction or obstructive shock is present or suspected.

Modification of fluid resuscitation is appropriate for the child with shock associated with diabetic ketoacidosis, burns, and some poisonings (particularly calcium channel blocker and β-adrenergic blocker overdoses).

Table 4 below provides a general guide to fluid bolus volumes and rates of delivery based on the underlying cause of shock.

Table 4. Guide to Fluid Boluses and Rates of Delivery Based on Underlying Cause of Shock

Type of Shock	Volume of Fluid	Rate of Delivery
Hypovolemic shock (non-DKA) **Distributive shock** **Obstructive shock**	20 mL/kg bolus (repeat PRN)	Deliver rapidly (over 5 to 10 min)
Cardiogenic shock (nonpoisonings)	5 to 10 mL/kg bolus (repeat PRN)	Deliver more slowly (over 10 to 20 min)
Diabetic ketoacidosis (DKA)	10 to 20 mL/kg	Deliver over 1 hour
Poisonings (eg, calcium channel blocker or β-adrenergic blocker)	5 to 10 mL/kg (repeat PRN)	Delivered more slowly (over 10 to 20 min)

Rapid Fluid Delivery

The minidrip IV systems used for routine pediatric fluid therapy do not deliver fluid boluses as rapidly as required for management of shock. To facilitate rapid fluid delivery, use the following:

- Adequate catheter diameter, especially if blood or colloid is needed
- Placement of an in-line 3-way stopcock in the IV tubing system
- A 35-mL to 60-mL syringe to push fluids through the stopcock
- A pressure bag (beware of risk of air embolism)
- Rapid infusion devices

Note: Depending on the size of the patient, entering a rapid fluid infusion rate on an infusion pump may not provide sufficiently rapid fluid delivery. For example, a 50-kg patient with septic shock should ideally receive 1 liter of crystalloid in 15 minutes rather than the hour required using an infusion pump.

Frequent Reassessment During Fluid Resuscitation

Frequent reassessment during fluid resuscitation is essential in effective shock management. To provide appropriate fluid therapy, you should

- assess the response to therapy after each fluid bolus
- determine the need for further fluid boluses
- assess for pulmonary edema during and after fluid resuscitation

Improvement in clinical condition may be indicated by improved perfusion, improved blood pressure, slowing heart rate (toward normal), decreased respiratory rate (toward normal), increased urinary output, and improved mental status.

If the clinical condition does not improve, identification of the cause of shock will help you determine the next interventions. For example, persistently delayed capillary refill despite initial fluid administration may be an indication of ongoing hemorrhage or other fluid loss. Deterioration of the child's condition after fluid therapy may signal cardiogenic or obstructive shock. Increased work of breathing may indicate pulmonary edema.

Indication for Blood Products

Blood and blood products are not the first choice for immediate volume expansion in children with shock. Blood is recommended for replacement of volume loss in pediatric trauma victims with inadequate perfusion despite administration of 2 to 3 boluses of 20 mL/kg of isotonic crystalloid. Under these circumstances packed red blood cells (PRBCs) 10 mL/kg should be ordered by a physician and administered as soon as available.

Priorities for transfusion include the following blood products in order:

- Crossmatched
- Type-specific
- Type O

Fully crossmatched blood is the first choice. Because most blood banks require approximately 1 hour for the crossmatching process, crossmatched blood is generally not available for use in emergencies. Crossmatched blood may be used for patients who are rapidly stabilized with crystalloid but who have ongoing blood losses.

Unmatched type-specific blood is indicated if ongoing blood loss results in hypotension despite administration of crystalloid. Most blood banks can supply type-specific blood within 10 minutes. Type-specific blood is ABO and Rh compatible, but unlike fully crossmatched blood, incompatibilities of other antibodies may exist.

Type O blood is used if the need for blood is immediate to avoid cardiac arrest. To avoid Rh sensitization, O-negative RBCs are preferred in females of childbearing age.

Complications of Rapid Administration of Blood Products

Rapid infusion of cold blood or blood products, particularly in large volume, may produce several complications, including[7]

- hypothermia
- myocardial dysfunction
- ionized hypocalcemia

Hypothermia may adversely affect cardiovascular function and compromise several metabolic functions, including metabolism of citrate, which is present in stored blood. Inadequate citrate clearance in turn causes ionized hypocalcemia. The combined effects of hypothermia and ionized hypocalcemia can result in significant myocardial dysfunction.

To minimize these problems, blood and blood products should be warmed if possible before or during rapid IV administration, using an approved commercial blood-warming device. Calcium should be available and in some cases should be administered empirically during rapid transfusions.

Glucose

Introduction

Monitor blood glucose concentration as a component of shock management. Hypoglycemia is a common finding in critically ill children,[8] and it can result in brain injury if not recognized and effectively treated. In a study of children who received resuscitative care in the emergency department for altered consciousness, status epilepticus, respiratory failure, cardiac failure, or cardiac arrest, 18% were hypoglycemic.[8]

Glucose Monitoring

Measure serum glucose concentration in all infants and children with coma, shock, or respiratory failure. Glucose can be measured with a bedside device or central laboratory analysis. The serum glucose concentration can be measured from samples of capillary blood, venous serum, or arterial whole blood.

Small infants and chronically ill children have limited stores of glycogen that may be rapidly depleted during episodes of cardiac distress, resulting in hypoglycemia. Infants receiving non–glucose-containing IV fluids are at increased risk for developing hypoglycemia.[9]

In all critically ill or injured children, perform a rapid glucose test to rule out hypoglycemia as a cause of shock or a contributing factor to poor clinical status.

Hyperglycemia, commonly seen in seriously ill or injured children, may result from a relative insulin-resistant state induced by high levels of endogenous catecholamines and hydrocortisone. Although correction of hyperglycemia with insulin infusion improves outcome in critically ill adult patients, there is insufficient data to recommend this treatment approach in critically ill children. In general, it is recommended to avoid hyperglycemia if possible and consider correcting hyperglycemia in high-risk groups, such as brain injured children.

Diagnosis of Hypoglycemia

Hypoglycemia may be difficult to recognize. Infants and children may be asymptomatic even though they are hypoglycemic (ie, asymptomatic hypoglycemia). Other children may have clinical signs of hypoglycemia (ie, poor perfusion, diaphoresis, tachycardia, hypothermia, irritability or lethargy, and hypotension) that are nonspecific and are also present with hypoxemia, ischemia, or shock.

In addition to the measured glucose concentration thresholds listed below, symptomatic hypoglycemia is defined by the presence of clinical symptoms such as altered mental status, sweating, tachycardia, or decreased perfusion. Although single values are not applicable to every patient, the following lowest acceptable glucose concentrations can be used to define hypoglycemia[10]:

Age	Consensus Definition of Hypoglycemia
Preterm neonates Term neonates	≤45 mg/dL
Infants Children Adolescents	≤60 mg/dL

The lower reported range of normal glucose is typically related to sample measurements obtained in nonstressed, fasting infants and children and may be difficult to correlate to the glucose concentration required by a stressed, critically ill, or injured child.

Management of Hypoglycemia

If the glucose concentration is low with minimal symptoms, glucose may be administered orally (eg, orange juice or other glucose-containing fluid). If the level is very low or the patient is symptomatic, glucose should be given intravenously (dextrose is the same as glucose). IV dextrose is commonly administered as $D_{25}W$ (2 to 4 mL/kg) or $D_{10}W$ (5 to 10 mL/kg, or 0.5 to 1 g/kg). Reassess the serum glucose concentration after dextrose administration.

Do not infuse dextrose-containing fluids for volume resuscitation in shock. Doing so can cause hyperglycemia, increased serum osmolality, and an osmotic diuresis, which can exacerbate hypovolemia and shock. Electrolyte imbalances (eg, hyponatremia) can also develop.

Management of Specific Categories of Shock

Introduction

Effective management of shock targets treatment to the etiology of the shock. For purposes of the PALS Provider Course, shock is categorized into 4 types, based on the underlying cause. This classification method, however, oversimplifies the physiologic state seen in individual patients. Some children with shock have elements of hypovolemic, distributive, and cardiogenic shock with one type being most dominant. Any child with severe shock will develop characteristics of myocardial dysfunction and maldistribution of blood flow. For a more comprehensive discussion of shock by etiology, see Chapter 4: Recognition of Shock.

Management of the following types of shock is discussed in this section:

- Hypovolemic shock
- Distributive shock
- Cardiogenic shock
- Obstructive shock

Management of Hypovolemic Shock

Introduction

Fluid resuscitation is the mainstay of therapy for hypovolemic shock. Children with hypovolemic shock who receive an appropriate volume of fluid within the first hour of resuscitation have the best chance for survival and recovery. Timely administration of fluid is key to preventing the deterioration of a relatively stable patient with compensatory hypovolemic shock to a patient with refractory hypotensive shock.

> *Avoid the common errors of inadequate or delayed administration of fluid resuscitation for hypovolemic shock.*

Other components in effective management of hypovolemic shock are

- identifying the type of volume loss (nonhemorrhagic versus hemorrhagic)
- replacing the deficit in intravascular and extracellular volume
- prevention of ongoing losses (eg, bleeding)
- restoring acid-base balance
- correcting metabolic derangements

Determining Adequate Fluid Resuscitation

Adequate fluid resuscitation in hypovolemic shock is determined by

- extent of volume depletion
- type of volume loss (eg, blood, electrolyte-containing fluid, or electrolyte-and-protein-containing fluid)

The extent of volume depletion may be underestimated and undertreated. In many cases volume depletion is compounded by inadequate fluid intake. The following clinical parameters can be assessed to help determine the percentage of dehydration[11]:

• General appearance	• Skin elasticity	• Presence of tears
• Pulse quality	• Urinary output	• Mucous membrane moisture
• Appearance of eyes (ie, normal vs sunken)	• Heart rate	• Respiratory rate and depth
	• Capillary refill time	

Generally, dehydration in children becomes clinically evident with approximately 4% dehydration (ie, 4% loss in body weight) corresponding to a fluid deficit of 40 mL/kg.[12] Therefore, treating a child with clinically evident dehydration with a single 20 mL/kg bolus of isotonic crystalloid may be insufficient. Conversely, it is usually unnecessary to completely correct the estimated deficit within the first hour. After perfusion is restored and the child is no longer in shock, the total fluid deficit may be corrected over the next 24 to 48 hours.

Although all forms of hypovolemic shock are initially treated similarly with rapid infusion of isotonic crystalloid, early identification of the type of volume loss will optimize further treatment. Fluid losses can be classified as hemorrhagic and nonhemorrhagic, including electrolyte-containing fluids (eg, diarrhea, vomiting, and osmotic diuresis associated with DKA), and electrolyte-and-protein-containing fluids (eg, losses associated with burns and peritonitis).

Nonhemorrhagic Hypovolemic Shock

Common sources of nonhemorrhagic fluid losses are gastrointestinal (ie, vomiting and diarrhea), urinary (eg, diabetic ketoacidosis), and capillary leak (eg, burns). Hypovolemia caused by nonhemorrhagic fluid losses is generally classified in terms of percent loss of body weight (Table 5).

Correlation of blood pressure and fluid deficits is imprecise. As a general rule, however, hypotensive shock may be observed in children with fluid deficits of 50 to 100 mL/kg, but it is more consistently observed with deficits of 100 mL/kg or more.

Treatment

Infuse 20 mL/kg boluses of isotonic crystalloid rapidly to effectively treat children with hypovolemic shock secondary to dehydration. If the child fails to improve after at least 3 boluses (ie, 60 mL/kg) of isotonic crystalloid, this indicates that

- the extent of fluid losses may be underestimated
- the type of fluid replacement may need to be altered (eg, the need for colloid or blood)
- there are ongoing fluid losses (eg, occult bleeding)
- the etiology of the shock may be more complex or different from your initial assumption

Ongoing fluid losses (eg, diarrhea, diabetic ketoacidosis, burns) must be replaced in addition to repletion of existing fluid deficits.

Colloid is not routinely indicated in the initial treatment of hypovolemic shock. Albumin and other colloids, however, have been used successfully for volume replacement in patients with large "third-space" losses or albumin deficits.[14,15]

Table 5. Stages and Signs of Dehydration[13]

Severity of Dehydration	Infant EWL (mL/kg)	Adolescent EWL (mL/kg)	Clinical Signs	Problems in Assessment
Mild	5% (50)	3% (30)	• Dry mucous membranes • Oliguria	• Oral mucosa may be dry in chronic mouth breathers • Frequency and amount of urine are difficult to assess during diarrhea, especially in girls
Moderate	10% (100)	5% to 6% (50 to 60)	• Poor skin turgor • Sunken fontanel • Marked oliguria • Tachycardia • Quiet tachypnea	• Affected by sodium concentration • Increased sodium concentration better maintains intravascular volume • Fontanel open only in infants • Oliguria is affected by fever, sodium concentration, underlying disease
Severe	15% (150)	7% to 9% (70 to 90)	• Marked tachycardia • Weak to absent distal pulses • Narrow pulse pressure • Quiet tachypnea • Hypotension and altered mental status (late findings)	Clinical signs are affected by fever, sodium concentration, underlying disease

EWL indicates estimated weight loss, and mL/kg refers to the estimated corresponding fluid deficit normalized to body weight.

Hemorrhagic Hypovolemic Shock

Hemorrhagic hypovolemic shock is classified based on estimated percentage of total blood volume loss (Table 6). The dividing line between compensated (Class I and II) and hypotensive (Class III and IV) hemorrhagic shock correlates with a loss of blood volume of approximately 30%.

Treatment

Fluid resuscitation in hemorrhagic shock begins with rapid infusion of isotonic crystalloid in boluses of 20 mL/kg. Because isotonic crystalloids are distributed throughout the extracellular water (25% in the intravascular space and 75% in the extravascular space), it may be necessary to give 3 boluses of 20 mL/kg (or a total of 60 mL/kg of fluid) to replace a 25% loss of blood volume. In other words, approximately 3 mL of crystalloid is needed for every 1 mL of blood lost. If the child remains hemodynamically unstable despite 2 to 3 isotonic crystalloid boluses of 20 mL/kg, consider a transfusion of PRBCs.

For blood replacement use PRBCs in 10 mL/kg boluses. To minimize adverse effects, warm the blood if a blood warming device is available. Whole blood (20 mL/kg) can be given in place of PRBCs, but it is harder and more time-consuming to obtain, and the risk of transfusion reaction is significantly increased.

Indications for transfusion in hemorrhagic shock include

- crystalloid-refractory hypotension or poor perfusion
- significant known blood loss

Crystalloid-refractory hemorrhagic shock is defined as persistent hypotension despite administration of 60 mL/kg crystalloid.[14] For children with acute hemorrhage, administer blood for a hemoglobin concentration less than 7 mg/dL because this level of anemia increases the risk of tissue hypoxia.

Table 6. Categorization of Hemorrhage and Shock in Pediatric Trauma Patients Based on Systemic Signs of Decreased Organ and Tissue Perfusion.

System	Mild Hemorrhage, Compensated Shock, Simple Hypovolemia (<30% blood volume loss)	Moderate Hemorrhage, Decompensated Shock, Marked Hypovolemia (30%-45% blood volume loss)	Severe Hemorrhage, Cardiopulmonary Failure, Profound Hypovolemia (>45% blood volume loss)
Cardiovascular	Mild tachycardia Weak peripheral pulses, strong central pulses Low-normal blood pressure (SBP >70 mm Hg + [2 × age in y]) Mild acidosis	Moderate tachycardia Thready peripheral pulses, weak central pulses Frank hypotension (SBP <70 mm Hg + [2 × age in y]) Moderate acidosis	Severe tachycardia Absent peripheral pulses, thready central pulses Profound hypotension (SBP <50 mm Hg) Severe acidosis
Respiratory	Mild tachypnea	Moderate tachypnea	Severe tachypnea
Neurologic	Irritable, confused	Agitated, lethargic	Obtunded, comatose
Integumentary	Cool extremities, mottling Poor capillary refill (>2 seconds)	Cool extremities, pallor Delayed capillary refill (>3 seconds)	Cold extremities, cyanosis Prolonged capillary refill (>5 seconds)
Excretory	Mild oliguria, increased specific gravity	Marked oliguria, increased blood urea nitrogen	Anuria

SBP indicates systolic blood pressure.

Used/Reproduced with permission from American College of Surgeons' Committee on Trauma, from *Advanced Trauma Life Support® for Doctors (ATLS®) Student Manual, 1997 (6th) Edition,* American College of Surgeons. Chicago: First Impressions, 1997.

Pharmacologic Support

Vasoactive agents are not indicated in the management of hypovolemic shock. Failure to respond to fluid therapy suggests that the extent of volume loss has been underestimated, the type of volume loss has been incorrectly identified, ongoing losses are occurring (eg, bleeding), or the type of shock is more complex (eg, septic or obstructive shock).

Moribund children with profound hypovolemic shock and hypotension may require short term administration of vasoactive agents such as epinephrine to restore cardiac contractility and vascular tone until adequate fluid resuscitation is provided.

Acid-Base Balance

Respiratory alkalosis secondary to tachypnea that does not completely correct the metabolic (lactic) acidosis produced by hypovolemic shock may be seen early. With long-standing or severe shock, the patient may lose respiratory drive or respiratory muscle strength so that the pH will fall without the compensatory respiratory alkalosis.

Persistent acidosis with poor perfusion is an indication of inadequate resuscitation or ongoing blood loss (in hemorrhagic shock). Routine use of sodium bicarbonate to treat metabolic acidosis secondary to hypovolemic shock is not recommended. As long as fluid resuscitation improves perfusion and end-organ function, metabolic acidosis is well tolerated and will gradually correct. If the metabolic acidosis is due to significant bicarbonate losses from renal or gastrointestinal losses (ie, a nonanion gap metabolic acidosis), the child may benefit from bicarbonate administration because it is difficult to compensate for ongoing bicarbonate loss.

Summary

Follow the initial management principles outlined in Table 3 in addition to the following considerations specific to hypovolemic shock (Table 7):

Table 7. Management of Hypovolemic Shock: Specific Treatment Considerations

Initiate fluid resuscitation as quickly as possible. • *In all patients,* infuse isotonic crystalloid (NS or LR) in 20 mL/kg boluses rapidly. • In *patients with crystalloid-refractory hemorrhagic shock,* give transfusion of 10 mL/kg PRBCs. • If loss of protein-containing fluids is documented or suspected by low albumin concentrations, consider use of colloid-containing fluids if the patient fails to respond to crystalloid resuscitation.
Correct metabolic derangements.
Identify type of volume loss (hemorrhagic or nonhemorrhagic) to determine best treatment.
Control external hemorrhage with direct pressure if present; measure and replace ongoing losses (eg, continued diarrhea).
Consider ancillary studies: • Complete blood cell count (CBC) • Type and crossmatch • ABG with particular attention to the base deficit • Electrolyte panel to calculate the anion gap • Serum or plasma lactate concentration • Chest x-ray

Management of Distributive Shock

Introduction

Management of distributive shock is aimed at expanding intravascular volume to correct hypovolemia and fill the expanded vascular space resulting from venodilation. If the child remains hypotensive or poorly perfused despite rapid fluid administration and the diastolic pressure is low with a wide pulse pressure, vasoconstrictors are indicated.

In this section we discuss specific management of the following types of distributive shock:

- Septic shock
- Anaphylactic shock
- Neurogenic shock

Management of Septic Shock

Introduction

The clinical, hemodynamic, and metabolic changes observed in septic shock result from the host's response to an infection with the release or activation of inflammatory mediators. The primary goals in the initial management of septic shock are

- restoration of hemodynamic stability
- identification and control of infection

Fundamental principles of management include increasing tissue oxygen delivery by optimizing cardiac output and arterial oxygen content and minimizing oxygen consumption.

Early recognition of the child with septic shock is key to initiation of resuscitation and prevention of cardiac arrest.

Overview of Septic Shock Algorithm

The recommended treatment approach to restore hemodynamic stability for septic shock in children is outlined in the PALS Septic Shock Algorithm (Figure), which outlines a 3-tiered treatment plan:

- Initiate treatment, including aggressive isotonic fluid administration, during the first hour for all patients with septic shock.
- Treat for fluid-refractory septic shock if the child does not respond to initial treatment.
- Anticipate the presence of adrenal insufficiency and provide stress dose hydrocortisone if the child does not respond to fluid administration and requires vasoactive drug support.

Initial Treatment

For a child in septic shock, adequate treatment during the first hour is critical to achieving a positive outcome. Early intubation and mechanical ventilation may be indicated. The initial components of management of septic shock are[4-6,9,16-19]

- rapid, aggressive fluid administration
- identification and correction of metabolic derangements (eg, hypoglycemia, hypocalcemia)
- rapid administration of antibiotics after cultures are obtained
- anticipation of possible need for vasopressors and stress-dose hydrocortisone
- laboratory studies such as lactate concentration, base deficit, and venous oxygen saturation to identify the severity of shock and monitor the response to fluid therapy

Begin aggressive fluid administration for initial hemodynamic support. Inadequate intravascular volume rapidly leads to low stroke volume and hypotension. A child in septic shock typically requires a large volume of fluid to restore perfusion. *Rapidly infuse 3 or 4 boluses (of 20 mL/kg each) of isotonic crystalloid.* Titrate to clinical indicators of tissue perfusion and cardiac output, including heart rate, peripheral pulses and skin temperature, urine output, capillary refill, and level of consciousness.

Pulmonary edema may develop in some children during fluid administration in septic shock. But the incidence of either cardiogenic or noncardiogenic pulmonary edema is more frequent with inadequate fluid resuscitation. Fluid should generally be given rapidly even though there is an increase in capillary permeability. If significant pulmonary edema develops, the child may require mechanical ventilatory support with supplementary oxygen and PEEP.

Hypoglycemia and ionized hypocalcemia are metabolic derangements commonly seen in septic shock. Identify and correct these conditions immediately because they may contribute to myocardial dysfunction.

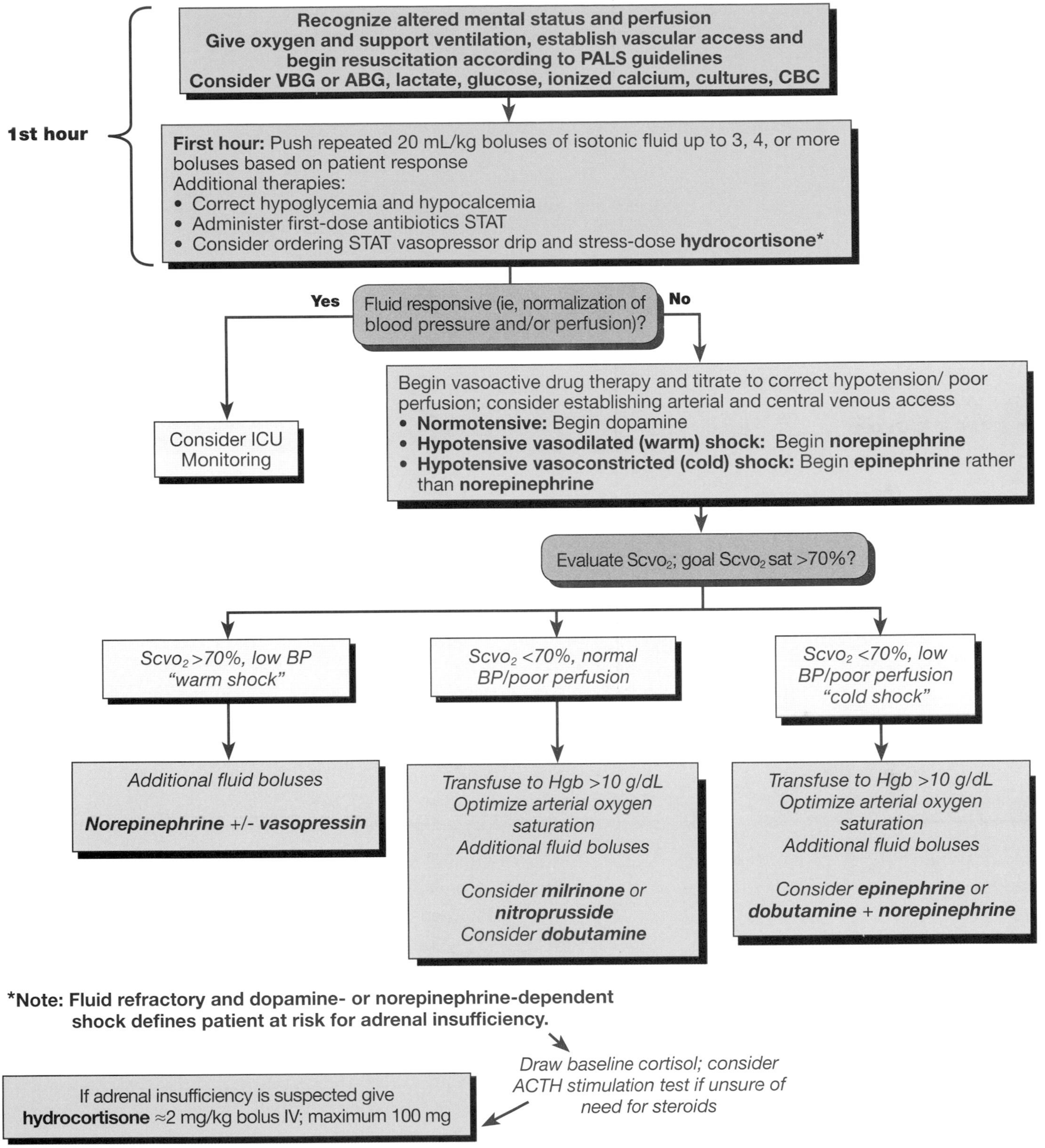

Figure. PALS Septic Shock Algorithm. Modified from Parker MM, Hazelzet JA, Carcillo JA. Pediatric considerations. Crit Care Med. 2004;32:S591-S594.

Draw blood samples for culture and sensitivity; administer the first-dose antibiotics as soon as possible. For severe sepsis do not delay antimicrobial therapy to obtain spinal fluid cultures. When possible, also obtain arterial or central venous samples, or both, for blood gas analysis and measurement of lactate concentration. If a venous sample is obtained, request measurement of the venous oxygen saturation because this can help identify the presence of a perfusion deficit.

Anticipate the possible need for vasopressors and stress-dose hydrocortisone. Order these drugs from the pharmacy early so that they will be at the bedside and immediately available if the child is fluid refractory or has the potential for adrenal insufficiency.

After initial treatment the next intervention is determined by blood pressure and perfusion. If blood pressure and perfusion are returning to normal, then consider transferring the child to an intensive care setting for monitoring. If blood pressure and perfusion are not normalizing, then proceed to the next level in the algorithm and treat the child for fluid-refractory septic shock.

Managing Fluid-Refractory Septic Shock

If severe shock persists despite rapid, aggressive administration of isotonic crystalloid in the first hour, start treatment for fluid-refractory septic shock as follows:

- Establish arterial and central venous access if not already in place.
- Administer vasopressors or vasoactive therapy to improve tissue perfusion and blood pressure.
- Administer additional fluid boluses of 20 mL/kg isotonic crystalloid and consider giving a colloid-containing fluid.
- Optimize arterial oxygen saturation (SaO_2) and oxygen-carrying capacity by transfusion if the hemoglobin concentration is below 10 g/dL.

Pharmacologic therapy is directed by the type of septic shock as defined by blood pressure, adequacy of tissue perfusion, and SvO_2.

Vasodilation or vasoconstriction is sometimes not evident from just the exam—some cold patients are vasodilated but poorly perfused because of low stroke volume and poor cardiac function.

The reasons for specific drug selection according to type of shock are described below.

Warm[16]

Norepinephrine is the vasoactive agent of choice for the child with fluid-refractory septic shock who presents in vasodilated (warm) shock with poor perfusion or hypotension. Norepinephrine is chosen for its potent α-adrenergic vasoconstricting effects. It is also chosen for its action to increase cardiac contractility with little change in heart rate, which can restore blood pressure by increasing systemic vascular resistance, venous tone, and stroke volume.

An infusion of *vasopressin* may be useful in the setting of norepinephrine-refractory shock. Vasopressin antagonizes the mechanisms of sepsis-mediated vasodilation and acts synergistically with endogenous or exogenous catecholamines in stabilizing blood pressure, but it lacks any effect on cardiac contractility.[17,18]

Normotensive

Dopamine is the preferred vasoactive agent for the child with fluid-refractory septic shock who presents with impaired perfusion but who is not hypotensive. Dopamine is best used in children with a wide pulse pressure consistent with a low systemic vascular resistance because it helps increase vascular smooth tone. It also has positive inotropic effects, but it is not as effective as epinephrine or norepinephrine as an inotropic agent. If the child's perfusion does not rapidly improve with a dopamine infusion, start an epinephrine or norepinephrine infusion. Based on the child's pulse pressure and clinical examination, use epinephrine if the child has normal to high vascular resistance; use norepinephrine if the child has low vascular resistance.

Vasodilators may be useful for improving tissue perfusion in normotensive children who have high systemic vascular resistance despite fluid resuscitation and initiation of inotropic support.

If poor perfusion persists despite use of dopamine, consider adding milrinone or nitroprusside to the treatment regimen. Milrinone is a phosphodiesterase inhibitor that has both inotropic and vasodilating effects. Nitroprusside is a pure vasodilator.

You may also consider dobutamine. Dobutamine provides both inotropic and vasodilating effects, but it often causes significant tachycardia and may produce substantial decreases in systemic vascular resistance.

Cold

Epinephrine is the preferred vasoactive agent to treat cold shock. Epinephrine has potent inotropic effects that improve stroke volume. Depending on the infusion dose, epinephrine can lower systemic vascular resistance at low infusion doses (from its β-adrenergic effects) or raise systemic vascular resistance at higher infusion rates (from its α-adrenergic action) to support both blood pressure and tissue perfusion. Infusion doses of epinephrine in the range of 0.3 µg/kg per minute or higher usually produce a predominant α-adrenergic action. Based on its effective use in adults with septic shock, the combination of dobutamine and norepinephrine may also be considered. The norepinephrine infusion counterbalances the tendency for dobutamine to cause excessive falls in systemic vascular resistance and appears to better restore splanchnic perfusion.

Correction of Adrenal Insufficiency

Fluid-refractory and dopamine-dependent or norepinephrine-dependent septic shock defines the patient at risk for adrenal insufficiency. In this case obtain a baseline cortisol level. In the absence of prospective data defining adrenal insufficiency based on cortisol level, adrenal insufficiency may be assumed at a random cortisol level of less than 18 µg/dL (496 nmol/L).

If the diagnosis of adrenal insufficiency is in doubt, an adrenocorticotropic hormone (ACTH) stimulation test can be performed to confirm the presence of the condition. An increase in cortisol of ≤9 µg/dL (248 nmol/L) after a 30-minute or 60-minute ACTH stimulation test is sufficient to confirm the diagnosis of adrenal insufficiency.[20]

If adrenal insufficiency is confirmed or suspected, give hydrocortisone 2 mg/kg IV bolus (maximum dose 100 mg).

Therapeutic End Points

The use of vasoactive agents in septic shock should be titrated to therapeutic end points, particularly

- good distal pulses and perfusion
- an adequate blood pressure
- an SvO_2 greater than 70%
- improving metabolic acidosis and lactate concentration

Strict adherence to end points is recommended to avoid excessive vasoconstriction in key organs.

Management of Anaphylactic Shock

Introduction

Management of anaphylactic shock focuses on the treatment of life-threatening cardiorespiratory problems and reversal or blockade of the mediators released as part of the uncontrolled allergic response.[21-24] Because angioedema (tissue swelling resulting from a marked increase in capillary permeability) may result in complete upper airway obstruction, early airway intervention is indicated. Provide assisted ventilation if necessary. The mainstay of therapy is administration of epinephrine to reverse hypotension and the release of histamine and other allergic mediators. Fluid resuscitation may also be helpful to restore blood pressure.

Specific Treatment Considerations

Consider the initial general management of shock outlined in Table 3 in addition to the following specific treatments for anaphylactic shock as indicated (Table 8).

Table 8. Management of Anaphylactic Shock: Specific Treatment Considerations

Rapidly administer pharmacologic support in the symptomatic child. • Epinephrine — L-epinephrine or epinephrine autoinjector (pediatric or adult, depending on the child's size) — This is the most important agent in the treatment of anaphylaxis — An infusion may be needed with severe anaphylaxis • Albuterol — Administer albuterol PRN for bronchospasm by intermittent nebulizer or continuous nebulizer • Antihistamines — H_1 blocker (ie, diphenhydramine) — Consider H_2 blocker — Note: The combination of both an H_1 and H_2 blocker may be more effective than either antihistamine given alone • Corticosteroids — Methylprednisolone or equivalent corticosteroid
For intramuscular epinephrine and fluid-refractory hypotension, use vasopressors as indicated • Epinephrine infusions, titrate as needed

Observation is indicated for identification and treatment of late-phase symptoms, which may occur several hours after acute-phase symptoms.[23] The likelihood of late-phase symptoms increases in proportion to the severity of acute-phase symptoms.

Management of Neurogenic Shock

Introduction

The child in neurogenic shock typically presents with hypotension, bradycardia, and sometimes hypothermia. Minimal response to fluid resuscitation is commonly observed. The blood pressure is characterized by a low diastolic blood pressure with wide pulse pressure because of the loss of vascular tone. Children with spinal shock may be more sensitive to variations in temperature and may require supplementary warming or cooling.

Specific Treatment Considerations

The initial management principles for shock outlined in Table 3 may be considered in addition to the following specific treatments for neurogenic shock as indicated (Table 9).

Table 9. Management of Neurogenic Shock: Specific Treatment Considerations

Position the patient flat or head-down to improve venous return.
For fluid-refractory hypotension, use vasopressors (eg, norepinephrine, epinephrine) as indicated.
Provide supplementary warming or cooling as needed.

Management of Cardiogenic Shock

Introduction

Cardiogenic shock is a condition of inadequate tissue perfusion resulting from myocardial dysfunction. The initial presentation of cardiogenic shock may resemble hypovolemic shock, so identifying a cardiogenic etiology can be difficult. If you suspect cardiogenic shock, consider a slow (10 to 20 minutes) fluid challenge (ie, 5 to 10 mL/kg bolus) while carefully monitoring the child for response. If the child does not improve or the child's condition deteriorates, including deterioration in respiratory function or development of pulmonary edema, cardiogenic shock is likely. Evidence of venous congestion (eg, distended jugular veins or hepatomegaly) and cardiomegaly (per chest x-ray) is also suggestive of a cardiac etiology of shock.

Main Objectives

The main objectives in the management of cardiogenic shock are to improve the effectiveness of cardiac function and overall cardiac output by increasing the efficiency of ventricular emptying and to minimize interventions or host responses that increase metabolic demand.

Many children with cardiogenic shock have high preload and do not require additional fluid therapy. Others may require a cautious fluid bolus to increase preload. The most effective way to increase stroke volume is to reduce afterload (systemic vascular resistance) rather than giving an inotropic agent, which may increase cardiac contractility but also will increase myocardial oxygen demand. It is also helpful to attempt to reduce oxygen demand. Specific management includes

- cautious fluid administration and monitoring
- laboratory and nonlaboratory studies
- pharmacologic support

Consultations with pediatric critical care or pediatric cardiology should be initiated at the earliest opportunity for facilitating a diagnosis (eg, echocardiogram), guiding ongoing therapy, and transfer to definitive care.

Cautious Fluid Administration and Monitoring

Adequate intravascular volume in the setting of cardiogenic shock may be assessed by seeing a large heart on chest x-ray. More objective data about the preload of the heart can be obtained with an echocardiogram. If objective data or the patient's history (eg, vomiting and poor intake) are consistent with inadequate preload, then a *cautious fluid bolus may be given*. Frequently assess respiratory function during fluid therapy, anticipating the development of pulmonary edema and deterioration in pulmonary function. Administer supplementary oxygen, and be prepared to provide assisted ventilation. BiPAP reduces the need for mechanical ventilation by decreasing the work of breathing and improving oxygenation.

Consider establishing central venous access. Central venous access will facilitate measurement of central venous pressure as an index of the preload status, provide access for multiple infusions, and allow for monitoring of central venous oxygen saturation as an objective measurement of the adequacy of tissue perfusion relative to the patient's metabolic demand. Invasive monitoring with a pulmonary artery catheter, which is performed in the pediatric intensive care unit, is not critical to the diagnosis of cardiogenic shock but may be helpful in guiding fluid resuscitation and vasoactive infusions, particularly if determination of left ventricular preload is needed.

Laboratory Studies

Laboratory studies should be obtained to assess the impact of shock on end-organ function. No single laboratory study is completely sensitive or specific for cardiogenic shock. Appropriate studies often include

- an ABG to determine the magnitude of metabolic acidosis and adequacy of oxygenation and ventilation
- hemoglobin concentration to ensure that the oxygen-carrying capacity is adequate
- lactate concentration and central venous oxygen saturation as indicators of the adequacy of cardiac output, cardiac enzymes, and thyroid function

Nonlaboratory studies often include the following:

Study	Use
Chest x-ray	Provides information about cardiac size, pulmonary vascular markings and presence of pulmonary edema, and coexistent pulmonary pathology
ECG	May detect arrhythmia, myocardial injury pattern, ischemic heart disease, or evidence of drug toxicity
Echocardiogram	May be diagnostic, revealing congenital heart disease, akinetic or dyskinetic ventricular wall motion, or valvular dysfunction; also provides objective measurement of ventricular chamber volume (ie, preload)

Pharmacologic Support

Typical pharmacologic support consists of diuretics and vasodilators. Diuretics are indicated when the patient has evidence of pulmonary edema or systemic venous congestion. Vasodilators are typically given by continuous infusion. Milrinone is the preferred drug in many centers.

Increased metabolic demand, particularly increased myocardial oxygen demand, plays a role in the vicious cycle of cardiogenic shock. Reducing metabolic demand is a critical component in the management of cardiogenic shock and can be achieved through the use of ventilatory support and antipyretics. Administration of analgesics, sedatives, or both may be helpful. Give these agents in small doses and monitor the child carefully. Analgesics and sedatives reduce the endogenous stress response that may have an effect on the child's ability to maintain borderline cardiovascular function.

Infants and children with cardiogenic shock may require drug therapy to increase cardiac output by improving contractility; most will receive agents to reduce vascular resistance. This therapy includes vasodilators, inotropes, and phosphodiesterase enzyme inhibitors (also referred to as inodilators). For a detailed discussion of these agents, see "Pharmacologic Support" in "General Management of Shock."

Summary

Follow the initial management principles for shock outlined in Table 3 in addition to the following considerations specific to cardiogenic shock (Table 10).

Table 10. Management of Cardiogenic Shock: Specific Treatment Considerations

• Administer fluid resuscitation cautiously. • Give 5 to 10 mL/kg isotonic crystalloid infusion. • Deliver slowly (over 10 to 20 minutes), repeat PRN. • Administer supplementary oxygen and consider need for BiPAP or mechanical ventilation. • Assess for pulmonary edema. • Be prepared to assist ventilation. • Obtain expert consultation early.
Order laboratory and nonlaboratory studies to determine underlying cause.
Administer pharmacologic support (eg, vasodilators, phosphodiesterase enzyme inhibitors, inotropes, analgesics, antipyretics).

Management of Obstructive Shock

Introduction

Management of obstructive shock is specific to the type of obstruction. This section discusses management of the following:

- Cardiac tamponade
- Tension pneumothorax
- Ductal-dependent congenital heart lesions
- Massive pulmonary embolism

Main Objectives

The early clinical presentation of obstructive shock may resemble hypovolemic shock. A reasonable initial approach may include administering a fluid challenge (10 to 20 mL/kg isotonic crystalloid). Rapid identification of obstructive shock by secondary and tertiary assessments is critical to effective treatment. The main objectives in the management of obstructive shock are

- correction of the cause of obstruction to cardiac output
- restoration of tissue perfusion

Because children with obstructive shock can rapidly progress to cardiac failure and arrest, immediate recognition and correction of the underlying cause of the obstruction can be life-saving.

General Management Principles

In addition to considerations specific to the etiology of the obstruction, follow the initial management principles outlined in the section "Fundamentals of Shock Management."

Specific Management of Cardiac Tamponade

Cardiac tamponade is caused by accumulation of fluid, blood, or air in the pericardial space that results in impaired systemic venous return, impaired ventricular filling, and reduced cardiac output. Favorable outcome depends on urgent diagnosis and immediate treatment.

Children with cardiac tamponade may improve with fluid administration to augment cardiac output and tissue perfusion until pericardial drainage can be performed.

Correction of Obstruction to Cardiac Output

Consult appropriate specialists (eg, pediatric critical care, pediatric cardiology, pediatric surgery). Elective pericardial drainage (pericardiocentesis) should be performed by specialists who are trained and skilled in the procedure, often guided by echocardiography or fluoroscopy. Emergency pericardiocentesis may be performed in the setting of impending or actual pulseless arrest when there is a strong suspicion of pericardial tamponade.

Specific Management of Tension Pneumothorax

Tension pneumothorax is characterized by the accumulation of air under pressure in the pleural space. The pleural air that is under increased pressure prevents the lung from expanding properly and applies pressure on the heart and great veins. Favorable outcome depends on urgent diagnosis and immediate treatment.

Correction of Tension Pneumothorax

Treatment of a tension pneumothorax is immediate needle decompression followed by thoracostomy for chest tube placement as soon as possible. A trained provider can quickly perform an emergent needle decompression by inserting an 18- to 20-gauge over-the-needle catheter over the top of the child's third rib in the midclavicular line. A gush of air is a sign that needle decompression has been successful, indicating relief of the buildup of pressure in the pleural space. Please refer to the procedure on the student CD: *"Tension Pneumothorax."*

Ductal-Dependent Lesions

Ductal-dependent lesions are congenital cardiac abnormalities that generally present in the first weeks of life. Immediate treatment with continuous infusion of prostaglandin E_1 to restore ductal patency may be life-saving.

Correction of Obstruction to Cardiac Output

Prostaglandin E_1 restores ductal patency by vasodilation.

Other Management Actions

Other management actions for ductal-dependent lesions consist of the following:

- Ventilatory support with oxygen administration
- Consult with appropriate specialist
- Use of echocardiography for diagnosis and to direct therapy
- Administration of inotropic agents to improve myocardial contractility
- Judicious fluid administration to improve cardiac output
- Correction of metabolic derangements, including metabolic acidosis

Specific Management of Massive Pulmonary Embolism

Massive pulmonary embolism is a sudden block in the main or branch pulmonary artery. This block is usually from a blood clot that has traveled to the lung from some other part of the body, but it can result from other substances, including fat, air, amniotic fluid, catheter fragment, or injected matter.

Treatment of a Massive Pulmonary Embolism

Initial treatment is supportive, including administration of oxygen, ventilatory assistance, and fluid therapy if the child is poorly perfused. Consult a specialist who can perform echocardiography, computed tomography (CT) scan with intravenous contrast, or angiography to confirm the diagnosis. Anticoagulants (eg, heparin, enoxaparin) are the definitive treatment for most children with pulmonary embolism who are not in shock. Because anticoagulants do not act immediately to relieve obstruction, use of thrombolytic agents (eg, urokinase, streptokinase, alteplase) may be considered in children with severe cardiovascular compromise.

Other Management Actions

CT angiography is the diagnostic test of choice because it is rapidly obtained and does not require an invasive angiogram. Additional diagnostic studies that might be useful include an ABG, CBC, D-dimer, ECG, chest x-ray, ventilation-perfusion scan, and echocardiography.[25-32]

References

1. Samotowka M, Ivy M, Burns GA. Endpoints of resuscitation. *Trauma Q.* 1997;13:231-245.
2. Finfer S, Bellomo R, Boyce N, et al. A comparison of albumin and saline for fluid resuscitation in the intensive care unit. *N Engl J Med.* 2004;350(22):2247-2256.
3. Griffel MI, Kaufman BS. Pharmacology of colloids and crystalloids. *Crit Care Clin.* 1992;8(2):235-253.
4. Powell KR, Sugarman LI, Eskenazi AE, et al. Normalization of plasma arginine vasopressin concentrations when children with meningitis are given maintenance plus replacement fluid therapy. *J Pediatr.* 1990;117(4):515-522.
5. Carcillo JA, Davis AL, Zaritsky A. Role of early fluid resuscitation in pediatric septic shock. *JAMA.* 1991;266(9):1242-1245.
6. Ceneviva G, Paschall JA, Maffei F, et al. Hemodynamic support in fluid-refractory pediatric septic shock. *Pediatrics.* 1998;102(2):e19.
7. Nacht A. The use of blood products in shock. *Crit Care Clin.* 1992;8(2):255-291.

8. Losek JD. Hypoglycemia and the ABC'S (sugar) of pediatric resuscitation. *Ann Emerg Med.* 2000;35(1):43-46.

9. Parker MM, Hazelzet JA, Carcillo JA. Pediatric considerations. *Crit Care Med.* 2004;32(11 suppl):S591-S594.

10. Cornblath M, Hawdon JM, Williams AF, et al. Controversies regarding definition of neonatal hypoglycemia: suggested operational thresholds. *Pediatrics.* 2000;105(5):1141-1145.

11. Gorelick MH, Shaw KN, Murphy KO. Validity and reliability of clinical signs in the diagnosis of dehydration in children. *Pediatrics.* 1997;99(5):E6.

12. Mackenzie A, Barnes G, Shann F. Clinical signs of dehydration in children. *Lancet.* 1989;2(8663):605-607.

13. Zaritsky A, Dieckmann R, the EMSC Taskforce. EMSC definitions and pediatric assessment approaches. In preparation.

14. De Bruin WJ, Greenwald BM, Notterman DA. Fluid resuscitation in pediatrics. *Crit Care Clin.* 1992;8(2):423-438.

15. Haupt MT, Kaufman BS, Carlson RW. Fluid resuscitation in patients with increased vascular permeability. *Crit Care Clin.* 1992;8(2):341-353.

16. Landry D RJ. Pro/con: vasopressin in the treatment of vasodilatory shock. Paper presented at: 33rd Critical Care Congress; February 23, 2004; Orlando, Fla.

17. Holmes CL, Walley KR, Chittock DR, et al. The effects of vasopressin on hemodynamics and renal function in severe septic shock: a case series. *Intensive Care Med.* 2001;27(8):1416-1421.

18. Patel BM, Chittock DR, Russell JA, et al. Beneficial effects of short-term vasopressin infusion during severe septic shock. *Anesthesiology.* 2002;96(3):576-582.

19. Carcillo JA, Fields AI. [Clinical practice parameters for hemodynamic support of pediatric and neonatal patients in septic shock.] *J Pediatr (Rio J).* 2002;78(6):449-466.

20. Pizarro CF, Troster EJ, Damiani D, et al. Absolute and relative adrenal insufficiency in children with septic shock. *Crit Care Med.* 2005;33(4):855-859.

21. Dibs SD, Baker MD. Anaphylaxis in children: a 5-year experience. *Pediatrics.* 1997;99(1):E7.

22. Korenblat P, Lundie MJ, Dankner RE, et al. A retrospective study of epinephrine administration for anaphylaxis: how many doses are needed? *Allergy Asthma Proc.* 1999;20(6):383-386.

23. Lee JM, Greenes DS. Biphasic anaphylactic reactions in pediatrics. *Pediatrics.* 2000;106(4):762-766.

24. Sampson HA, Munoz-Furlong A, Campbell RL, et al. Second symposium on the definition and management of anaphylaxis: summary report—Second National Institute of Allergy and Infectious Disease/Food Allergy and Anaphylaxis Network symposium. *J Allergy Clin Immunol.* 2006;117(2):391-397.

25. Beitzke A, Zobel G, Zenz W, et al. Catheter-directed thrombolysis with recombinant tissue plasminogen activator for acute pulmonary embolism after fontan operation. *Pediatr Cardiol.* 1996;17(6):410-412.

26. David M, Andrew M. Venous thromboembolic complications in children. *J Pediatr.* 1993;123(3):337-346.

27. Dollery CM. Pulmonary embolism in parenteral nutrition. *Arch Dis Child.* 1996;74(2):95-98.

28. Kossel H, Bartsch H, Philippi W, et al. Pulmonary embolism and myocardial hypoxia during extracorporeal membrane oxygenation. *J Pediatr Surg.* 1999;34(3):485-487.

29. Kossoff EH, Poirier MP. Peripherally inserted central venous catheter fracture and embolization to the lung. *Pediatr Emerg Care.* 1998;14(6):403-405.

30. Vichinsky EP, Neumayr LD, Earles AN, et al. Causes and outcomes of the acute chest syndrome in sickle cell disease. National Acute Chest Syndrome Study Group. *N Engl J Med.* 2000;342(25):1855-1865.

31. Monagle P, Michelson AD, Bovill E, et al. Antithrombotic therapy in children. *Chest.* 2001;119(1 suppl):344S-370S.

32. Monagle P, Chan A, Massicotte P, et al. Antithrombotic therapy in children: the Seventh ACCP Conference on Antithrombotic and Thrombolytic Therapy. *Chest.* 2004;126(3 suppl):645S-687S.

Chapter 6

Recognition and Management of Bradyarrhythmias and Tachyarrhythmias

Overview

Introduction

Cardiac rhythm disturbances (arrhythmias) occur as a result of abnormalities in, or insults to, the cardiac conduction system or heart tissues. In the advanced life support setting, an arrhythmia in a child can be broadly classified according to the observed heart rate or effect on perfusion:

Heart Rate	Classification
Slow	Bradyarrhythmia
Fast	Tachyarrhythmia
Arrest	Pulseless arrest

This chapter discusses the recognition and management of abnormal rhythms with pulses, broadly sorting them into 2 groups: bradyarrhythmias and tachyarrhythmias. See Chapter 7 for a discussion of arrest rhythms.

Evaluating Heart Rate and Rhythm

Consider the following in evaluating the heart rate and rhythm in any seriously ill or injured child:

- the child's typical heart rate and baseline rhythm
- the child's level of activity and clinical condition (including baseline myocardial function)

Children with congenital heart disease often have one or more rhythm abnormalities; you must also interpret their cardiac rate and rhythm in light of those baseline abnormalities. Children with poor baseline myocardial function will often be less tolerant of arrhythmias than children with good myocardial function.

Learning Objectives

After studying this chapter you should be able to

- recognize unstable conditions requiring urgent intervention, such as those that produce shock with hypotension, poor end-organ perfusion (especially altered consciousness), and conditions with high risk for deterioration to arrest
- differentiate supraventricular tachycardia (SVT) from sinus tachycardia (ST)
- describe initial steps to stabilize the child who is unstable as the result of an arrhythmia
- describe indications for vagal maneuvers used for treatment of SVT with adequate perfusion
- describe when and how to provide electrical therapy for arrhythmias with a pulse: synchronized cardioversion attempts or pacing
- select appropriate medications for treatment of symptomatic bradycardia (rhythms that are too slow) and tachycardia (rhythms that are too fast)
- give an example of a child with an arrhythmia and know when to seek expert consultation

Bradyarrhythmias

Introduction

Bradyarrhythmias are the most common prearrest rhythms in children. They are often associated with conditions such as hypoxemia, hypotension, and acidosis.

Bradycardia

Bradycardia is defined as a heart rate that is slow compared with normal heart rates for the patient's age. See Table 2: Normal Heart Rates by Age in Chapter 1.

A *relative bradycardia* is defined as a heart rate that is too slow for the child's level of activity and clinical condition.

Clinically significant bradycardia is defined as a heart rate of less than the normal rate for age associated with poor systemic perfusion. A heart rate less than 60/min with poor perfusion is an indication to begin chest compressions.

Primary and Secondary Bradycardia

Bradycardia may be classified as

- primary bradycardia
- secondary bradycardia

Primary bradycardia is the result of congenital and acquired heart conditions that directly slow the spontaneous depolarization rate of the heart's normal pacemaker cells or slow conduction through the heart's conduction system. Causes of primary bradycardia include intrinsic problems with the heart pacemaker (eg, congenital abnormality), postsurgical injury to the pacemaker or conduction system, cardiomyopathy, and myocarditis.

Secondary bradycardia is the result of conditions that alter the normal function of the heart (ie, slow the sinus node pacemaker or slow conduction through the atrioventricular [AV] junction). Causes of secondary bradycardia include hypoxia, acidosis, hypotension, hypothermia, and drug effects.

Recognition of Bradyarrhythmias

Symptoms of Bradyarrhythmias

Bradyarrhythmias may present with nonspecific symptoms, such as change in level of consciousness, lightheadedness, dizziness, syncope, and fatigue. An extremely slow heart rate can be life threatening. The cardinal signs of instability associated with bradyarrhythmias are

- shock with hypotension
- poor end-organ perfusion
- altered consciousness
- sudden collapse

A very slow heart rate can cause shock from inadequate cardiac output. The child is potentially unstable if deterioration to shock or cardiac arrest is likely.

> ***Symptomatic bradycardia requiring urgent treatment is defined as a heart rate slower than normal for the patient's age associated with evidence of shock (eg, poor systemic perfusion, hypotension, altered consciousness) and/or respiratory distress or failure.***

Tissue hypoxia, often due to hypoxemia, is the leading cause of symptomatic bradycardia in children.

ECG Characteristics of Bradycardia

The ECG characteristics of bradycardia include

Heart rate	Slow compared with normal rates for the patient's age
P waves	May or may not be visible
QRS complex	Narrow or wide (depending on location of intrinsic cardiac pacemaker and location of any injury to the conduction system)
P wave and QRS complex	May be unrelated (ie, AV dissociation)

Refer to the student CD for a discussion of basic ECG interpretation.

Examples of Bradyarrhythmias

Examples of bradyarrhythmias[1] include

- sinus bradycardia
- sinus node arrest with atrial, junctional or idioventricular escape rhythms
- AV block

Sinus Bradycardia

Sinus bradycardia (Figure 1A) is commonly an incidental finding in otherwise healthy persons, particularly in young adults, sleeping patients, and well-conditioned athletes. It normally develops as a physiologic consequence of reduced metabolic demand (eg, during sleep, rest, or hypothermia) or increased stroke volume (eg, in the well-conditioned athlete). The most common pathologic cause of symptomatic sinus bradycardia is hypoxia. Other pathologic causes include poisoning, electrolyte disorders, infection, sleep apnea, drug effects, hypoglycemia, hypothyroidism, and increased intracranial pressure.

Sinus Node Arrest

Sinus node arrest is characterized by absent pacemaker activity in the sinus node. Under such circumstances, a subsidiary pacemaker in the atrium, AV junction, or ventricles may initiate cardiac depolarization, resulting in the following rhythms:

- Atrial escape rhythm
- Junctional escape rhythm
- Idioventricular escape rhythm

An atrial escape rhythm arises during episodes of bradycardia when the impulse arises from a subsidiary nonsinus atrial pacemaker. It is characterized by a late P wave of different morphology.

A junctional escape rhythm (Figure 1B) is a relatively slow narrow-complex rhythm. The rhythm originates in the AV node, which has the intrinsic ability to initiate depolarization of the myocardium (automaticity). This ability allows the tissue to initiate and depolarize the myocardium if other pacemaker tissues (that normally have faster spontaneous rates of depolarization) fail. This escape mechanism produces a narrow QRS complex because the ventricle is depolarized through the normal conduction pathway. The QRS complexes are also uniform in appearance. Retrograde P waves representing depolarization of the atria arising from the AV node may or may not be present.

An idioventricular escape rhythm (Figure 1C) is a slow, wide-complex rhythm. The rhythm originates in the ventricles, which also have intrinsic automaticity allowing them to initiate depolarization of the myocardium during periods of significant bradycardia or high-grade AV block. The ventricular depolarization rate is typically between 30 to 40/min but may be as low as 15/min. If atrial activity is present, there is no relation between atrial and ventricular activity due to heart block.

AV Block

AV block is a disturbance of electrical conduction through the AV node. AV block is classified as the following:

- First degree—characterized by a prolonged PR interval representing slowed conduction through the AV node (Figure 2A)
- Second degree—some but not all atrial impulses are conducted to the ventricle. This block can be further characterized as Mobitz type I or Mobitz type II second-degree block. Mobitz type I block (also known as Wenckebach phenomenon) typically occurs at the AV node and is characterized by progressive prolongation of the PR interval until an atrial impulse is not conducted to the ventricles (Figure 2B). As a result one P is not followed by a QRS complex. In Mobitz type II second-degree block (Figure 2C), the block occurs below the level of the AV node and is characterized by consistent inhibition of a specific proportion of atrial impulses, usually a 2:1 atrial to ventricular rate.
- Third degree—none of the atrial impulses is conducted to the ventricle. This block may also be referred to as complete heart block or complete AV block (Figure 2D).

Type	Cause	Characteristics	Symptoms
First degree	• Intrinsic AV nodal disease • Enhanced vagal tone • Myocarditis • Electrolyte disturbances (eg, hyperkalemia) • Myocardial infarction • Drugs (eg, calcium channel blockers, β-adrenergic blockers, digoxin) • Acute rheumatic fever (May also be found in healthy persons)	Prolonged PR interval	Typically occurs without symptoms
Second-degree Mobitz type I (Wenckebach phenomenon)	• Drugs (eg, calcium channel and β-adrenergic blockers, digoxin) • Any condition that stimulates parasympathetic tone • Myocardial infarction (May also be found in healthy persons)	Progressive prolongation of the PR interval until a P wave is blocked and the cycle is repeated	Rarely causes dizziness
Second-degree Mobitz type II	• Typically results from organic lesion in the conduction pathway • Rarely caused by increased parasympathetic tone or drugs • Acute coronary syndrome	Some but not all P waves are conducted to the ventricle (PR interval is typically prolonged but constant). Most often every other P-wave is conducted (2:1 block)	May cause • sensed irregularities of heart beat • presyncope (ie, feeling faint and lightheaded) • syncope
Third degree	• Extensive conduction system disease or injury (usually from surgery) • Myocardial infarction • Congenital block • Myocarditis • Can also result from increased parasympatholytic tone or toxic drug effects	• No relationship between P waves and QRS complex • No atrial impulses reach ventricles • Ventricular rhythm is maintained by subsidiary pacemaker	Symptomatic condition; most frequently reported symptoms are • fatigue • presyncope • syncope

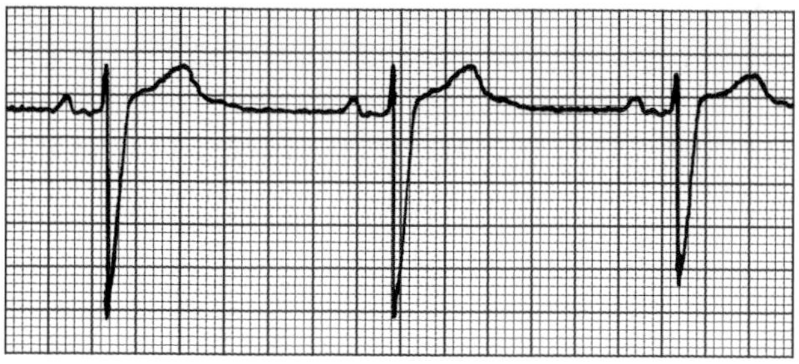

A

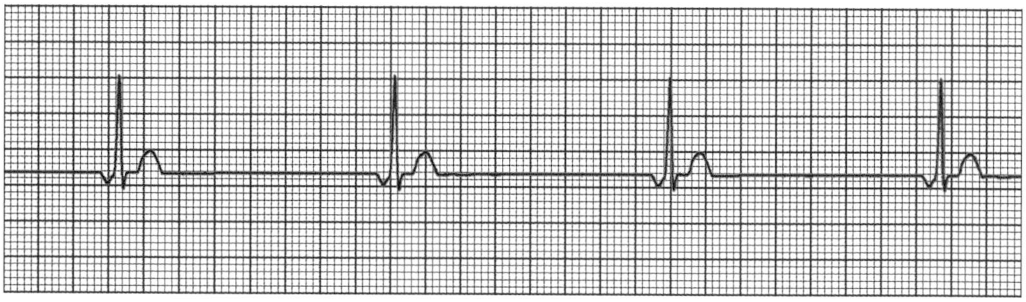

B

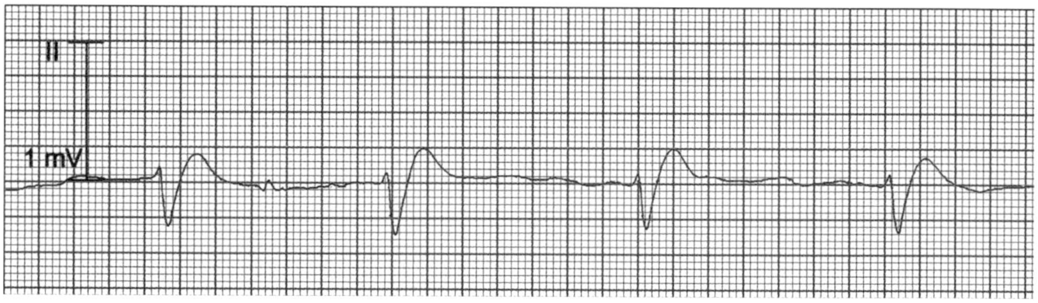

C

Figure 1. Bradycardia. **A**, Sinus bradycardia. **B**, Junctional escape rhythm. **C**, Idioventricular escape rhythm.

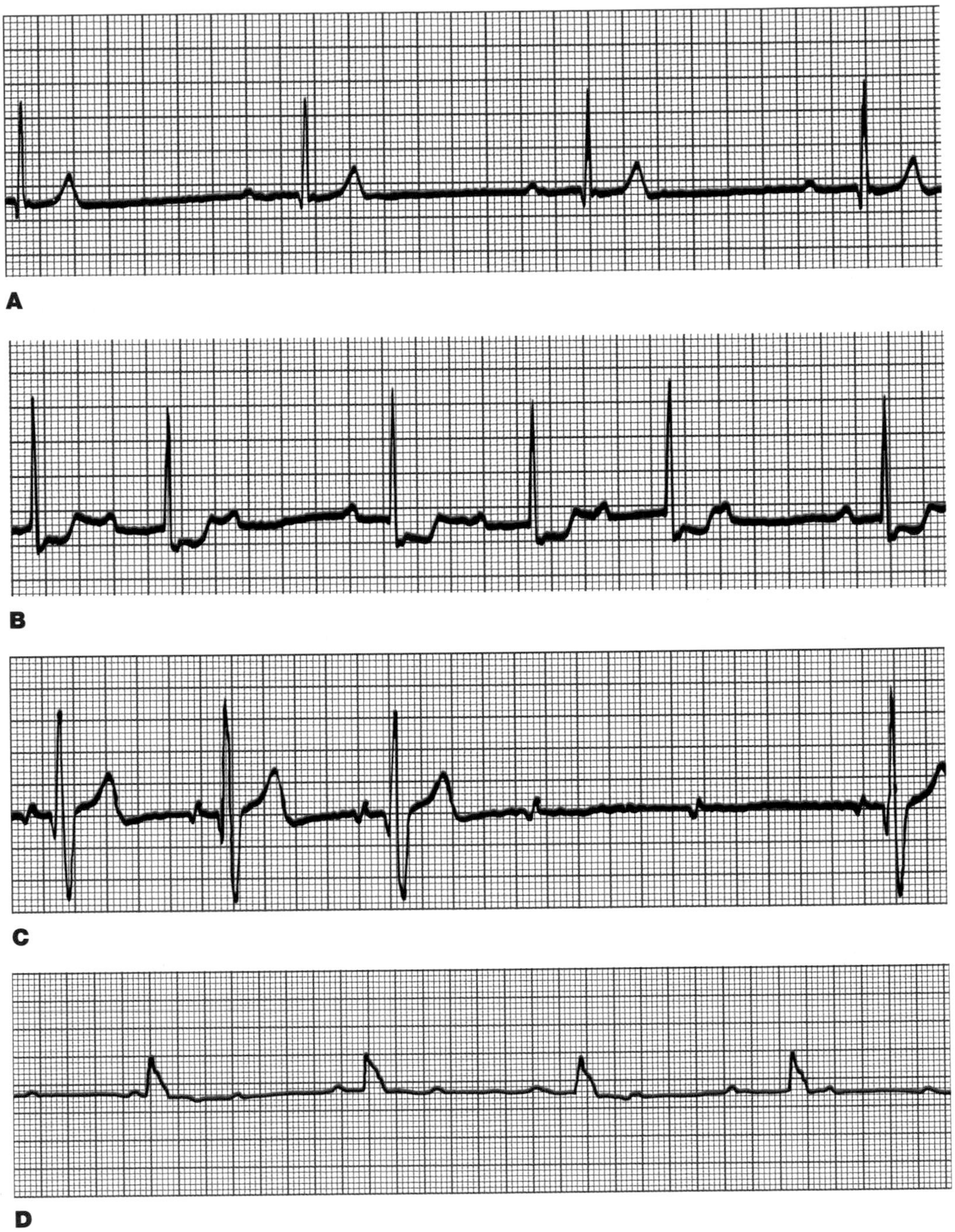

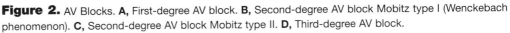

Figure 2. AV Blocks. **A,** First-degree AV block. **B,** Second-degree AV block Mobitz type I (Wenckebach phenomenon). **C,** Second-degree AV block Mobitz type II. **D,** Third-degree AV block.

Management of Bradyarrhythmias: Pediatric Bradycardia With a Pulse Algorithm

Overview (Box 1)

The Pediatric Bradycardia Algorithm (Figure 3) outlines the steps for assessment and management of the child presenting with symptomatic bradycardia (bradycardia with cardiorespiratory compromise). Symptomatic bradycardia is defined as a heart rate less than the normal rate for age associated with evidence of shock (eg, poor systemic perfusion, hypotension, altered consciousness) and/or respiratory distress or failure.

Initiate Management (Box 2)

Once you recognize a bradyarrhythmia resulting in shock or life-threatening hemodynamic instability, initial management may include the following:

Airway	Support the airway (position child or allow child to assume a position of comfort) or open the airway (perform manual airway maneuver).
Breathing	• Provide oxygen in high concentration—use a nonrebreathing system if available. • Assist ventilation as indicated (eg, bag-mask ventilation). • Attach a pulse oximeter to assess oxygenation.
Circulation	• Assess perfusion. • Perform chest compressions as indicated (ie, HR <60/min with poor perfusion). • Attach a monitor/defibrillator (with transcutaneous pacing capability if available). • Check electrode pad position and skin contact to ensure that there are no artifacts and that the ECG tracing is accurate. • Record a 12-lead ECG if available. (Note: Although a 12-lead ECG may be useful, a precise diagnosis of the bradyarrhythmia is not immediately required.) • Establish vascular access. • Obtain appropriate laboratory studies (eg, potassium, glucose, ionized calcium, magnesium, blood gas for pH, toxicology screen).

The child with a bradyarrhythmia may benefit from evaluation by a pediatric cardiologist. This consultation should not delay initiation of emergency treatment if indicated.

Do not delay therapy if severe symptoms are present.

Reassess (Box 3)

Reassess to determine if bradycardia is causing cardiorespiratory compromise.

Cardiorespiratory compromise?	Management
NO	Go to Box 5A. Plan to support ABCs, administer supplementary oxygen as needed, and observe the child. Consider expert consultation and other interventions listed above in Box 2.
YES	Go to Box 4. Perform chest compressions with ventilations (CPR).

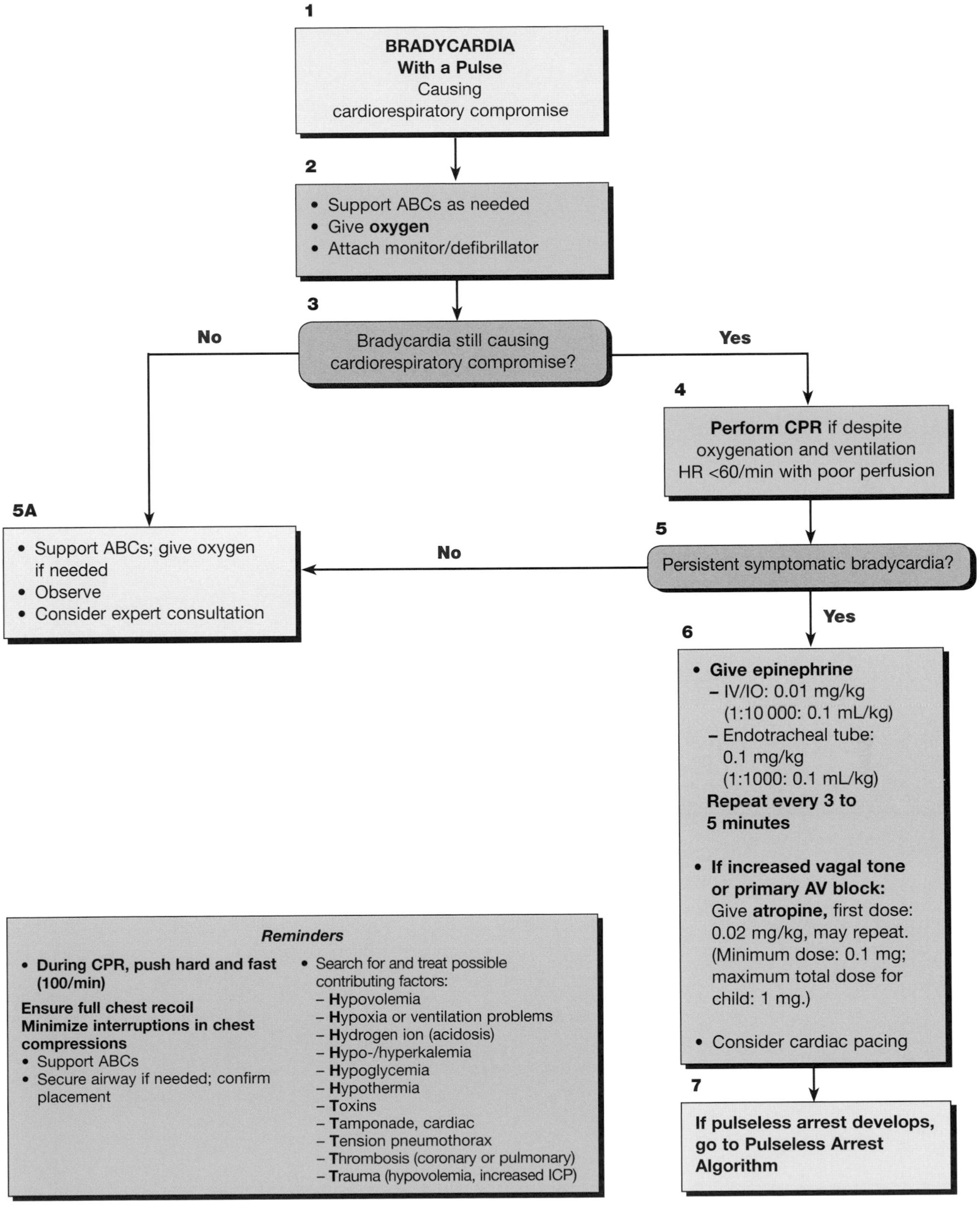

Figure 3. Pediatric Bradycardia With a Pulse Algorithm.

Perform CPR (Box 4)

If bradycardia is associated with cardiorespiratory compromise and if heart rate is less than 60/min despite effective oxygenation and ventilation, perform chest compressions with ventilations.

During CPR push hard and fast at a rate of 100 compressions per minute. Ensure full chest recoil. Try to minimize interruptions in chest compressions.

Reassess (Box 5)

Reassess if bradycardia persists and is causing cardiorespiratory compromise.

Cardiorespiratory compromise?	Management
NO	Go to Box 5A. Plan to support ABCs, administer supplementary oxygen as needed, and observe the child. Consider expert consultation.
YES	Go to Box 6. Administer pharmacologic agents and consider cardiac pacing.

Administer Pharmacologic Agents (Box 6)

If bradycardia is associated with cardiorespiratory compromise, administer epinephrine and consider atropine.

Epinephrine

Epinephrine is indicated for persistent symptomatic bradycardia despite effective oxygenation and ventilation. The efficacy of epinephrine and other catecholamines may be reduced by acidosis and hypoxia.[2,3] This makes support of the airway, ventilation, oxygenation, and perfusion (with chest compressions) essential. A continuous epinephrine infusion may be useful, particularly if the patient has responded to bolus infusions of epinephrine.

IV/IO	0.01 mg/kg (1:10 000: 0.1 mL/kg)
Endotracheal tube	0.1 mg/kg (1:1000: 0.1 mL/kg)
Repeat every 3 to 5 minutes as needed.	

For persistent bradycardia, consider a continuous infusion of epinephrine (0.1 to 0.3 μg/kg per minute) or dopamine (2 to 20 μg/kg per minute). Titrate the infusion dose to clinical response.

Atropine

For bradycardia caused by increased vagal tone, cholinergic drug toxicity (eg, organophosphates), or AV block, administer atropine rather than epinephrine as indicated by the patient's symptoms. If the patient fails to respond to atropine, then epinephrine may be used. Atropine sulfate is a parasympatholytic drug that accelerates sinus or atrial pacemakers and enhances AV conduction.

IV/IO	First dose—0.02 mg/kg; minimum 0.1 mg (maximum single dose of 0.5 mg for a child and 1 mg for an adolescent)[4] May repeat dose in 5 minutes (maximum total dose of 1 mg for a child and 2 mg for an adolescent) Note: Larger doses may be required for organophosphate poisoning[5]
Endotracheal tube Note: IV/IO access is preferred, but if it is not available, you can administer atropine by endotracheal tube.[6] Because absorption by the endotracheal route is unreliable, a larger dose (2 to 3 times the IV dose for drugs other than epinephrine) may be required.[5]	0.04 to 0.06 mg/kg

Atropine or atropine-like drugs are often used prophylactically in young children to prevent vagally mediated bradycardia during endotracheal intubation attempts.

Note that small doses of atropine may produce paradoxical bradycardia[4]; for this reason a minimum dose of 0.1 mg is recommended. Tachycardia may follow administration of atropine, but atropine-induced tachycardia is generally well tolerated in the pediatric patient.

Symptomatic AV block due to intrinsic disease is an indication for using atropine (and pacing) preferentially over epinephrine. Intrinsic AV block (called "primary" AV block in the algorithm) is a form of AV block that results from primary causes of bradycardia. These are conditions related to heart disease such as intrinsic cardiac conditions (eg, cardiomyopathy, myocarditis) and postsurgical cardiac conditions, rather than from treatable causes such as transient hypoxia or drug therapy.

The rationale for the preferential use of atropine in the treatment of primary AV block is that the combination of epinephrine and a chronically abnormal and often ischemic myocardium can lead to ventricular arrhythmias. Atropine may be beneficial in the treatment of symptomatic second- or third-degree AV block at the level of the AV node. The healthcare provider should recognize, however, that symptomatic AV block may not respond to atropine, and the child may require pacing. First-degree AV block generally does not require treatment.

Consider Cardiac Pacing (Box 6)

Cardiac pacing may be life-saving in selected cases of bradycardia caused by complete heart block or abnormal sinus node function.[7-9] For example, pacing is indicated for AV block following surgical correction of congenital heart disease.

Pulseless Arrest (Box 7)

If pulseless arrest develops, provide CPR and refer to the Pediatric Pulseless Arrest Algorithm (in Chapter 7).

Identifying and Treating Underlying Causes

Identify and treat potentially reversible causes and special circumstances that can cause bradyarrhythmias. The 2 most common potentially reversible causes are hypoxia and increased vagal tone. Following heart transplantation the heart is "denervated," so it will have an unpredictable response to sympathomimetic drug administration. For the same reason, anticholinergics may not be effective. Early cardiac pacing may be indicated.

Potentially reversible causes can be recalled using some of the H's and T's as follows:

Reversible Cause	Treatment
Hypoxia	Give supplementary oxygen in high concentration.
Hypothermia	Treat with warming techniques. Avoid hyperthermia if the patient has experienced a cardiac arrest.
Hyperkalemia	Restore normal potassium concentrations.
Heart block	Consider atropine for AV block, along with chronotropic drugs, electrical pacing, and expert consultation.
Toxins/poisons/ drugs	Treat with a specific antidote as indicated and provide supportive care. The more important toxicologic causes of bradyarrhythmias include — cholinesterase inhibitors (organophosphates, carbamates, and nerve agents) — calcium channel blockers — β-adrenergic blockers — digoxin and other cardiac glycosides — clonidine and other centrally acting α_2-adrenergic agonists — opioids — succinylcholine
Trauma	Head trauma — Provide oxygenation and ventilation. If signs of impending herniation develop, provide hyperventilation.

Tachyarrhythmias

Introduction

Tachyarrhythmias represent a variety of fast *abnormal* rhythms originating either in the atria or the ventricles of the heart.

Tachycardia

Tachycardia is defined as a heart rate that is fast compared with normal heart rates for the patient's age. See Table 2: Normal Heart Rates by Age in Chapter 1.

A *relative tachycardia* is a heart rate that is too fast for the child's level of activity and clinical condition.

Tachycardia may be a normal response to stress or fever (ie, sinus tachycardia). Tachyarrhythmias may or may not cause acute compromise in the child's condition. Certain fast rhythms can lead to shock and deteriorate further to cardiac arrest. Appropriate recognition and management of tachyarrhythmias are important to prevent morbidity and mortality in children.

Recognition of Tachyarrhythmias

Tachyarrhythmias may cause nonspecific signs and symptoms that differ according to the age of the patient. Clinical findings may include palpitations, lightheadedness, dizziness, fatigue, and syncope. In infants the tachyarrhythmia may be undetected for long periods (eg, for hours at home) until cardiac output is significantly impaired and the infant develops signs of congestive heart failure, such as poor feeding, rapid breathing, and irritability. Episodes of extremely rapid heart rate are life threatening if they significantly compromise cardiac output. In this chapter we discuss tachycardia with detectable pulses.

The cardinal signs of instability associated with tachyarrhythmias are

- respiratory distress/failure, often due to pulmonary edema (lung tissue disease)
- shock with hypotension or poor end-organ perfusion
- altered consciousness
- sudden collapse with rapid detectable pulses

The rhythm is unstable if it causes signs or symptoms of poor tissue perfusion. To a point, when the heart rate increases, cardiac output increases. Extremely rapid heart rates can, however, produce a fall in cardiac output when there is insufficient time for diastolic filling and stroke volume falls substantially. Coronary artery perfusion occurs chiefly during diastole; a very rapid heart rate decreases the time for diastole and reduces coronary artery perfusion. A fast heart rate also increases myocardial oxygen demand. A very fast heart rate combined with inadequate cardiac output and poor myocardial perfusion can lead to cardiogenic shock.

Classification

Tachycardic rhythms may be generally classified according to the width of the QRS complex, either narrow complex or wide complex:

Narrow Complex	Wide Complex
• Sinus tachycardia • Supraventricular tachycardia • Atrial flutter	• Ventricular tachycardia • Supraventricular tachycardia with aberrant intraventricular conduction

Sinus Tachycardia

Introduction

Sinus tachycardia (ST) is defined as a rate of sinus node discharge faster than normal for the patient's age. ST typically develops in response to the body's need for increased cardiac output or oxygen delivery. When ST is present, the heart rate is not fixed; it varies with activity and other factors influencing oxygen demand (eg, the child's temperature). ST is a nonspecific clinical sign rather than a true arrhythmia (Figure 4).

Common causes of ST include tissue hypoxia, hypovolemia (hemorrhagic and nonhemorrhagic fluid loss), fever, metabolic stress, injury, pain, anxiety, toxins/poisons/drugs, and anemia. Cardiac tamponade, tension pneumothorax, and thromboembolism are less common causes of ST.

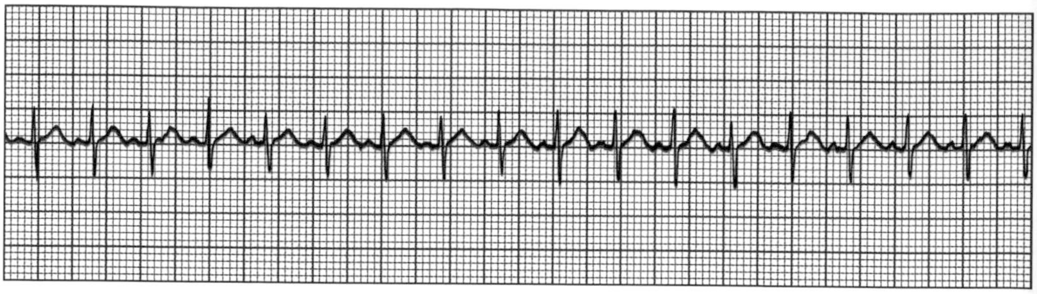

Figure 4. ST (heart rate 180/min) in a febrile 10-month old infant.

ECG Characteristics of ST

The ECG characteristics of ST include the following:

Heart rate	Beat to beat variability with changes in activity or stress level • Usually <220/min in infants • Usually <180/min in children
P waves	Present/normal
PR interval	Constant, normal duration
R-R interval	Variable
QRS complex	Narrow

Supraventricular Tachycardia

Introduction

Supraventricular tachycardia (SVT) is an abnormally fast rhythm originating above the ventricles. It is most commonly caused by a reentry mechanism that involves an accessory pathway or the AV conduction system. SVT is the most common tachyarrhythmia producing cardiovascular compromise during infancy.

Outdated terms for SVT include *paroxysmal atrial tachycardia* (PAT) and *paroxysmal supraventricular tachycardia* (PSVT). SVT was labeled "paroxysmal" because it starts and stops without warning.

Mechanism

SVT is caused by one of the following mechanisms:

- Accessory pathway reentry
- AV nodal reentry
- Ectopic atrial focus

Accessory Pathway Reentry

SVT in children most commonly involves an abnormal rhythm circuit that allows a wave of depolarization to travel in a circle, between the atria and ventricles. It includes either a reentry mechanism within the AV node, or it involves the AV node as an accessory pathway. A reentrant circuit is established as a wave of depolarization is conducted to the ventricle through the AV node and then back to the atrium using an accessory pathway.

Accessory pathway SVT is the most common cause of nonsinus tachycardia in children. A common example of a condition that produces SVT via an accessory pathway is Wolff-Parkinson-White (WPW) syndrome, in which ventricular pre-excitation (producing a "delta wave" on the ECG) is visible during sinus rhythm.

AV Nodal Reentry

SVT may also result from reentry using dual pathways (fast and slow) within the AV node. When regular conduction through the typical "fast" pathway is blocked following a premature atrial contraction (because the "fast" pathway is temporarily refractory), the wave of depolarization proceeds along a different pathway (ie, down the "slow" pathway). At the point when the depolarization completes the slow pathway, conduction in the fast pathway is no longer blocked because the tissue has now recovered its ability to conduct. As a result the wave of depolarization can now proceed back along the fast pathway, completing a circuit of conduction back into the atria and starting the cycle again.

Ectopic Atrial Focus

In a small number of children with SVT, particularly following cardiac surgical repairs, the tachyarrhythmia results from an ectopic focus in the atria, which depolarizes at a faster rate than the SA node. Names for this type of SVT include ectopic atrial tachycardia (EAT), atrial ectopic tachycardia (AET), or automatic tachycardia. An ectopic focus may also arise in the AV node, leading to junctional ectopic tachycardia (JET). Again, JET is most commonly seen following surgical repair in infants.

Clinical Presentation of SVT

SVT (Figure 5) is a rapid, regular rhythm that often appears abruptly and may be intermittent. Cardiopulmonary function during episodes of SVT is affected by the child's age, duration of SVT, prior ventricular function, and ventricular rate.

In infants very rapid rates may go undetected for long periods until cardiac output is significantly impaired. This deterioration in cardiac function results from the combination of increased myocardial oxygen demand and limitation in myocardial oxygen delivery. Myocardial oxygen delivery is reduced because coronary artery perfusion time is compromised during the short diastolic phase associated with very rapid heart rates.

If baseline myocardial function is impaired (eg, in a child with congenital heart disease or cardiomyopathy), SVT can produce signs of shock in a relatively short time.

Symptoms

SVT is often diagnosed in infants because of symptoms of congestive heart failure. SVT usually presents differently in older children.

Common signs and symptoms of SVT in infants include poor feeding, rapid breathing, irritability, unusual sleepiness, pale or blue skin color, and vomiting.

Common signs and symptoms of SVT in older children include palpitations, shortness of breath, chest pain or discomfort, dizziness, lightheadedness, and fainting.

SVT is initially well tolerated in most infants and older children. It can, however, lead to congestive heart failure and clinical evidence of shock, particularly if baseline myocardial function is impaired (eg, a child with congenital heart disease or cardiomyopathy). It can ultimately cause cardiovascular collapse.[10,11]

Signs

Using the primary assessment model, SVT may be recognized by its effect on systemic perfusion. SVT with cardiorespiratory compromise can produce the signs and symptoms noted below.

Airway	
Breathing	• Tachypnea • Increased work of breathing • Rales (or "wheezing" in infants) may be present if congestive heart failure develops • Grunting if congestive heart failure is present
Circulation	• Tachycardia beyond the normal range for ST and characterized by fixed rate or abrupt onset • Hypotension may be present • Delayed capillary refill time • Weak peripheral pulses • Cool extremities • Diaphoretic, mottled, gray or cyanotic skin • Jugular venous distention (difficult to appreciate in young children)—only if CHF develops
Disability	• Diminished level of consciousness • Irritability
Exposure	Defer evaluation of temperature until you support ABCs

ECG Characteristics of SVT

The ECG characteristics of SVT include the following:

Heart rate	No beat to beat variability with activity • Usually >220/min in infants • Usually >180/min in children
P waves	Absent or abnormal
PR interval	Since P waves are usually absent, cannot determine PR interval. If ectopic atrial tachycardia, may see short PR interval
R-R interval	Often constant
QRS complex	Usually narrow; wide complex uncommon

Narrow-Complex SVT

In more than 90% of children with SVT, the QRS complex is narrow (Figure 5), ie, ≤0.08 sec.[12]

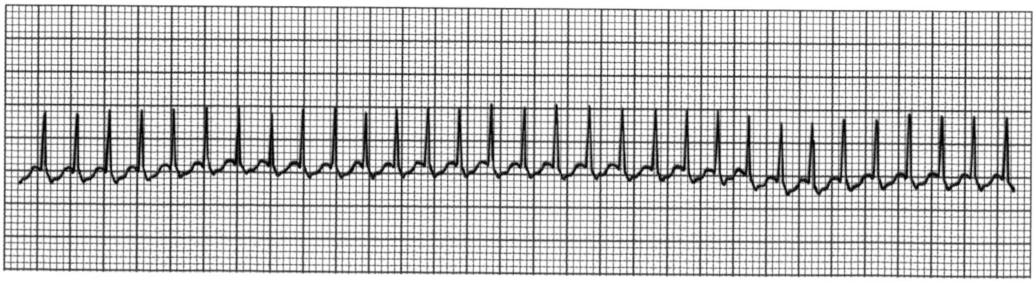

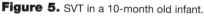

Figure 5. SVT in a 10-month old infant.

Wide-Complex SVT

SVT with aberrant conduction producing a wide QRS complex (ie, >0.08 sec) is uncommon. This form of SVT most often occurs due to rate-related bundle branch block within the ventricles or preexisting bundle branch block. It may also be caused by an unusual accessory pathway in which electrical impulses are conducted to the ventricles through the accessory tract (rather than along the usual route through the AV node) and return to the atrium through the AV node.

Correct diagnosis of SVT with aberrant conduction and differentiation from VT require careful analysis of at least one 12-lead ECG that may be supplemented by information from an esophageal lead. Both SVT and VT can cause hemodynamic instability, so evidence of shock is not helpful in differentiating SVT with aberrant conduction from VT.

Of note, one case series of 32 patients suggested that wide-complex tachycardia in infants, children, and adolescents is more likely to be supraventricular than ventricular in origin.[13] However, unless the child is known to have aberrant conduction, the provider should generally presume that a wide-complex tachycardia is VT.

Comparison of ST and SVT

It may be difficult to differentiate SVT as the *primary cause of shock* from ST representing an *appropriate compensatory response* to a shock state of another etiology. The following characteristics may aid in differentiation of ST and SVT, noting that signs of heart failure and other symptoms may be absent early after the onset of SVT.

Characteristic	ST	SVT
History	Gradual onset compatible with ST (eg, history of fever, pain, dehydration, hemorrhage)	Abrupt onset or termination Infant: congestive heart failure (CHF) symptoms Child: palpitations
Physical exam	Signs of underlying cause of ST (eg, fever, hypovolemia, anemia)	Signs of CHF (eg, rales, hepatomegaly, edema)
Heart rate	Infant: usually <220/min Child: usually <180/min	Infant: usually >220/min Child: usually >180/min
Monitor	Variability in heart rate with changes in level of activity or stimulation; slowing of heart rate with rest or treatment of underlying cause (eg, administration of IV fluids for hypovolemia)	Minimal variability in heart rate with changes in level of activity or stimulation
ECG	P waves present/normal/ upright in leads I/aVF	P waves absent/abnormal/ inverted (negative) in leads II/III/aVF
Chest x-ray	Usually small heart and clear lungs unless cause of ST is pneumonia or underlying heart disease	Signs of CHF (eg, pulmonary edema) may be present

P waves may be difficult to identify in both ST and SVT once the ventricular rate exceeds 200/min.

Atrial Flutter

Atrial flutter is an uncommon narrow-complex tachyarrhythmia in children. It is characterized by a reentry circuit within the atria that allows a wave of depolarization to travel in a circle within the atria. Often a constant proportion of these depolarization waves are transmitted through the AV node, resulting in ventricular depolarization. Flutter waves often occur at a rate of around 350 to 400/min, resulting in ventricular depolarization at 175 to 200/min with 2:1 conduction or 115 to 130/min if 3:1 conduction. A reentrant circuit typically is present in children with enlarged atria or with anatomic barriers resulting from cardiac surgery (eg, atriotomy scars or surgical anastomoses). Classically a "sawtooth" pattern of the P waves is present on the ECG. As noted above, because the AV node is not part of the reentrant circuit, AV conduction may be variable, and the ventricular rate may be irregular.

Ventricular Tachycardia

Introduction

Ventricular tachycardia (VT) is a wide-complex tachyarrhythmia generated within the ventricles (Figure 6). VT is uncommon in children. When VT with pulses is present, the ventricular rate may vary from near normal to more than 200/min. Rapid ventricular rates often compromise stroke volume and cardiac output, and they may deteriorate into pulseless VT or VF.

Most children who develop VT have underlying heart disease (or have had surgical intervention for heart disease), prolonged QT syndrome, or myocarditis/cardiomyopathy. Other causes of VT in children include electrolyte disturbances (eg, hyperkalemia, hypocalcemia, hypomagnesemia) and drug toxicity (eg, tricyclic antidepressants, cocaine).

ECG Characteristics of Ventricular Tachycardia

The ECG characteristics of VT include the following:

Ventricular rate	At least 120/min and regular
QRS complex	Wide (>0.08 sec)
P waves	Often not identifiable; when present, may not be related to the QRS (AV dissociation); at slower rates, atria may be depolarized in a retrograde manner, and there will be a 1:1 ventricular-to-atrial association
T waves	Typically opposite in polarity from QRS

It may be difficult to differentiate SVT with aberrant conduction from VT. Fortunately, aberrant conduction is present in less than 10% of children with SVT. In general, the healthcare provider should initially assume that a wide-complex rhythm is VT unless the child is known to have aberrant conduction.[14]

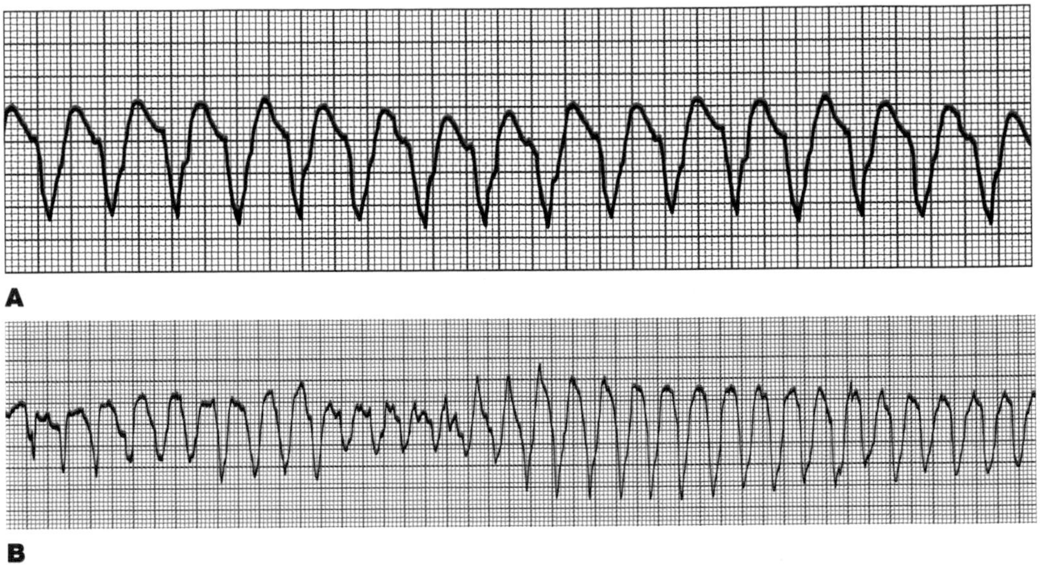

Figure 6. Ventricular tachycardia. **A,** Monomorphic; **B,** Polymorphic (torsades de pointes)

Polymorphic VT, Including Torsades de Pointes

Pulseless VT may be monomorphic (QRS complexes are uniform in appearance) or polymorphic (QRS complexes vary in appearance). Torsades de pointes ("to turn on a point") is a distinctive form of polymorphic VT. In torsades the QRS complexes change in polarity and amplitude, appearing to rotate around the ECG isoelectric line (Figure 6B). The ventricular rate can range from 150 to 250/min. Torsades de pointes can be seen in conditions associated with a markedly prolonged baseline QT interval, including congenital conditions and drug toxicity. The prolonged QT interval is identified during sinus rhythm; it cannot be evaluated during the tachycardia. A rhythm strip may show the patient's baseline QT prolongation because torsades de pointes sometimes occurs in bursts that are not sustained.

Conditions and agents that predispose to torsades de pointes include

- long QT syndromes (often inherited conditions)
- hypomagnesemia
- antiarrhythmic drug toxicity (ie, Class IA quinidine, procainamide, diisopyramide; Class IC encainide, flecainide; Class III sotalol, amiodarone)
- other drug toxicities (eg, tricyclic antidepressants, calcium channel blockers, phenothiazines)

It is important to recognize that VT, including torsades de pointes, can deteriorate to VF. The long QT syndromes are associated with sudden death due to either primary VF or torsades de pointes. Polymorphic VT not associated with a prolonged QT interval during sinus rhythm is treated as generic VT.

Management of Tachyarrhythmias

Initial Management Questions

Answer the following questions to direct your initial management of a critically ill or injured patient with a rapid heart rate seen on the monitor:

Does the patient have a pulse (or signs of circulation)?

Pulse or Signs of Circulation	Management
Absent	Initiate the Pediatric Pulseless Arrest Algorithm. Note: Since the accuracy of a pulse check is poor,[15-21] recognition of cardiac arrest may require that you identify *the absence of signs of circulation* (ie, the child is unresponsive, has no breathing other than agonal gasps). With invasive monitoring of arterial pressure, absence of arterial waveform is observed.
Present	Proceed with the tachycardia algorithms.

Is perfusion adequate or poor?

Perfusion	Management
Poor	Initiate the Algorithm for Pediatric Tachycardia With Pulses and Poor Perfusion for emergency treatment.
Adequate	Initiate the Algorithm for Pediatric Tachycardia With Adequate Perfusion. Consider consulting a pediatric cardiologist.

Is the rhythm narrow complex or wide complex?

Rhythm	Management
Narrow Complex	Consider the differential of sinus tachycardia versus supraventricular tachycardia.
Wide Complex	Consider the differential of SVT versus VT but treat as presumed VT unless the child has known aberrant conduction.

Initial Management Priorities

Once you recognize an arrhythmia resulting in shock or life-threatening hemodynamic instability, initial management priorities include the following:

- Support the ABCs and oxygenation as needed.
- Establish monitoring: attach monitor/defibrillator and pulse oximeter.
- Establish vascular access.
- Obtain laboratory studies (eg, potassium, glucose, ionized calcium, magnesium, blood gas to assess pH and cause of pH changes) as appropriate (do not delay urgent intervention for these studies).
- Assess neurologic status.
- Treat hypothermia.
- Anticipate need for appropriate medications depending on the type of rhythm disturbance (ie, supraventricular versus ventricular).

You should simultaneously seek to identify and treat reversible causes.

> ***Many children with tachyarrhythmias should be evaluated by a pediatric cardiologist. This consultation should not delay initiation of emergency treatment.***

Emergency Interventions

Introduction

Specific emergency interventions used to treat tachyarrhythmias with pulses are dictated by the severity of the child's condition. Treatments also vary based on the width of the observed QRS complex (narrow versus wide). Interventions include the following:

- Vagal maneuvers (if the child with a narrow-complex tachycardia is stable or while preparations are made for synchronized cardioversion)
- Synchronized cardioversion
- Pharmacologic therapy
- Expert consultation

Vagal Maneuvers

In normal infants and children, the heart rate falls when the vagus nerve is stimulated. In patients with SVT, vagal stimulation may terminate the tachycardia by slowing conduction through the AV node. Several maneuvers stimulate vagal activity. The success rates of these maneuvers in terminating tachyarrhythmias vary, depending on the child's age, level of cooperation, and underlying condition.

Be sure to support the patient's airway, breathing, and circulation. If possible, obtain a 12-lead ECG before and after the maneuver; record and monitor the ECG continuously during the maneuver. *If the patient is stable* and the rhythm does not convert, you may repeat the attempt. *If the second attempt fails,* select another method or provide pharmacologic therapy. *If the patient is unstable,* attempt vagal maneuvers only while making preparations for pharmacologic or electrical cardioversion. Do not delay definitive treatment to perform vagal maneuvers. See the student CD for a detailed description of vagal maneuvers.

Cardioversion

Electrical cardioversion can be frightening and painful for a child. Whenever possible, establish vascular access and provide procedural sedation before cardioversion, particularly when the cardioversion is elective. If the patient's condition is unstable, do not delay synchronized cardioversion to achieve vascular access. Sedation in the setting of an arrhythmia carries significant risk. When procedural sedation is given in this setting, providers must carefully select medications in order to minimize the risk of a cardiac arrest.

This section discusses the following important concepts regarding cardioversion:

- Definition of synchronized cardioversion
- Potential problems with synchronized shocks
- Indications for the use of synchronized cardioversion
- Energy doses

Synchronized Cardioversion

Modern defibrillators are capable of delivering 2 types of shocks: unsynchronized and synchronized. Unsynchronized shocks are high-dose shocks used to attempt defibrillation for victims of cardiac arrest. Synchronized shocks are shocks of lower dose used for cardioversion.

Synchronized cardioversion uses a sensor to deliver a shock that is synchronized with a specified duration after the peak of the QRS complex (highest point of the R wave). The initial shock dose used for synchronized cardioversion is lower than that used for (unsynchronized) attempted defibrillation. When the synchronize option of the defibrillator/cardioverter is engaged, the shock is delivered a few milliseconds after the R wave. When you press the SHOCK button, the defibrillator/cardioverter may seem to pause before it delivers a shock because it is waiting to synchronize shock delivery with the next QRS complex. This avoids the delivery of a shock on the T wave (during cardiac repolarization). Such delivery is undesirable because it could precipitate VF.

Potential Problems

In theory synchronization is simple. The operator pushes the SYNC button on the face of the defibrillator, charges the device, and delivers the shock. In practice, however, there are potential problems. For example:

- The SYNC button must be activated each time before synchronized cardioversion is attempted. The device will default to deliver an unsynchronized shock immediately after delivery of the synchronized shock.
- If the R-wave peaks of a tachycardia are undifferentiated or of low amplitude, the monitor sensors may be unable to identify an R-wave peak and therefore will not deliver the shock.
- Synchronization can take extra time (eg, if it is necessary to attach separate ECG electrodes or if the operator is unfamiliar with the equipment).

Indications

Synchronized cardioversion is used for

- unstable patients with tachyarrhythmias (SVT, VT with pulses, atrial flutter) who have a perfusing rhythm and evidence of cardiovascular compromise, such as poor perfusion, hypotension, or heart failure
- elective cardioversion at the direction of a pediatric cardiologist in children with stable SVT, atrial flutter, or VT

Energy Doses

Low-energy shocks should always be delivered as synchronized shocks. For synchronized cardioversion, use a first dose of 0.5 to 1 J/kg for SVT or VT with a pulse that causes cardiovascular instability or is unresponsive to initial measures. Increase the dose to 2 J/kg if the initial dose is ineffective. The experienced provider who uses 0.5 J/kg for the first shock may increase the shock dose more gradually (eg, 0.5 J/kg, then 1 J/kg, then all remaining shocks at 2 J/kg). If the rhythm does not convert to sinus rhythm, reevaluate the diagnosis of SVT versus ST.

Cardioversion is unlikely to be effective for treatment of atrial ectopic tachycardias because these rhythms have an automatic focus arising from cells that are depolarizing at a rapid rate. Delivery of a shock generally cannot stop these rhythms and may increase the rate of the tachyarrhythmia.

Resources

See the student CD for details on performing cardioversion.

Pharmacologic Therapy

Common Agents

The Table reviews common agents used in the management of tachyarrhythmias.

Table. Pharmacologic Therapy Used in the Algorithm for Management of Tachyarrhythmias

Drug	Indications/Precautions	Dosage/Administration
Adenosine	**Indications** • Drug of choice for treatment of SVT • Effective for SVT caused by reentry at the AV node (both accessory pathway and AV nodal reentry mechanisms) • May be helpful in distinguishing atrial flutter from SVT • Not effective for treatment of atrial flutter, atrial fibrillation, or tachycardias caused by mechanisms other than reentry at the AV node **Mechanism of Action** • Blocks conduction through the AV node temporarily (for about 10 seconds) **Precautions** • A common cause of adenosine cardioversion "failure" is that the drug is administered too slowly or with inadequate IV flush • A brief period (10 to 15 seconds) of bradycardia (asystole or third-degree heart block) may ensue following adenosine administration	**Dosage** • With continuous ECG monitoring, administer 0.1 mg/kg (maximum initial dose 6 mg) as a rapid IV bolus • If the drug is effective, you will see a conversion of rhythm within 15 to 30 seconds of the bolus (Figure 7) • If there is no effect, you may give one dose of 0.2 mg/kg; maximum second dose: 12 mg). This dose is more likely to be needed when the drug is given into a peripheral (rather than central) vein.[22,23] **Administration** • Because adenosine has a very short half-life (less than 10 seconds), administer as rapidly as possible • Drug is rapidly taken up by vascular endothelial cells and red blood cells and metabolized by an enzyme on the surface of red blood cells (adenosine deaminase) • To enhance delivery to site of action in the heart, use a rapid flush technique • Adenosine may be given by the IO route according to experimental data and a case report[24,25]

<table>
<tr><th>Drug</th><th>Indications/Precautions</th><th>Dosage/Administration</th></tr>
<tr><td>Amiodarone</td><td>Indications<ul><li>Effective in the treatment of a wide variety of atrial and ventricular tachyarrhythmias in children[26-40]</li><li>May be considered in the treatment of hemodynamically stable SVT refractory to vagal maneuvers and adenosine[26-36]</li><li>Safe and effective for hemodynamically unstable VT in children[27,29,31,33,34,41-43]</li></ul>Mechanism of Action<ul><li>Inhibits α- and β-adrenergic receptors, producing vasodilation and AV nodal suppression (this slows conduction through the AV node)</li><li>Inhibits the outward potassium current, so it prolongs the QT duration</li><li>Inhibits sodium channels, which slows conduction in the ventricles and prolongs QRS duration</li></ul>Precautions<ul><li>Drug effects may be beneficial in some patients but may also increase the risk for polymorphic VT (torsades de pointes)[44] by prolonging the QT interval</li><li>Rare but significant acute side effects of amiodarone include bradycardia, hypotension, and polymorphic VT[45,46]</li><li>Use with caution if hepatic failure is present</li><li>Because of the complex pharmacology of amiodarone, slow and incomplete oral absorption, long half-life, and potential for long-term adverse effects, a pediatric cardiologist or similarly experienced provider should direct long-term amiodarone therapy</li></ul></td><td>Dosage<ul><li>For both supraventricular and ventricular arrhythmias associated with poor perfusion, a loading dose infusion of 5 mg/kg over 20 to 60 minutes is recommended. Because this drug can cause hypotension and decrease cardiac contractility, a slower rate of delivery is recommended for treatment of a perfusing rhythm than for treatment of cardiac arrest. Providers must weigh the potential for causing hypotension against the need to achieve a rapid drug effect[30,33,39,47-49]</li><li>Repeat doses of 5 mg/kg may be given up to a maximum of 15 mg/kg per day as needed (should not exceed the maximum recommended adult cumulative daily dose of 2.2 g/24 hours).</li></ul>Administration<ul><li>Rapid administration of amiodarone may cause vasodilation and hypotension; may also cause heart block or polymorphic VT</li><li>Monitor blood pressure frequently during administration</li><li>Routine use in combination with another agent that prolongs the QT interval (eg, procainamide) is not recommended without expert consultation</li></ul></td></tr>
</table>

Drug	Indications/Precautions	Dosage/Administration
Procainamide	**Indications** • Can be used to treat a wide range of atrial and ventricular arrhythmias in children, including SVT and VT[33,50] • Can terminate SVT that is resistant to other drugs[51-66] • May be considered in the treatment of hemodynamically stable SVT refractory to vagal maneuvers and adenosine • Effective in the treatment of atrial flutter and atrial fibrillation[51,67] • May be used to treat or suppress VT[40,51,60,68-85] **Mechanism of Action** • A sodium channel blocking antiarrhythmic agent that prolongs the effective refractory period of both the atria and ventricles and depresses conduction velocity within the conduction system • By slowing intraventricular conduction, drug prolongs the QT, QRS, and PR intervals **Precautions** • Paradoxically shortens the effective refractory period of the AV node and increases AV nodal conduction; may cause an increased heart rate when used to treat ectopic atrial tachycardia and atrial fibrillation[56] • Can cause hypotension in children through its potent vasodilator effect[13,68,86,87] • Active metabolite may accumulate in patients with renal dysfunction	**Dosage** • Infuse the loading dose of 15 mg/kg over 30 to 60 minutes with continuous monitoring of the ECG and frequent blood pressure monitoring **Administration** • Must be given by slow infusion to avoid toxicity from heart block, hypotension, and prolongation of the QT interval (which predisposes to ventricular tachycardia or torsades de pointes tachycardia) • Monitor blood pressure frequently during administration • Procainamide, like amiodarone, may increase the risk of polymorphic VT (torsades de pointes). Routine use in combination with another agent (eg, amiodarone) that prolongs the QT interval is not recommended without expert consultation. **Other** Despite a long history of use, there is little data comparing the effectiveness of procainamide with other antiarrhythmic agents used in children[88,89]
Lidocaine	**Indications** • An alternative agent for treatment of stable VT Not used for narrow-complex supraventricular arrhythmias **Mechanism of Action** • A sodium channel blocker that decreases automaticity and suppresses wide-complex ventricular arrhythmias[90] **Precautions** • Lidocaine toxicity may be observed in patients with high plasma concentrations, which usually occurs in association with a persistently low cardiac output and hepatic or renal failure	**Dosage/Administration** • Provide a loading dose of 1 mg/kg of lidocaine • Consider an infusion of 20 to 50 µg/kg per minute • If there is a delay of more than 15 minutes between the bolus dose and the start of an infusion, consider giving a second bolus of 0.5 to 1 mg/kg to reestablish therapeutic concentrations

Drug	Indications/Precautions	Dosage/Administration
Magnesium sulfate	**Indications** Use for the treatment of torsades de pointes or VT with hypomagnesemia	**Dosage** 25 to 50 mg/kg IV/IO (maximum dose 2 grams), given over 10 to 20 minutes (faster for torsades with cardiac arrest)

Other Interventions

Many other interventions (eg, digoxin, short-acting β-blockers, overdrive pacing) have been used for treatment of SVT in children when expert consultation is available.

Verapamil, a calcium channel blocking agent, *should not be used routinely* to treat SVT in infants. Refractory hypotension and cardiac arrest have been reported after its administration.[91,92] Use verapamil with caution in children because it may cause hypotension and myocardial depression.[93] If used in children older than 1 year, infuse verapamil in a dose of 0.1 mg/kg.

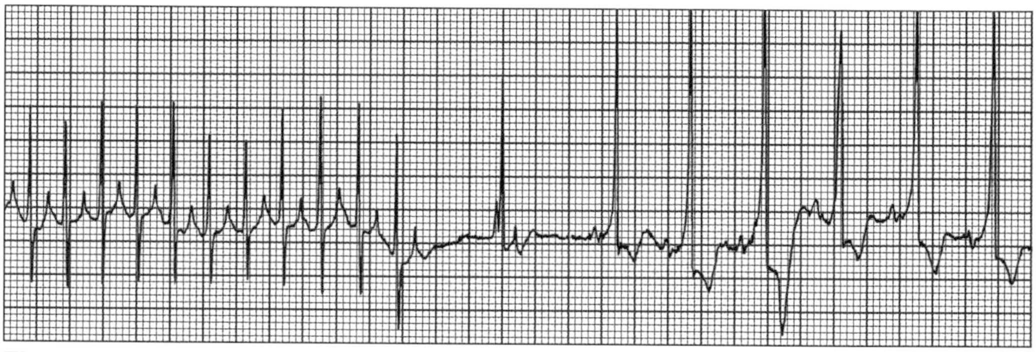

Figure 7. SVT converting to sinus rhythm with administration of adenosine.

Summary

Below is a summary of specific emergency interventions used to treat tachyarrhythmias *with pulses,* based on the width of the observed QRS complex (narrow versus wide).

Intervention	Narrow-Complex Tachyarrhythmia	Wide-Complex Tachyarrhythmia
Vagal maneuvers	Used for SVT	Used for SVT
Synchronized cardioversion	Used for • SVT • Atrial flutter (seek expert consultation)	Used for VT with a pulse
Pharmacologic therapy	Drugs used for SVT: • Adenosine • Amiodarone • Procainamide • Verapamil for children >1 year Drugs used for other SVT with a pulse (eg, atrial flutter): seek expert consultation	Drugs used for VT with a pulse: • Amiodarone • Procainamide • Lidocaine Drug used for torsades de pointes: • Magnesium sulfate Drugs used for SVT with abnormal/aberrant intraventricular conduction: • Adenosine • Amiodarone • Procainamide (seek expert consultation)

Pediatric Tachycardia With Adequate Perfusion Algorithm

Overview

The Pediatric Tachycardia With Adequate Perfusion Algorithm (Figure 8) outlines the steps for assessment and management of the child presenting with symptomatic tachycardia and adequate perfusion.

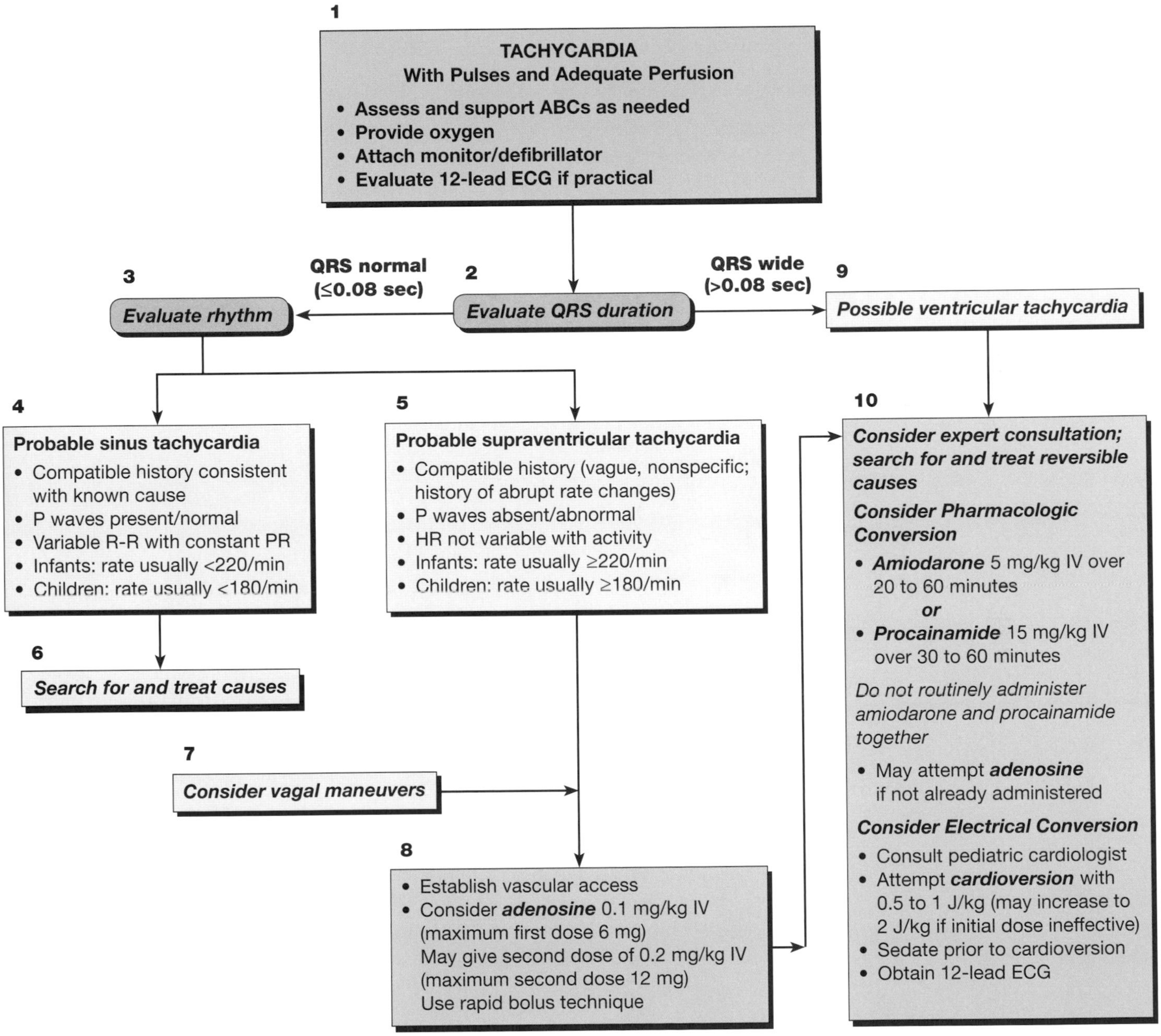
1
TACHYCARDIA
With Pulses and Adequate Perfusion
• Assess and support ABCs as needed
• Provide oxygen
• Attach monitor/defibrillator
• Evaluate 12-lead ECG if practical
2
Evaluate QRS duration
QRS normal (≤0.08 sec)
QRS wide (>0.08 sec)
3
Evaluate rhythm
9
Possible ventricular tachycardia
4
Probable sinus tachycardia
• Compatible history consistent with known cause
• P waves present/normal
• Variable R-R with constant PR
• Infants: rate usually <220/min
• Children: rate usually <180/min
5
Probable supraventricular tachycardia
• Compatible history (vague, nonspecific; history of abrupt rate changes)
• P waves absent/abnormal
• HR not variable with activity
• Infants: rate usually ≥220/min
• Children: rate usually ≥180/min
6
Search for and treat causes
7
Consider vagal maneuvers
8
• Establish vascular access
• Consider adenosine 0.1 mg/kg IV (maximum first dose 6 mg) May give second dose of 0.2 mg/kg IV (maximum second dose 12 mg) Use rapid bolus technique
10
Consider expert consultation; search for and treat reversible causes
Consider Pharmacologic Conversion
• Amiodarone 5 mg/kg IV over 20 to 60 minutes
or
• Procainamide 15 mg/kg IV over 30 to 60 minutes
Do not routinely administer amiodarone and procainamide together
• May attempt adenosine if not already administered
Consider Electrical Conversion
• Consult pediatric cardiologist
• Attempt cardioversion with 0.5 to 1 J/kg (may increase to 2 J/kg if initial dose ineffective)
• Sedate prior to cardioversion
• Obtain 12-lead ECG

Figure 8. Tachycardia With Adequate Perfusion Algorithm

Initial Management (Box 1)

When tachycardia is present but systemic perfusion is adequate, you have more time to evaluate the rhythm and the patient. Begin initial management steps (Box 1), which may include the following:

- Assess and support the airway, oxygenation, and ventilation as needed
- Provide oxygen by nonrebreathing mask as needed
- Evaluate the character of the pulse
- Attach a continuous ECG monitor/defibrillator and a pulse oximeter
- Obtain a 12-lead ECG if practical

Evaluate QRS Duration (Box 2)

Evaluate QRS duration to determine the type of arrhythmia.

Is QRS duration?	Probable Arrhythmia	Proceed in Algorithm
Normal for age (≤0.08 sec)	ST or SVT	Boxes 3, 4, 5, 6, 7 8
Wide for age (>0.08 sec)	VT	Boxes 9 and 10

Normal QRS, Then ST or SVT? (Boxes 3-5)

If QRS duration is normal for age, evaluate the rhythm and try *to determine if the rhythm represents ST or SVT* (Box 3).

Signs consistent with ST (Box 4) include

- history is compatible with ST, consistent with a known cause (eg, the patient has fever, dehydration, pain)
- P waves are present and normal
- heart rate varies with activity or stimulation
- R-R is variable but PR is constant
- heart rate <220/min for an infant or <180/min for a child

Signs consistent with SVT (Box 5) include

- no history compatible with ST (eg, no fever, dehydration, or other identifiable cause of ST); there is a history compatible with SVT or the history is vague or nonspecific
- P waves are absent or abnormal
- heart rate does not vary with activity or stimulation
- rate changes abruptly
- heart rate is >220/min for an infant or >180/min for a child

Treatment of ST (Box 6)

Treatment of ST is directed at the cause of the ST. Because sinus tachycardia is a symptom, you should not attempt to decrease heart rate by pharmacologic or electrical interventions. Instead you should search for and treat the cause. Continuous ECG monitoring will confirm a decrease in heart rate to more normal levels if treatment of the underlying cause is effective.

Treatment of SVT (Boxes 7-8)

Treatment of SVT is outlined in Boxes 7-8.

Vagal maneuvers
Consider vagal maneuvers (Box 7). In the stable patient with SVT, try the following:

- Put a bag of ice water over the face and eyes of the infant (without obstructing the airway).
- Ask the older child to try to blow through an obstructed straw.

Perform continuous ECG monitoring and recording before, during, and after attempted vagal maneuvers. Do not apply ocular pressure or provide carotid massage. See "Vagal Maneuvers" on the student CD for more information.

Adenosine
For SVT resistant to attempted vagal maneuvers, establish vascular access to administer adenosine (Box 8). Adenosine is the drug of choice for most common forms of SVT caused by a reentrant pathway involving the AV node.[11,22,23]

IV/IO	0.1 mg/kg (maximum first dose 6 mg) If first dose is ineffective, you may give one dose of 0.2 mg/kg (maximum second dose 12 mg)
Use a rapid bolus with a *rapid flush* 2-syringe technique	

Wide QRS, Possible VT? (Box 9)

If QRS duration is wide for age (>0.08 sec), the rhythm is either VT with a pulse or SVT with aberrant intraventricular conduction (Box 9). In infants and children, you should treat wide-complex tachycardia as presumed VT unless the child is known to have aberrant conduction.

Pharmacologic Conversion vs Electrical Conversion (Box 10)

If the child is hemodynamically stable with a wide-complex tachycardia, early consultation with a pediatric cardiologist or other physician with appropriate expertise is recommended.

Pharmacologic Conversion
Establish vascular access and consider administering ***one*** of the following medications:

Medication	Route	Dosage and Administration
Amiodarone	IV/IO	5 mg/kg over 20 to 60 minutes
Procainamide	IV/IO	15 mg/kg over 30 to 60 minutes
Lidocaine	IV/IO	1 mg/kg bolus
Infuse loading doses slowly in the stable patient to avoid hypotension. Monitor blood pressure frequently during administration.		

Do not routinely administer amiodarone and procainamide together or with other medications that prolong the QT interval without expert consultation. If these initial efforts do not terminate the rapid rhythm, reevaluate the rhythm.

Because a wide-complex tachycardia could be SVT with aberrant intraventricular conduction, consider giving an empiric dose of adenosine, which can be effective in treating SVT. It is important to recognize that adenosine is not effective in the treatment of VT.

Electrical Conversion

If either the SVT or the wide-complex tachycardia do not respond to pharmacologic therapy, consult a pediatric cardiologist. You may attempt synchronized cardioversion, but since the child is stable, you may wish to await expert consultation. For synchronized cardioversion use a first dose of 0.5 to 1 J/kg. Increase the dose to 2 J/kg if the initial dose is ineffective. The experienced provider who uses 0.5 J/kg for the first shock may increase the shock dose more gradually (eg, 0.5 J/kg, then 1 J/kg, then all remaining shocks at 2 J/kg). *Record and monitor the ECG continuously during any cardioversion.*

If the patient is conscious, provide procedural sedation before elective cardioversion. Obtain a 12-lead ECG after conversion.

Pediatric Tachycardia With Pulses and Poor Perfusion Algorithm

Overview

The Pediatric Tachycardia With Pulses and Poor Perfusion Algorithm (Figure 9) outlines the steps for assessment and management of the child presenting with symptomatic tachycardia and poor perfusion.

Initial Management (Box 1)

In a patient with tachycardia who has palpable pulses but signs of hemodynamic compromise (ie, poor perfusion, weak pulses), begin initial management steps (Box 1), which include the following:

- Attach a continuous ECG monitor/defibrillator and a pulse oximeter

Evaluate QRS Duration (Box 2)

Quickly evaluate QRS duration to determine type of arrhythmia. Although a 12-lead ECG may be useful, initial therapy does not require precise ECG diagnosis of the tachyarrhythmia causing poor perfusion. You can calculate QRS width from a rhythm strip.

Is QRS duration?	Probable Arrhythmia	Proceed in Algorithm
Normal for age (≤0.08 sec)	ST or SVT	Box 3, 4, 5, 6, 7, 8
Wide for age (>0.08 sec)	VT	Boxes 9, 10, and 11

Normal QRS, Then ST or SVT? (Boxes 3-5)

If QRS duration is normal for age, evaluate the rhythm and try *to determine if the rhythm* represents ST or SVT (Box 3).

Signs and symptoms consistent with ST (Box 4) include

- history is compatible with ST or consistent with a known cause (eg, the patient has fever, dehydration, pain)
- P waves are present and normal
- heart rate varies with activity or stimulation
- R-R is variable but PR is constant
- heart rate <200/min for an infant or <180/min for a child

Signs and symptoms consistent with SVT (Box 5) include

- history is compatible with SVT (vague, nonspecific) and is not consistent with a known cause of sinus tachycardia
- P waves are absent or abnormal
- heart rate does not vary with activity or stimulation
- rate changes abruptly
- heart rate is >220/min for an infant or >180/min for a child

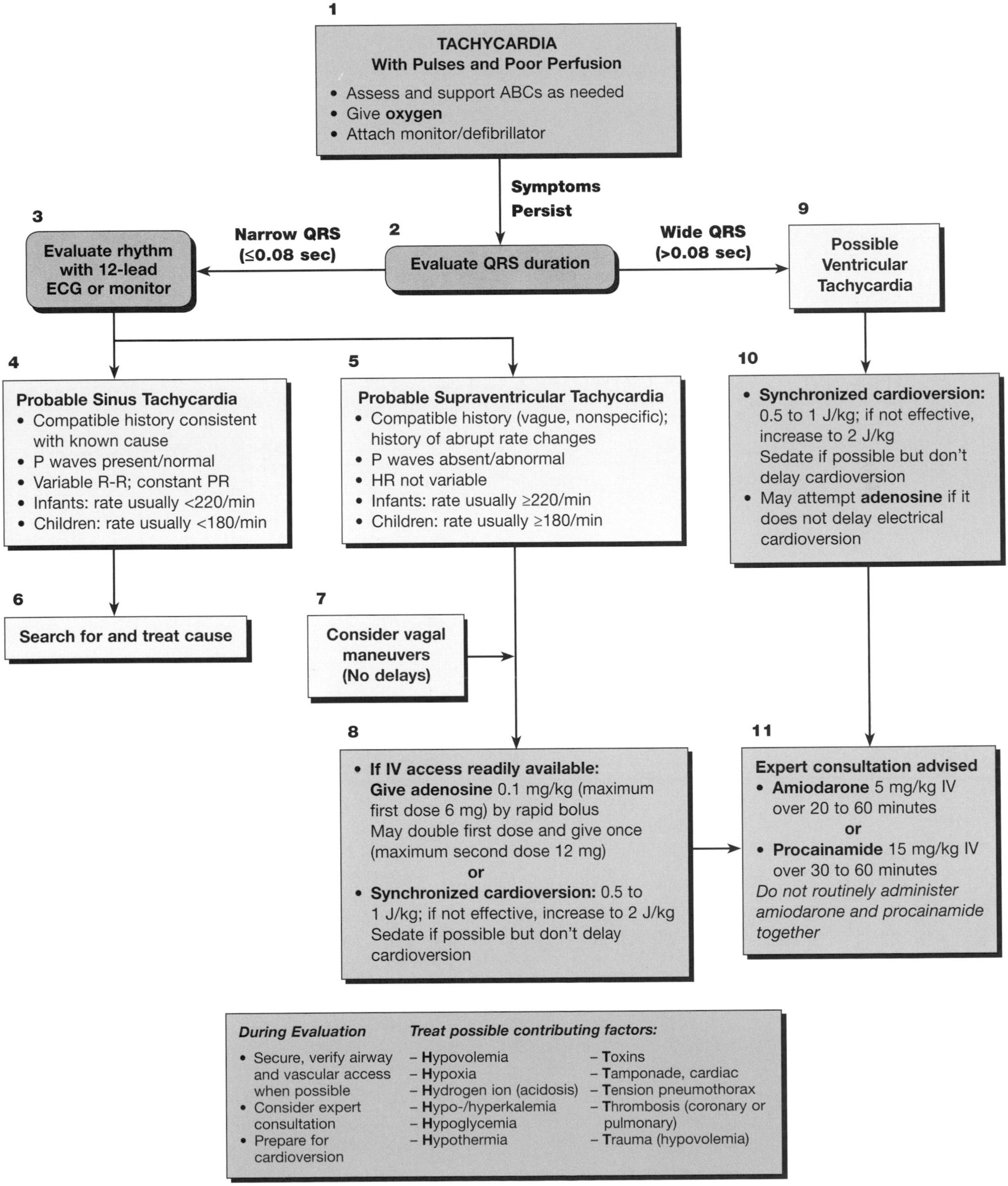
1
TACHYCARDIA
With Pulses and Poor Perfusion
• Assess and support ABCs as needed
• Give oxygen
• Attach monitor/defibrillator
Symptoms Persist
2
Evaluate QRS duration
Narrow QRS (≤0.08 sec)
Wide QRS (>0.08 sec)
3
Evaluate rhythm with 12-lead ECG or monitor
4
Probable Sinus Tachycardia
• Compatible history consistent with known cause
• P waves present/normal
• Variable R-R; constant PR
• Infants: rate usually <220/min
• Children: rate usually <180/min
5
Probable Supraventricular Tachycardia
• Compatible history (vague, nonspecific); history of abrupt rate changes
• P waves absent/abnormal
• HR not variable
• Infants: rate usually ≥220/min
• Children: rate usually ≥180/min
6
Search for and treat cause
7
Consider vagal maneuvers (No delays)
8
• If IV access readily available: Give adenosine 0.1 mg/kg (maximum first dose 6 mg) by rapid bolus May double first dose and give once (maximum second dose 12 mg)
or
• Synchronized cardioversion: 0.5 to 1 J/kg; if not effective, increase to 2 J/kg Sedate if possible but don't delay cardioversion
9
Possible Ventricular Tachycardia
10
• Synchronized cardioversion: 0.5 to 1 J/kg; if not effective, increase to 2 J/kg Sedate if possible but don't delay cardioversion
• May attempt adenosine if it does not delay electrical cardioversion
11
Expert consultation advised
• Amiodarone 5 mg/kg IV over 20 to 60 minutes
or
• Procainamide 15 mg/kg IV over 30 to 60 minutes
Do not routinely administer amiodarone and procainamide together
During Evaluation
• Secure, verify airway and vascular access when possible
• Consider expert consultation
• Prepare for cardioversion
Treat possible contributing factors:
– Hypovolemia
– Hypoxia
– Hydrogen ion (acidosis)
– Hypo-/hyperkalemia
– Hypoglycemia
– Hypothermia
– Toxins
– Tamponade, cardiac
– Tension pneumothorax
– Thrombosis (coronary or pulmonary)
– Trauma (hypovolemia)

Figure 9. Pediatric Tachycardia With Pulses and Poor Perfusion Algorithm.

Treatment of ST (Box 6)

Treatment of ST is directed at the cause of the ST. Because sinus tachycardia is a symptom, you should not attempt to decrease the heart rate by pharmacologic or electrical interventions. Instead search for and treat the cause. Continuous ECG monitoring will confirm a decrease in heart rate to more normal levels if treatment of the underlying cause is effective.

Treatment of SVT (Boxes 7 and 8)

Treatment of SVT with poor perfusion is outlined in Boxes 7 and 8.

Vagal maneuvers

Consider vagal maneuvers (Box 7), but ***do not delay chemical or electrical cardioversion in the unstable patient.***

- Put a bag of ice water over the face and eyes of the infant (without obstructing the airway).
- Ask the child to try to blow through an obstructed straw.

Perform continuous ECG monitoring and recording before, during, and after these attempted vagal maneuvers. Do not apply ocular pressure or provide carotid massage. See "Vagal Maneuvers" on the student CD for more information.

Adenosine

If vascular access (IV/IO) and medications are readily available, administer adenosine (Box 8).

IV/IO	0.1 mg/kg (maximum first dose 6 mg) If first dose is ineffective, you may give one dose of 0.2 mg/kg (maximum second dose 12 mg)
Use a rapid bolus with a *rapid* flush 2-syringe technique	

If IV/IO access is not readily available, provide synchronized cardioversion (Box 8).

Synchronized Cardioversion

If IV/IO access is not readily available, attempt synchronized cardioversion. Use a first dose of 0.5 to 1 J/kg. Increase the dose to 2 J/kg if the initial dose is ineffective. The experienced provider who uses 0.5 J/kg for the first shock may increase the shock dose more gradually (eg, 0.5 J/kg, then 1 J/kg, then all remaining shocks at 2 J/kg). *Record and monitor the ECG continuously during any cardioversion.* Provide procedural sedation if it will not delay cardioversion.

If neither intervention is effective, proceed to Box 11. It is advisable to obtain expert consultation.

Wide QRS, Possible VT (Box 9)

If QRS duration is wide for age (>0.08 second), the rhythm may be either VT or SVT with aberrant intraventricular conduction. Treat the rhythm as presumed VT unless the patient is known to have aberrant conduction (Box 9).

Treatment of Wide-Complex Tachycardia (Box 10)

For urgent treatment of a wide-complex tachycardia with pulses but poor perfusion, provide immediate synchronized cardioversion with 0.5 to 1 J/kg. Increase the dose to 2 J/kg if the initial dose is ineffective. The experienced provider who uses 0.5 J/kg for the first shock may increase the shock dose more gradually (eg, 0.5 J/kg, then 1 J/kg, then all remaining shocks at 2 J/kg). Provide sedation with analgesia if possible, but do not delay cardioversion in the unstable patient.

Because a wide-complex tachycardia could be SVT with aberrant intraventricular conduction, you can consider giving an empiric dose of adenosine (it can be effective in treating SVT) *if it does not delay cardioversion.* It is important to recognize that adenosine is not effective in the treatment of VT and should be used only when SVT with aberrant conduction is suspected.

If Wide-Complex Tachycardia Is Refractory (Box 11)

For wide-complex tachycardia refractory to initial management interventions, consultation with a pediatric cardiologist is advised.

Consider administration of ***one*** of the following medications:

Medication	Route	Dosage and Administration
Amiodarone	IV/IO	5 mg/kg over 20 to 60 minutes
Procainamide	IV/IO	15 mg/kg over 30 to 60 minutes

Amiodarone or procainamide can be used for the treatment of wide-complex SVT (unresponsive to adenosine) and VT in children. Do not routinely administer amiodarone and procainamide together or with other medications that prolong the QT interval unless you have expert consultation.

Actions During Evaluation (Green Box)

During evaluation of the tachycardia, perform the following actions as appropriate:

- Continue to support the ABCs and provide oxygen as needed.
- Verify that the continuous ECG monitor/defibrillator is attached.
- If the rhythm is consistent with SVT or VT with stable perfusion, consult a pediatric cardiologist.
- Prepare to provide synchronized cardioversion with appropriate procedural sedation.

Identify and treat potentially reversible causes and conditions, using the H's and T's as listed in the following table. Special attention should include electrolyte and toxin/drug causes in the setting of a wide-complex tachycardia.

Hypovolemia	**T**oxins/drugs (particularly tricyclic antidepressants)
Hypoxia	**T**amponade (cardiac)
Hydrogen ion (acidosis)	**T**ension pneumothorax
Hyper-/Hypokalemia and other metabolic disorders, including hypomagnesemia	**T**hrombosis (coronary or pulmonary)
Hypoglycemia	**T**rauma (hypovolemia)
Hypothermia	

References

1. Walsh CK, Krongrad E. Terminal cardiac electrical activity in pediatric patients. *Am J Cardiol.* 1983;51:557-561.

2. Huang YG, Wong KC, Yip WH, et al. Cardiovascular responses to graded doses of three catecholamines during lactic and hydrochloric acidosis in dogs. *Br J Anaesth.* 1995;74:583-590.

3. Preziosi MP, Roig JC, Hargrove N, et al. Metabolic acidemia with hypoxia attenuates the hemodynamic responses to epinephrine during resuscitation in lambs. *Crit Care Med.* 1993;21:1901-1907.

4. Dauchot P, Gravenstein JS. Effects of atropine on the electrocardiogram in different age groups. *Clin Pharmacol Ther.* 1971;12:274-280.

5. Lee PL, Chung YT, Lee BY, et al. The optimal dose of atropine via the endotracheal route. *Ma Zui Xue Za Zhi.* 1989;27:35-38.

6. Howard RF, Bingham RM. Endotracheal compared with intravenous administration of atropine. *Arch Dis Child.* 1990;65:449-450.

7. Cummins RO, Haulman JR, Quan L, et al. Near-fatal yew berry intoxication treated with external cardiac pacing and digoxin-specific FAB antibody fragments. *Ann Emerg Med.* 1990;19:38-43.

8. Kissoon N, Rosenberg HC, Kronick JB. Role of transcutaneous pacing in the setting of a failing permanent pacemaker. *Pediatr Emerg Care.* 1989;5:178-180.

9. Beland MJ, Hesslein PS, Finlay CD, et al. Noninvasive transcutaneous cardiac pacing in children. *Pacing Clin Electrophysiol.* 1987;10:1262-1270.

10. Olley PH. Cardiac arrhythmias. In: Keith JD, Rowe RD, Vald P, eds. *Heart Disease in Infancy and Childhood.* 3rd ed. New York: Macmillan Publishing Co., Inc.; 1978:279-280.

11. Gikonyo BM, Dunnigan A, Benson DW Jr. Cardiovascular collapse in infants: association with paroxysmal atrial tachycardia. *Pediatrics*. 1985;76:922-926.

12. Kugler JD, Danford DA. Management of infants, children, and adolescents with paroxysmal supraventricular tachycardia. *J Pediatr.* 1996;129:324-338.

13. Benson D Jr, Smith W, Dunnigan A, et al. Mechanisms of regular wide QRS tachycardia in infants and children. Am J Cardiol. 1982;49:1778-1788.

14. Garson A Jr. Medicolegal problems in the management of cardiac arrhythmias in children. *Pediatrics.* 1987;79:84-88.

15. Eberle B, Dick WF, Schneider T, et al. Checking the carotid pulse check: diagnostic accuracy of first responders in patients with and without a pulse. *Resuscitation.* 1996;33:107-116.

16. Owen CJ, Wyllie JP. Determination of heart rate in the baby at birth. *Resuscitation.* 2004;60:213-217.

17. Graham CA, Lewis NF. Evaluation of a new method for the carotid pulse check in cardiopulmonary resuscitation. *Resuscitation.* 2002;53:37-40.

18. Ochoa FJ, Ramalle-Gomara E, Carpintero JM, et al. Competence of health professionals to check the carotid pulse. *Resuscitation.* 1998;37:173-175.

19. Mather C, O'Kelly S. The palpation of pulses. *Anaesthesia.* 1996;51:189-191.

20. Lapostolle F, Le Toumelin P, Agostinucci JM, et al. Basic cardiac life support providers checking the carotid pulse: performance, degree of conviction, and influencing factors. *Acad Emerg Med.* 2004;11:878-880.

21. Moule P. Checking the carotid pulse: diagnostic accuracy in students of the healthcare professions. *Resuscitation.* 2000;44:195-201.

22. Losek JD, Endom E, Dietrich A, et al. Adenosine and pediatric supraventricular tachycardia in the emergency department: multicenter study and review. *Ann Emerg Med.* 1999;33:185-191.

23. Overholt ED, Rheuban KS, Gutgesell HP, et al. Usefulness of adenosine for arrhythmias in infants and children. *Am J Cardiol.* 1988;61:336-340.

24. Getschman SJ, Dietrich AM, Franklin WH, et al. Intraosseous adenosine. As effective as peripheral or central venous administration? *Arch Pediatr Adolesc Med.* 1994;148:616-619.

25. Friedman FD. Intraosseous adenosine for the termination of supraventricular tachycardia in an infant. *Ann Emerg Med.* 1996;28:356-358.

26. Burri S, Hug MI, Bauersfeld U. Efficacy and safety of intravenous amiodarone for incessant tachycardias in infants. *Eur J Pediatr.* 2003;162:880-884.

27. Cabrera Duro A, Rodrigo Carbonero D, Galdeano Miranda J, et al. [The treatment of postoperative junctional ectopic tachycardia]. *An Esp Pediatr.* 2002;56:505-509.

28. Celiker A, Ceviz N, Ozme S. Effectiveness and safety of intravenous amiodarone in drug-resistant tachyarrhythmias of children. *Acta Paediatr Jpn.* 1998;40:567-572.

29. Dodge-Khatami A, Miller O, Anderson R, et al. Impact of junctional ectopic tachycardia on postoperative morbidity following repair of congenital heart defects. *Eur J Cardiothorac Surg.* 2002;21:255-259.

30. Figa FH, Gow RM, Hamilton RM, et al. Clinical efficacy and safety of intravenous Amiodarone in infants and children. *Am J Cardiol.* 1994;74:573-577.

31. Hoffman TM, Bush DM, Wernovsky G, et al. Postoperative junctional ectopic tachycardia in children: incidence, risk factors, and treatment. *Ann Thorac Surg.* 2002;74:1607-1611.

32. Laird WP, Snyder CS, Kertesz NJ, et al. Use of intravenous amiodarone for postoperative junctional ectopic tachycardia in children. *Pediatr Cardiol.* 2003;24:133-137.

33. Perry JC, Fenrich AL, Hulse JE, et al. Pediatric use of intravenous amiodarone: efficacy and safety in critically ill patients from a multicenter protocol. *J Am Coll Cardiol.* 1996;27:1246-1250.

34. Soult JA, Munoz M, Lopez JD, et al. Efficacy and safety of intravenous amiodarone for short-term treatment of paroxysmal supraventricular tachycardia in children. *Pediatr Cardiol.* 1995;16:16-19.

35. Valsangiacomo E, Schmid ER, Schupbach RW, et al. Early postoperative arrhythmias after cardiac operation in children. *Ann Thorac Surg.* 2002;74:792-796.

36. Yap S-C, Hoomtje T, Sreeram N. Polymorphic ventricular tachycardia after use of intravenous amiodarone for postoperative junctional ectopic tachycardia. *Int J Cardiol.* 2000;76:245-247.

37. Juneja R, Shah S, Naik N, et al. Management of cardiomyopathy resulting from incessant supraventricular tachycardia in infants and children. *Indian Heart J.* 2002;54:176-180.

38. Michael JG, Wilson WR Jr, Tobias JD. Amiodarone in the treatment of junctional ectopic tachycardia after cardiac surgery in children: report of two cases and review of the literature. *Am J Ther.* 1999;6:223-227.

39. Perry JC, Knilans TK, Marlow D, et al. Intravenous amiodarone for life-threatening tachyarrhythmias in children and young adults. *J Am Coll Cardiol.* 1993;22:95-98.

40. Singh BN, Kehoe R, Woosley RL, et al. Multicenter trial of sotalol compared with procainamide in the suppression of inducible ventricular tachycardia: a double-blind, randomized parallel evaluation. Sotalol Multicenter Study Group. *Am Heart J.* 1995;129:87-97.

41. Rokicki W, Durmala J, Nowakowska E. [Amiodarone for long term treatment of arrhythmia in children]. *Wiad Lek.* 2001;54:45-50.

42. Strasburger JF, Cuneo BF, Michon MM, et al. Amiodarone therapy for drug-refractory fetal tachycardia. *Circulation.* 2004;109:375-379.

43. Beder SD, Cohen MH, BenShachar G. Time course of myocardial amiodarone uptake in the piglet heart using a chronic animal model. *Pediatr Cardiol.* 1998;19:204-211.

44. Mattioni TA, Zheutlin TA, Dunnington C, et al. The proarrhythmic effects of amiodarone. *Prog Cardiovasc Dis.* 1989;31:439-446.

45. Daniels CJ, Schutte DA, Hammond S, et al. Acute pulmonary toxicity in an infant from intravenous amiodarone. *Am J Cardiol.* 1998;80:1113-1116.

46. Gandy J, Wonko N, Kantoch MJ. Risks of intravenous amiodarone in neonates. *Can J Cardiol.* 1998;14:855-858.

47. Raja P, Hawker RE, Chaikitpinyo A, et al. Amiodarone management of junctional ectopic tachycardia after cardiac surgery in children. *Br Heart J.* 1994;72:261-265.

48. Scheinman MM, Levine JH, Cannom DS, et al. Dose-ranging study of intravenous amiodarone in patients with life- threatening ventricular tachyarrhythmias. The Intravenous Amiodarone Multicenter Investigators Group. *Circulation.* 1995;92:3264-3272.

49. Pongiglione G, Strasburger JF, Deal BJ, et al. Use of amiodarone for short-term and adjuvant therapy in young patients. *Am J Cardiol.* 1991;68:603-608.

50. Naccarelli GV, Wolbrette DL, Patel HM, et al. Amiodarone: clinical trials. *Curr Opin Cardiol.* 2000;15:64-72.

51. Boahene KA, Klein GJ, Yee R, et al. Termination of acute atrial fibrillation in the Wolff-Parkinson-White syndrome by procainamide and propafenone: importance of atrial fibrillatory cycle length. *J Am Coll Cardiol.* 1990;16:1408-1414.

52. Dodo H, Gow RM, Hamilton RM, et al. Chaotic atrial rhythm in children. *Am Heart J.* 1995;129:990-995.

53. Komatsu C, Ishinaga T, Tateishi O, et al. Effects of four antiarrhythmic drugs on the induction and termination of paroxysmal supraventricular tachycardia. *Jpn Circ J.* 1986;50:961-972.

54. Mandapati R, Byrum CJ, Kavey RE, et al. Procainamide for rate control of postsurgical junctional tachycardia. *Pediatr Cardiol.* 2000;21:123-128.

55. Mandel WJ, Laks MM, Obayashi K, et al. The Wolff-Parkinson-White syndrome: pharmacologic effects of procaine amide. *Am Heart J.* 1975;90:744-754.

56. Mehta AV, Sanchez GR, Sacks EJ, et al. Ectopic automatic atrial tachycardia in children: clinical characteristics, management and follow-up. *J Am Coll Cardiol.* 1988;11:379-385.

57. Rhodes LA, Walsh EP, Saul JP. Conversion of atrial flutter in pediatric patients by transesophageal atrial pacing: a safe, effective, minimally invasive procedure. *Am Heart J.* 1995;130:323-327.

58. Satake S, Hiejima K, Moroi Y, et al. Usefulness of invasive and non-invasive electrophysiologic studies in the selection of antiarrhythmic drugs for the patients with paroxysmal supraventricular tachyarrhythmia. *Jpn Circ J.* 1985;49:345-350.

59. Singh S, Gelband H, Mehta A, et al. Procainamide elimination kinetics in pediatric patients. *Clin Pharmacol Ther.* 1982;32:607-611.

60. Walsh EP, Saul JP, Sholler GF, et al. Evaluation of a staged treatment protocol for rapid automatic junctional tachycardia after operation for congenital heart disease. *J Am Coll Cardiol.* 1997;29:1046-1053.

61. Wang JN, Wu JM, Tsai YC, et al. Ectopic atrial tachycardia in children. *J Formos Med Assoc.* 2000;99:766-770.

62. Chen F, Wetzel G, Klitzner TS. Acute effects of amiodarone on sodium currents in isolated neonatal ventricular myocytes: comparison with procainamide. *Dev Pharmacol Ther.* 1992;19:118-130.

63. Fujiki A, Tani M, Yoshida S, et al. Electrophysiologic mechanisms of adverse effects of class I antiarrhythmic drugs (cibenzoline, pilsicainide, disopyramide, procainamide) in induction of atrioventricular re-entrant tachycardia. *Cardiovasc Drugs Ther.* 1996;10:159-166.

64. Bauernfeind RA, Swiryn S, Petropoulos AT, et al. Concordance and discordance of drug responses in atrioventricular reentrant tachycardia. *J Am Coll Cardiol.* 1983;2:345-350.

65. Hordof AJ, Edie R, Malm JR, et al. Electrophysiologic properties and response to pharmacologic agents of fibers from diseased human atria. *Circulation.* 1976;54:774-779.

66. Jawad-Kanber G, Sherrod TR. Effect of loading dose of procaine amide on left ventricular performance in man. *Chest.* 1974;66:269-272.

67. Hjelms E. Procainamide conversion of acute atrial fibrillation after open-heart surgery compared with digoxin treatment. *Scand J Thorac Cardiovasc Surg.* 1992;26:193-196.

68. Shih JY, Gillette PC, Kugler JD, et al. The electrophysiologic effects of procainamide in the immature heart. *Pediatr Pharmacol (New York).* 1982;2:65-73.

69. Meldon SW, Brady WJ, Berger S, et al. Pediatric ventricular tachycardia: a review with three illustrative cases. *Pediatr Emerg Care.* 1994;10:294-300.

70. Stanton MS, Prystowsky EN, Fineberg NS, et al. Arrhythmogenic effects of antiarrhythmic drugs: a study of 506 patients treated for ventricular tachycardia or fibrillation. *J Am Coll Cardiol.* 1989;14:209-215; discussion 216-217.

71. Hasin Y, Kriwisky M, Gotsman MS. Verapamil in ventricular tachycardia. *Cardiology.* 1984;71:199-206.

72. Hernandez A, Strauss A, Kleiger RE, et al. Idiopathic paroxysmal ventricular tachycardia in infants and children. *J Pediatr.* 1975; 86:182-188.

73. Horowitz LN, Josephson ME, Farshidi A, et al. Recurrent sustained ventricular tachycardia 3. Role of the electrophysiologic study in selection of antiarrhythmic regimens. *Circulation.* 1978;58:986-997.

74. Mason JW, Winkle RA. Electrode-catheter arrhythmia induction in the selection and assessment of antiarrhythmic drug therapy for recurrent ventricular tachycardia. *Circulation.* 1978;58:971-985.

75. Cain M, Martin T, Marchlinski FE, et al. Changes in ventricular refractoriness after an extrastimulus: effects of prematurity, cycle length and procainamide. *Am J Cardiol.* 1983;52:996-1001.

76. Swiryn S, Bauernfeind RA, Strasberg B, et al. Prediction of response to class I antiarrhythmic drugs during electrophysiologic study of ventricular tachycardia. *Am Heart J.* 1982;104:43-50.

77. Velebit V, Podrid P, Lown B, et al. Aggravation and provocation of ventricular arrhythmias by antiarrhythmic drugs. *Circulation.* 1982;65:886-894.

78. Roden D, Reele S, Higgins S, et al. Antiarrhythmic efficacy, pharmacokinetics and safety of N-acetylprocainamide in human subjects: comparison with procainamide. *Am J Cardiol.* 1980;46:463-468.

79. Naitoh N, Washizuka T, Takahashi K, et al. Effects of class I and III antiarrhythmic drugs on ventricular tachycardia-interrupting critical paced cycle length with rapid pacing. *Jpn Circ J.* 1998;62:267-273.

80. Kasanuki H, Ohnishi S, Hosoda S. Differentiation and mechanisms of prevention and termination of verapamil-sensitive sustained ventricular tachycardia. *Am J Cardiol.* 1989;64:46J-49J.

81. Kasanuki H, Ohnishi S, Tanaka E, et al. Clinical significance of Vanghan Williams classification for treatment of ventricular tachycardia: study of class IA and IB antiarrhythmic agents. *Jpn Circ J.* 1988;52:280-288.

82. Videbaek J, Andersen E, Jacobsen J, et al. Paroxysmal tachycardia in infancy and childhood. II. Paroxysmal ventricular tachycardia and fibrillation. *Acta Paediatr Scand.* 1973;62:349-357.

83. Sanchez J, Christie K, Cumming G. Treatment of ventricular tachycardia in an infant. *CMAJ.* 1972;107:136-138.

84. Gelband H, Steeg C, Bigger JJ. Use of massive doses of procaineamide in the treatment of ventricular tachycardia in infancy. *Pediatrics.* 1971;48:110-115.

85. Drago F, Mazza A, Guccione P, et al. Amiodarone used alone or in combination with propranolol: A very effective therapy for tachyarrhythmias in infants and children. *Pediatric Cardiology.* 1998;19:445-449.

86. Karlsson E, Sonnhag C. Haemodynamic effects of procainamide and phenytoin at apparent therapeutic plasma levels. *Eur J Clin Pharmacol.* 1976;10:305-310.

87. Kuga K, Yamaguchi I, Sugishita Y. Effect of intravenous amiodarone on electrophysiologic variables and on the modes of termination of atrioventricular reciprocating tachycardia in Wolff-Parkinson-White syndrome. *Jpn Circ J.* 1999;63:189-195.

88. Luedtke SA, Kuhn RJ, McCaffrey FM. Pharmacologic management of supraventricular tachycardias in children, part 2: atrial flutter, atrial fibrillation, and junctional and atrial ectopic tachycardia. *Ann Pharmacother.* 1997;31:1347-1359.

89. Luedtke SA, Kuhn RJ, McCaffrey FM. Pharmacologic management of supraventricular tachycardias in children. Part 1: Wolff-Parkinson-White and atrioventricular nodal reentry. *Ann Pharmacother.* 1997;31:1227-1243.

90. Chow MS, Kluger J, DiPersio DM, et al. Antifibrillatory effects of lidocaine and bretylium immediately postcardiopulmonary resuscitation. *Am Heart J.* 1985;110:938-943.

91. Epstein ML, Kiel EA, Victorica BE. Cardiac decompensation following verapamil therapy in infants with supraventricular tachycardia. *Pediatrics.* 1985;75:737-740.

92. Kirk CR, Gibbs JL, Thomas R, et al. Cardiovascular collapse after verapamil in supraventricular tachycardia. *Arch Dis Child.* 1987;62:1265-1266.

93. Rankin AC, Rae AP, Oldroyd KG, et al. Verapamil or adenosine for the immediate treatment of supraventricular tachycardia. *Q J Med.* 1990;74:203-208.

Chapter 7

Recognition and Management of Cardiac Arrest

Overview

Introduction

Cardiac arrest, also called cardiopulmonary arrest, is the cessation of circulation of blood as a result of absent or ineffective cardiac mechanical activity. Cessation of circulation and resulting organ and tissue ischemia can cause cell, organ, and patient death if not rapidly reversed. Clinically the patient is unresponsive, apneic, with no detectable pulse. Cerebral hypoxia causes the victim to lose consciousness and stop breathing, although agonal gasps may be observed during the first minutes of sudden arrest.

In contrast to cardiac arrest in adults, sudden cardiac arrest in children is uncommon. Cardiac arrest is more often caused by progression of respiratory distress, respiratory failure, or shock than by primary cardiac arrhythmias.[1] Such secondary cardiac arrest is typically associated with hypoxemia and acidosis and occurs most often in infants and young children, particularly those with underlying disease. Outcomes from respiratory failure or shock in children are generally good, but if pediatric cardiac arrest develops, outcome is generally poor.

Sudden collapse due to ventricular fibrillation (VF)/pulseless ventricular tachycardia (VT) is the presentation in about 5% to 15% of all pediatric prehospital cardiac arrests.[2-4] The incidence of VF as the initial recorded rhythm increases in cardiac arrest victims over 12 years of age and is especially likely if the child collapses suddenly.[5] In the hospital a shockable rhythm is present during some point in the attempted resuscitation of approximately 25% of children with cardiac arrest, with 10% having VF/VT as the initial arrest rhythm.[6]

Survival rates from pediatric cardiac arrest vary according to

- the location of the arrest
- the presenting rhythm

Survival to hospital discharge is higher if the arrest occurs in-hospital compared with out-of-hospital (2% to 10%). Intact neurologic outcome in survivors of pediatric cardiac arrest is also much higher if the arrest occurs in-hospital rather than out-of-hospital.[1,6-8]

Survival is higher (average survival about 25% to 33%) when VF or VT is the presenting rhythm than when a "nonshockable" rhythm is the presenting rhythm (average survival about 7% to 11%).[5,6] Although VF/VT is associated with better survival as the presenting rhythm, when VF/VT develops during cardiac arrest in hospitalized children, it is associated with a worse outcome than observed with nonshockable rhythms (11% versus 27% survival to discharge).[9]

Because the outcomes from cardiac arrest are poor, *appropriate focus should be placed on prevention of cardiac arrest* by

- prevention of disease processes and injuries that can lead to cardiac arrest
- early recognition and management of respiratory distress, respiratory failure, and shock before deterioration to cardiac arrest

Learning Objectives

After completing this chapter you should be able to

- recall the common causes of cardiac arrest in children in both the in-hospital and out-of-hospital environments
- define and recognize the common arrest rhythms, state whether each rhythm is shockable versus nonshockable, and summarize recommended treatment steps (including electrical and pharmacologic therapy) according to the Pediatric Pulseless Arrest Algorithm
- describe the clinical pathway leading to cardiac arrest and recognize the clinical signs of cardiopulmonary failure and cardiac arrest
- recall the potential reversible causes of cardiac arrest (H's and T's) and their specific management

Presentations of Cardiac Arrest

Introduction

The two presentations of cardiac arrest in children are

- hypoxic/asphyxial arrest
- sudden cardiac arrest

Hypoxic/Asphyxial Arrest

Although the term *asphyxia* may be confused with suffocation, it refers to a condition leading to a lack of oxygen to the tissues. Although this group of arrests may be called *hypoxic arrest*, the term *asphyxial arrest* has been commonly used for many years. Asphyxial arrest is the most common pathophysiologic mechanism of cardiac arrest in infants and in children through adolescence. It is the terminal event of progressive tissue hypoxia and acidosis caused by respiratory failure, shock, or cardiopulmonary failure. Regardless of the initiating event or disease process, the final common pathway preceding asphyxial arrest is the development of cardiopulmonary failure (Figure 1).

This course emphasizes the importance of recognizing and treating respiratory distress, respiratory failure, and shock before the development of cardiopulmonary failure and cardiac arrest. Early recognition and treatment are crucial to saving the lives of seriously ill or injured children.

Sudden Cardiac Arrest

Sudden cardiac arrest (SCA) is uncommon in children. When it does occur, SCA is most often associated with an arrhythmia, specifically VF or pulseless VT. Predisposing conditions or causes for sudden cardiac arrest may include the following:

- Hypertrophic cardiomyopathy
- Anomalous coronary artery (from the pulmonary artery)
- Long QT syndrome
- Myocarditis
- Drug intoxication (eg, digoxin, ephedra, cocaine)
- Commotio cordis (ie, sharp blow to the chest)

Primary prevention of some episodes of pediatric cardiac arrest may be possible with cardiovascular screening (eg, for long QT syndrome) and treatment of predisposing problems (eg, myocarditis or anomalous coronary artery). The key secondary intervention to prevent death from SCA is timely and effective resuscitation. Prompt treatment of SCA in children will be possible only if coaches, trainers, parents, and the general public are aware that SCA can occur in children. Prompt treatment can be provided only if trained bystanders are present at the scene of an arrest to activate the emergency response system, provide high-quality CPR, and use an AED as soon as one is available. See the student CD for more information on pediatric SCA.

Pathway to Cardiac Arrest

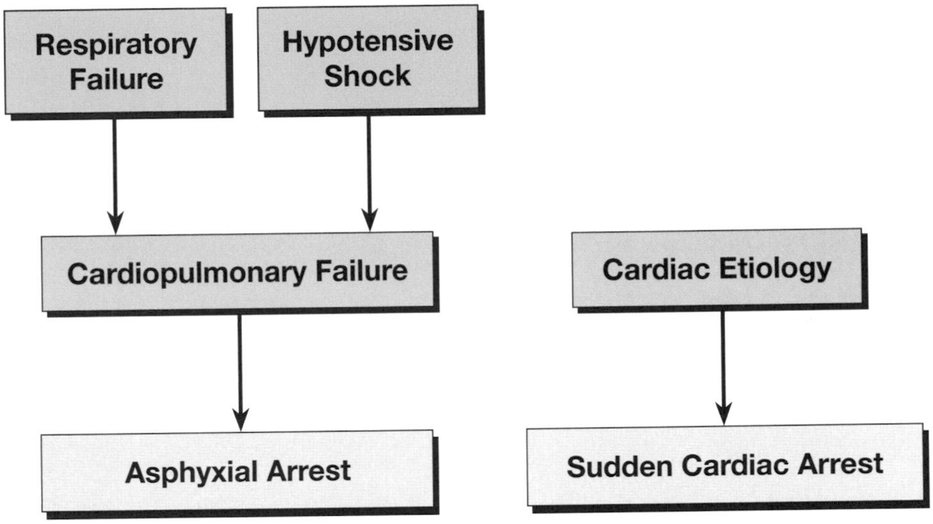

Figure 1. Pathway to cardiac arrest.

Causes of Cardiac Arrest

Causes of Cardiac Arrest

The causes of cardiac arrest in children vary based on the child's age and underlying health and whether the location of the event is

- out-of-hospital
- in-hospital

Most out-of-hospital cardiac arrests in infants and children occur at or near home. Trauma is the predominant cause of death in children from 6 months of age through young adulthood. Causes of traumatic arrest include airway compromise, tension pneumothorax, hemorrhagic shock, and massive head injury. Sudden infant death syndrome (SIDS) is a leading cause of death in infants under 6 months of age. The frequency of SIDS has decreased in recent years with the "back to sleep" campaign, which instructs parents to place infants on their back to sleep. See the student CD for more information on SIDS.

The most common immediate causes of pediatric cardiac arrest are respiratory failure and hypotension. Arrhythmia is a less common cause.

Figure 2 summarizes common causes of in-hospital and out-of-hospital cardiac arrest, categorized according to respiratory, shock, or sudden cardiac etiologies.

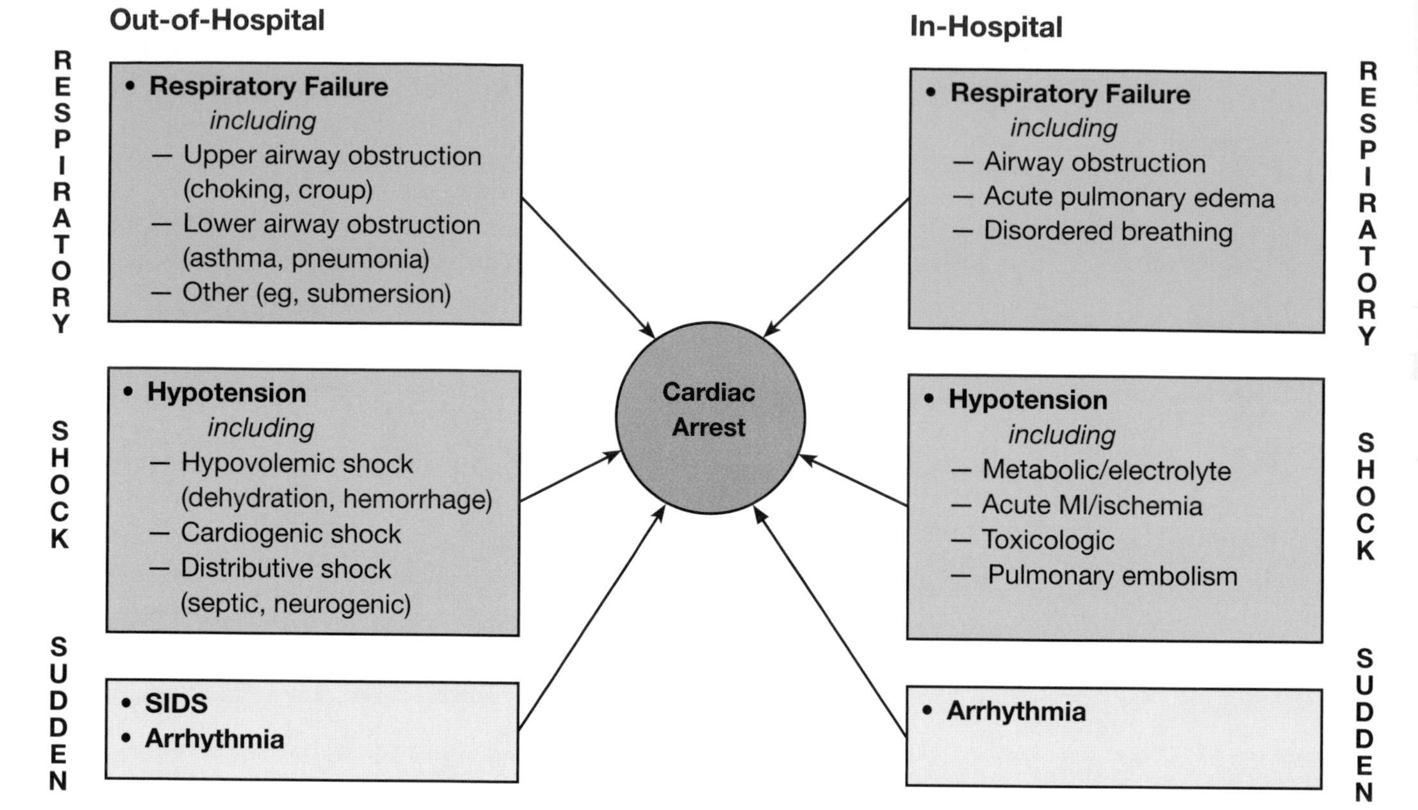

Figure 2. Causes of pediatric cardiac arrest.

Recognition of Cardiopulmonary Failure

Regardless of the initiating event or disease process, children in respiratory distress, respiratory failure, or shock develop cardiopulmonary failure immediately preceding cardiac arrest. Cardiopulmonary failure is defined as the combination of respiratory failure and shock (usually hypotensive). It is characterized by inadequate oxygenation, ventilation, and tissue perfusion. Clinically the patient is cyanotic, gasping, or breathing irregularly and is bradycardic. The child in cardiopulmonary failure may be only minutes from cardiac arrest. Once the child develops cardiopulmonary failure, the process may be difficult to reverse.

You must promptly recognize and treat cardiopulmonary failure before it deteriorates to cardiac arrest. Using the primary assessment model, look for evidence of cardiopulmonary failure, which may include some or all of the following signs:

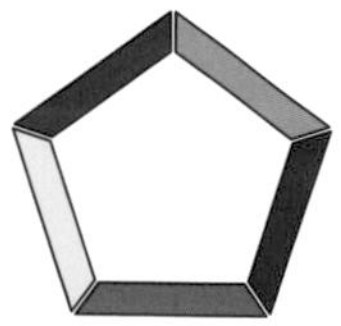

	Signs
Airway	Possible upper airway obstruction due to decreased level of consciousness
Breathing	• Bradypnea (ie, slow respiratory rate) • Irregular, ineffective respirations (decreased breath sounds or gasping)
Circulation	• Bradycardia • Delayed capillary refill time (typically >5 seconds) • Weak central pulses • Absence of peripheral pulses • Hypotension (usually) • Cool extremities • Mottled or cyanotic skin

	Signs
Disability	Diminished level of consciousness
Exposure	Deferred while addressing life-threatening condition

Detect and treat respiratory failure and shock before the child deteriorates to cardiopulmonary failure and cardiac arrest.

Recognition of Cardiac Arrest

Introduction

Cardiac arrest is recognized by

- absence of signs of cardiorespiratory function (no movement, no breathing or response to rescue breaths, no pulse)
- arrest rhythm on the cardiac monitor (Note: Monitoring is not mandatory for recognition of cardiac arrest)

Clinical Signs

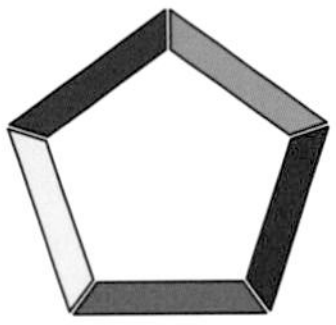

Using the primary assessment model, clinical signs of cardiac arrest are the following:

Airway	
Breathing	Apnea or agonal gasps
Circulation	No detectable pulses
Disability	Unresponsiveness
Exposure	

Children in cardiac arrest do not have detectable pulses. Studies have shown that healthcare providers have an error rate of about 35%[10-16] when they try to determine the presence or absence of pulses. Since the accuracy of a pulse check is poor, the recognition of cardiac arrest may be determined by the *absence* of other clinical signs, including

- breathing (note that agonal gasps are not adequate breathing)
- movement in response to stimulation (eg, response to rescue breathing)

Arrest Rhythms

Cardiac arrest is associated with one of the following rhythms, also known as arrest rhythms:

- asystole
- pulseless electrical activity (PEA): requires assessment of pulse and is not an identifiable rhythm; most often slow but may be fast or have a normal rate
- VF
- pulseless VT (including torsades de pointes; requires pulse assessment)

Asystole and PEA are the most common initial arrest rhythms detected in children with both out-of-hospital and in-hospital cardiac arrest, particularly in children younger than about 12 years of age.[6,8] Asystole may be preceded by narrow–QRS-complex bradycardia that may then deteriorate to a slow, wide QRS complex without a pulse (ie, pulseless electrical activity).[1,7] VF and pulseless VT are more likely to be observed in pediatric victims of sudden collapse.

Asystole

Asystole is cardiac standstill associated with no discernable electrical activity. It is represented by a straight (flat) line on the ECG (Figure 3). Causes of asystole and PEA may include submersion, hypothermia, sepsis, or poisoning (eg, sedative-hypnotics, narcotics) leading to hypoxia and acidosis.

You must clinically confirm that the child with asystole on the monitor is unresponsive, has no breathing, and has no pulse because a "flat line" on the ECG can also be caused by a loose ECG lead.

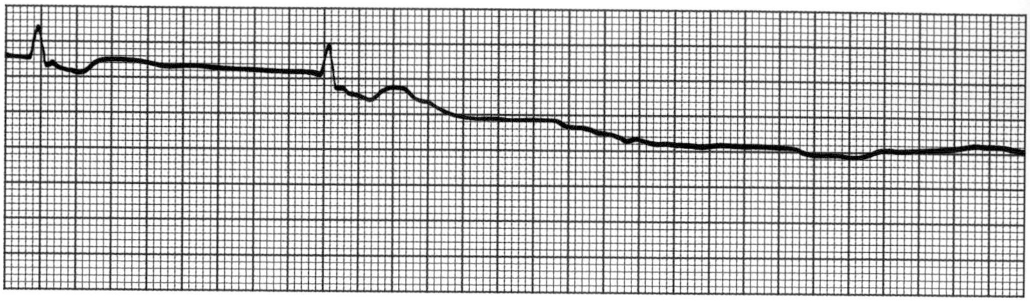

Figure 3. Agonal rhythm progressing to asystole.

Pulseless Electrical Activity

Pulseless electrical activity (PEA) refers to any organized electrical activity observed on an ECG or cardiac monitor in a patient with no palpable pulse. This definition specifically excludes VF, VT, and asystole. Although some aortic pulsations may be detected by an arterial waveform or Doppler study, if the patient has PEA, you cannot palpate (detect) central pulses.

PEA may be caused by reversible conditions such as severe hypovolemia or cardiac tamponade. You may be able to successfully treat PEA if you can quickly treat the underlying condition. Unless you can identify and treat the cause of the PEA, the rhythm will likely deteriorate to asystole.

You can recall potential reversible causes of cardiac arrest (including PEA) in children using the H's and T's mnemonic described later in this chapter.

The ECG may display normal or wide QRS complexes or other abnormalities, including

- low-amplitude or high-amplitude T waves
- prolonged PR and QT intervals
- AV dissociation or complete heart block

Reassess the monitored rhythm and note the rate and width of the QRS complexes.

The ECG may provide clues to the etiology of the cardiac arrest. QRS complexes may initially appear normal, particularly in problems of short duration. Examples include significant hypovolemia (eg, hemorrhage), massive pulmonary embolism, tension pneumothorax, or cardiac tamponade. Wide-complex, slow-rhythm PEA is more often seen in processes of longer duration, particularly those characterized by severe tissue hypoxia and acidosis.

Ventricular Fibrillation

VF is a form of pulseless arrest. When VF is present, the heart has no organized rhythm and no coordinated contractions (Figure 4). Electrical activity is chaotic. The heart quivers and does not pump blood. VF is often preceded by a brief period of VT.

Primary VF is uncommon in children. In studies of pediatric cardiac arrest, VF was the initial rhythm in 5% to 15% of out-of hospital[17] and 10% of in-hospital[6] cardiac arrests. Overall prevalence may be higher because VF may occur early during an arrest and quickly deteriorate to asystole.[9,18,19] VF has been reported in up to 25% of pediatric in-hospital arrests at some point during the resuscitation.

Causes of out-of-hospital VF in children are medical illness (especially cardiac conditions), poisonings, electrical or lightning shocks, submersion accidents, and trauma.[20]

Survival in patients with VF or pulseless VT as the *initial* arrest rhythm is better than in patients with asystole or PEA.[6,17] Outcomes may be further improved by prompt recognition and treatment (ie, CPR and defibrillation) of VF.

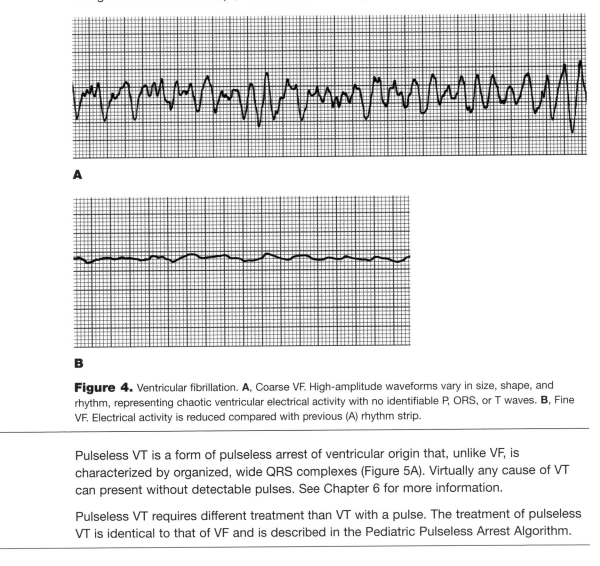

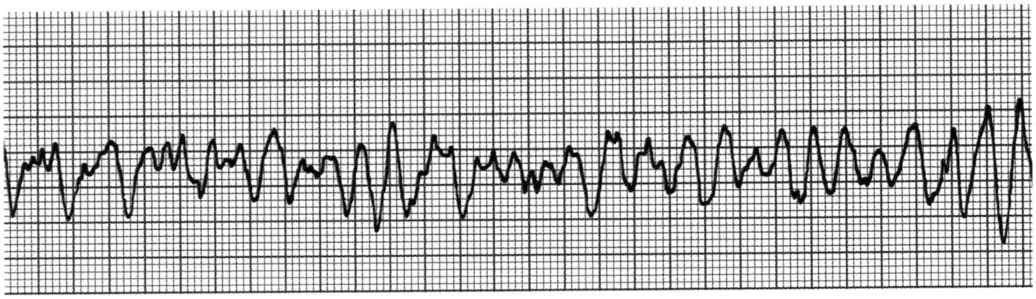

A

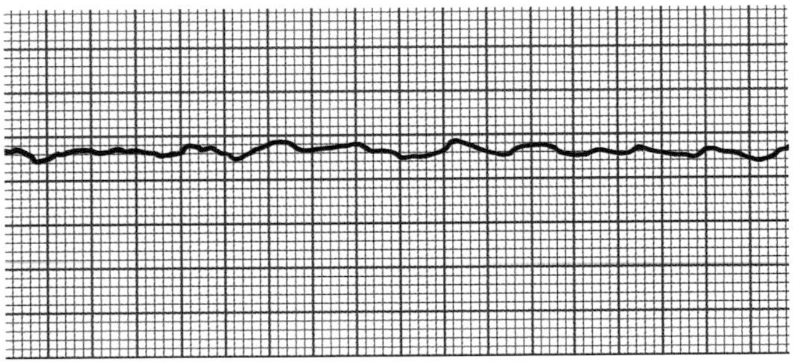

B

Figure 4. Ventricular fibrillation. **A**, Coarse VF. High-amplitude waveforms vary in size, shape, and rhythm, representing chaotic ventricular electrical activity with no identifiable P, ORS, or T waves. **B**, Fine VF. Electrical activity is reduced compared with previous (A) rhythm strip.

Pulseless VT

Pulseless VT is a form of pulseless arrest of ventricular origin that, unlike VF, is characterized by organized, wide QRS complexes (Figure 5A). Virtually any cause of VT can present without detectable pulses. See Chapter 6 for more information.

Pulseless VT requires different treatment than VT with a pulse. The treatment of pulseless VT is identical to that of VF and is described in the Pediatric Pulseless Arrest Algorithm.

Torsades de Pointes

Pulseless VT may be monomorphic (ventricular complexes appear uniform) or polymorphic (ventricular complexes appear different in form). Torsades de pointes ("to turn on a point") is a distinctive form of polymorphic VT. In torsades the QRS complexes change in polarity and amplitude, appearing to rotate around the ECG isoelectric line (Figure 5B). This arrhythmia is seen in conditions distinguished by a long baseline QT interval, including congenital conditions and drug toxicity. See Chapter 6 for more information.

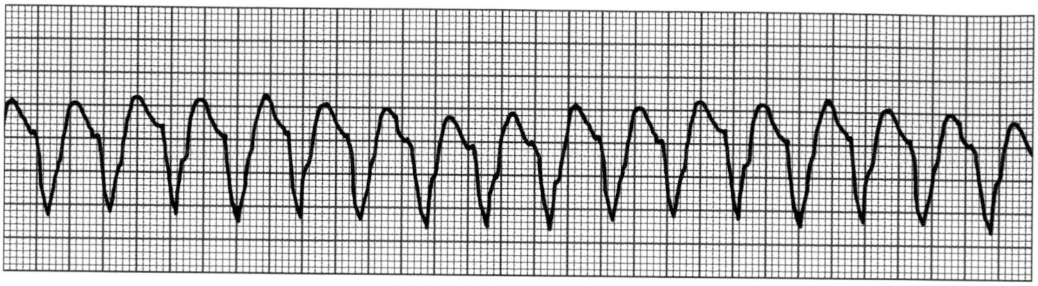

A

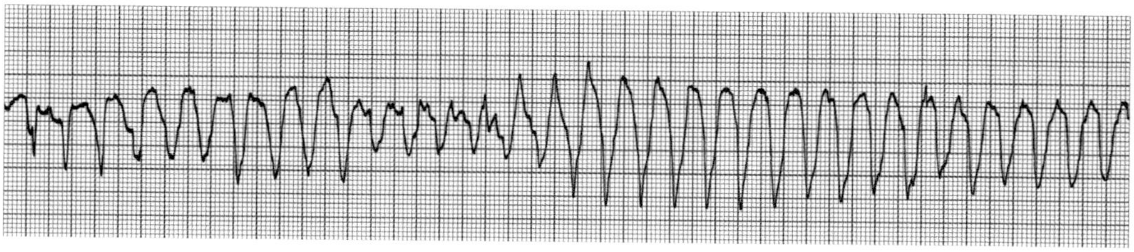

B

Figure 5. Ventricular tachycardia. **A,** VT in a child with muscular dystrophy and known cardiomyopathy. The ventricular rhythm is rapid and regular at a rate of 158/min (greater than the minimum 120/min characteristic of VT). The QRS is wide (greater than 0.06 second), and there is not evidence of atrial depolarization. **B,** Torsades de pointes in a child with hypomagnesemia.

Management of Cardiac Arrest

Introduction

High-quality CPR is the foundation of basic and advanced life support for the management of cardiac arrest. Until the defibrillator arrives, a team member should perform high-quality chest compressions. Remember to push hard, push fast, allow complete chest recoil, and try to minimize interruptions in chest compressions.

> *Chest compressions should ideally be interrupted only for ventilation (until an advanced airway is placed), rhythm check, and shock delivery.*

Management priorities are tailored to the cause of the arrest. If you are a lone rescuer, you will need to choose a sequence of action; if multiple rescuers are present, several activities can occur at the same time.

If you are a lone rescuer for an *unwitnessed* pediatric arrest in the out-of-hospital setting, treat the arrest as asphyxial in origin. Initiate immediate CPR and perform cycles of chest compressions and ventilations for about 2 minutes before leaving the child to activate the emergency response system (ERS) and to get an AED for the child (if available). If someone else activates the ERS and brings the AED, use the AED for the child after about 5 cycles (about 2 minutes) of CPR.

If you are a lone rescuer in the out-of-hospital setting and you witness a child collapse *suddenly*, treat the collapse as a primary cardiac rhythm disturbance. Activate the ERS, get the AED (if available), return to the child, and begin the steps of CPR. Use the AED as soon as you determine that the child has no pulse.

For an in-hospital arrest there will likely be help available. Send someone to activate the ERS and get the code cart (with monitor/defibrillator) while you begin CPR. Attach the monitor/defibrillator as soon as it is available. The lone rescuer for an unwitnessed arrest will rarely be in a location where a code cannot quickly be activated. If this is the case, perform 2 minutes of CPR before leaving the child to activate the ERS and get the code cart with monitor/defibrillator.

Please review the fundamentals of basic life support (BLS) in Table 1. These recommendations are based on the *2005 AHA Guidelines for CPR and ECC. Remember that the best advanced life support interventions will be ineffective if BLS is of poor quality.*

Basic Life Support

Introduction

BLS includes recognition of signs of cardiac arrest, performance of high-quality CPR, and defibrillation with an AED. Performance of high-quality CPR is integral to effective advanced life support efforts. Table 1 summarizes these important concepts.

Table 1. Summary of BLS ABCD Maneuvers for Infants, Children, and Adults
(Newborn/Neonatal Information Not Included) *Note:* Maneuvers used only by healthcare providers are indicated by "HCP."

Maneuver	Adult **Lay rescuer: ≥8 years** **HCP:** Adolescent and older	Child **Lay rescuers: 1 to 8 years** **HCP: 1 year to adolescent**	Infant **Under 1 year of age**
ACTIVATE Emergency Response Number (lone rescuer)	Activate when victim found unresponsive **HCP:** if asphyxial arrest likely, call after 5 cycles (2 minutes) of CPR	Activate after performing 5 cycles of CPR For sudden, witnessed collapse, activate after verifying that victim unresponsive	
AIRWAY	Head tilt–chin lift (HCP: suspected trauma, use jaw thrust)		
BREATHS Initial	2 breaths at 1 second/breath	2 effective breaths at 1 second/breath	
HCP: Rescue breathing without chest compressions	10 to 12 breaths/min (approximately 1 breath every 5 to 6 seconds)	12 to 20 breaths/min (approximately 1 breath every 3 to 5 seconds)	
HCP: Rescue breaths for CPR with advanced airway	8 to 10 breaths/min (approximately 1 breath every 6 to 8 seconds)		
Foreign-body airway obstruction	Abdominal thrusts		Back slaps and chest thrusts
CIRCULATION **HCP:** Pulse check (≤10 sec)	Carotid (**HCP** can use femoral in child)		Brachial or femoral
Compression landmarks	Center of chest, between nipples		Just below nipple line

(continued)

Maneuver	Adult **Lay rescuer: ≥8 years** **HCP:** Adolescent and older	Child **Lay rescuers: 1 to 8 years** **HCP: 1 year to adolescent**	Infant **Under 1 year of age**
Compression method Push hard and fast Allow complete recoil	**2 Hands:** Heel of 1 hand, other hand on top	**2 Hands:** Heel of 1 hand with second on top or **1 Hand:** Heel of 1 hand only	1 rescuer: 2 fingers **HCP**, 2 rescuers: 2 thumb–encircling hands
Compression depth	$1\frac{1}{2}$ to 2 inches	Approximately $\frac{1}{3}$ to $\frac{1}{2}$ the depth of the chest	
Compression rate	Approximately 100/min		
Compression-ventilation ratio	30:2 (1 or 2 rescuers)	30:2 (single rescuer) **HCP**: 15:2 (2 rescuers)	
DEFIBRILLATION			
AED	Use adult pads. Do not use child pads/child system. **HCP:** For out-of-hospital response may provide 5 cycles/2 minutes of CPR before shock if response > 4 to 5 minutes and arrest not witnessed.	**HCP:** Use AED as soon as available for sudden collapse and in-hospital. **All:** After about 2 minutes of CPR (out-of-hospital). Use child pads/child system for child 1 to 8 years if available. If child pads/system not available, use adult AED and pads.	No recommendation for infants <1 year of age

Chest Compressions After Advanced Airway Placed

Try to limit interruptions in chest compressions except to provide ventilation (until an advanced airway is placed), perform a rhythm check, or deliver a shock. Once an advanced airway is in place, do the following:

- Replace "cycles" of alternating compressions and ventilations with *continuous* chest compressions (rate of about 100/min) and a ventilation rate of about 8 to 10 breaths/min (1 breath every 6 to 8 seconds)
- Interrupt continuous chest compressions ideally only for rhythm check and shock delivery

Compression-to-Ventilation Ratio for 1 and 2 Rescuers

A universal compression-to-ventilation ratio of 30:2 for lone rescuers is recommended for all victims of cardiac arrest from infants to adults. The ratio is modified to 15:2 for infants and children if 2 rescuers are present.

High compression-to-ventilation ratios ensure a greater number of uninterrupted chest compressions within a CPR series. This results in higher sustained coronary and cerebral arterial blood flow. When chest compressions are interrupted, blood flow stops. Every time chest compressions begin again, the first few compressions are not as effective as the later compressions.

During cardiac arrest, blood flow to the lungs is only about 25% to 33% of normal. This means that the victim needs less ventilation (ie, fewer breaths and smaller volume) than normal to match perfusion with oxygenation and elimination of carbon dioxide.

Ventilation, however, is important for victims of asphyxial arrest, the most common form of pediatric cardiac arrest. If 2 rescuers are available, pediatric victims are believed to have the best chance of survival at a compression-to-ventilation ratio of 15:2 (compared with the 30:2 ratio for lone rescuers).

Pediatric Advanced Life Support in Cardiac Arrest

Introduction

The goal of therapeutic interventions in cardiac arrest is return of spontaneous circulation (ROSC), defined as restoration of a spontaneous and perfusing heart rhythm. ROSC is detected by resumption of organized cardiac electrical activity on the monitor and corresponding clinical evidence of perfusion (eg, palpable pulses, measurable blood pressure).

Advanced Management

Once the defibrillator arrives and is attached, advanced management may include the following:

- Assessment of rhythm (shockable versus nonshockable)
- Delivery of shocks as needed
- Establishment of vascular access
- Provision of pharmacologic therapy
- Insertion of an advanced airway

Remember that the success of any resuscitation is built on a strong base of high-quality CPR, good teamwork, and shock delivery for any shockable rhythm.

Rhythm Assessment and Shock Delivery

Identifying the rhythm as shockable versus nonshockable determines the applicable pathway of the Pediatric Pulseless Arrest Algorithm (Figure 6). The algorithm outlines the recommended sequence of CPR, shocks, and drug administration based on this determination. The rescuer should note that although the algorithm depicts actions sequentially, in reality many actions (eg, compressions and drug administration) are typically performed simultaneously when multiple rescuers are present.

Vascular Access

Historically in advanced life support, drugs were administered either via the intravenous (IV) or endotracheal (ET) route. New science and consensus opinion have reprioritized access routes. The intraosseous (IO) route is now preferred to the ET route when IV access is not available. General priorities for vascular access during PALS are as follows:

1. IV route
2. IO route
3. ET route

Limit the time you spend trying to obtain venous access in the seriously ill or injured child. If you cannot achieve reliable IV access quickly, establish IO access.

Intravenous Route

Obtaining peripheral IV access is preferred in most instances for drug and fluid administration rather than attempting central venous access.

Although a central line is more secure than a peripheral line, central line access is not needed during most resuscitation attempts. It is undesirable to attempt central line access if it requires interruption of chest compressions. In addition, CPR can cause complications during central line insertion, such as vascular laceration, hematomas, and bleeding. If a central line is in place during CPR, it is the preferred route for drug administration. Central venous administration of medications provides a more rapid onset and higher peak concentrations than peripheral venous injection.[21]

Establishing a peripheral line does not require interruption of CPR, but drug delivery to the central circulation may be delayed.

If a drug is given by the peripheral venous route, administer it as follows to improve drug delivery to the central circulation:

- Give the drug by bolus injection.
- Give the drug during compressions.
- Follow with a 5-mL flush of normal saline to move the drug from the peripheral to the central circulation.

Intraosseous Route

Drugs and fluids during resuscitation can be delivered safely and effectively via the IO route if IV access is not available. Important points about IO access are

- IO access can be established in all age groups
- IO access often can be achieved in 30 to 60 seconds
- the IO route of administration is preferred to the ET route
- any drug or fluid that is administered IV can be given IO

IO cannulation provides access to a noncollapsible marrow venous plexus, which serves as a rapid, safe, and reliable route for administration of drugs and resuscitation fluids. The technique uses a rigid needle, preferably a specially designed IO or bone marrow needle. Although an IO needle with a stylet is preferred to prevent obstruction of the needle with cortical bone during insertion, butterfly needles,[22] standard hypodermic needles, and spinal needles can be inserted successfully and used effectively. See the student CD for more information on IO access.

Endotracheal Route

IV and IO routes of administration are preferred to the ET route of administration. When considering administration of drugs via the ET route during CPR, keep these concepts in mind:

- Lipid-soluble drugs such as lidocaine, epinephrine, atropine, and naloxone ("LEAN") may be given by the ET route. Vasopressin is also lipid-soluble and can be administered by the ET route, although there are no human studies to provide dosing guidelines.
- The optimal dose of most drugs given by the ET route is unknown.
- Drug absorption from the tracheobronchial tree is unpredictable,[23-26] so drug levels and drug effects will be unpredictable.
- Drug administration into the trachea results in lower blood levels than the same dose given via IV or IO routes. In fact, animal data suggests that the lower epinephrine concentrations achieved when the drug is delivered by the ET route may produce transient but detrimental β-adrenergic–mediated vasodilation.
- The typical ET dose of drugs other than epinephrine is 2 to 3 times the IV dose. The recommended ET dose of epinephrine is 10 times the IV dose.

If a drug is given by the ET route, administer it as follows:

- Instill in the ET tube (briefly hold compressions during installation)
- Follow with a minimum of 5 mL normal saline flush; may use smaller volume in neonates

Provide 5 positive-pressure ventilations after the drug is instilled.

Defibrillation

Defibrillation does not restart the heart. A defibrillation shock "stuns" the heart by depolarizing all of the myocardial cells. If a shock is successful, it terminates VF. This allows the heart's natural pacemaker cells to resume an organized rhythm. The return of an organized rhythm alone, however, does not ensure survival. The organized rhythm must ultimately produce effective cardiac mechanical activity that results in ROSC, defined by the presence of palpable central pulses.

When attempting defibrillation, deliver 1 shock. Follow with immediate CPR, beginning with chest compressions.

A single shock with a biphasic defibrillator is associated with a first-shock efficacy rate of 85% to 94% for VF arrest of short duration in adults. This success rate refers to the elimination of VF, but elimination of VF does not always lead to ROSC. In a recent study of 64 adult patients with out-of-hospital VF, none had a perfusing rhythm immediately after shock delivery.[27] If shock delivery abolishes VF, CPR is still needed because most victims have asystole or PEA immediately after shock delivery. Chest compressions are needed to maintain blood flow to the heart and brain until cardiac contractility resumes. There is no evidence that performance of chest compressions on a patient with spontaneous cardiac activity is harmful.

If VF is not eliminated by a shock, the heart is probably ischemic, and resumption of chest compressions is likely to be of greater value to the patient than delivery of another shock. Chest compressions will deliver a small but critical amount of blood flow to the coronary circulation.

In the out-of-hospital or unmonitored setting, do not waste time looking for a shockable rhythm or palpating a pulse immediately after shock delivery; neither is likely to be present. Resume high-quality CPR beginning with chest compressions. In in-hospital units with continuous monitoring (eg, electrocardiography, hemodynamics), this sequence may be modified at a physician's direction.

See the manual defibrillation procedure on the student CD.

Pharmacologic Therapy

The objectives of administration of medications during cardiac arrest are to

- increase coronary and cerebral perfusion pressures and blood flow
- stimulate spontaneous or more forceful myocardial contractility
- accelerate heart rate
- correct and treat the cause of metabolic acidosis
- suppress or treat arrhythmias

Drugs that may be used during treatment of cardiac arrest are listed in Table 2.

Table 2. Pharmacologic Agents That May Be Relevant During Resuscitation of Pediatric Cardiac Arrest

Vasopressors	
Epinephrine	The α-adrenergic–mediated vasoconstriction of *epinephrine* increases aortic diastolic pressure and thus coronary perfusion pressure, a critical determinant of successful resuscitation.[28,29] Although epinephrine has been used universally in resuscitation, there is little evidence to show that it improves survival in humans. Both beneficial and toxic physiologic effects of epinephrine administration during CPR have been shown in animal and human studies.[30] There is no survival benefit from routine use of *high-dose epinephrine* (0.1 to 0.2 mg/kg or 0.1 to 0.2 mL/kg of 1:1000 solution), and it may be harmful, particularly in asphyxial arrest.[31-34] High-dose epinephrine may be considered for special resuscitation circumstances. See Chapter 9 for more information.
Vasopressin	There is insufficient evidence to recommend for or against the routine use of *vasopressin* during cardiac arrest in children. Vasopressin given after lack of response to epinephrine may result in return of spontaneous circulation during pediatric cardiac arrest.[35-37] In a recent clinical trial in adult patients with asystole, the combination of epinephrine and vasopressin improved ROSC and survival to hospital discharge but did not improve intact neurologic survival when compared with giving epinephrine alone.[38-42]
Antiarrhythmics	
Amiodarone	*Amiodarone* may be considered as part of the treatment of shock-refractory or recurrent VF/VT. Amiodarone has α-adrenergic and β-adrenergic blocking activity; affects sodium, potassium, and calcium channels; slows AV conduction; prolongs the AV refractory period and QT interval; and slows ventricular conduction (widens the QRS). Adult studies showed increased survival to hospital admission but not to hospital discharge when amiodarone was compared with placebo or lidocaine for shock-resistant VF.[43-45] One study in children demonstrated the effectiveness of amiodarone for life-threatening ventricular arrhythmias,[46,47] but there have been no published studies on the use of amiodarone for pediatric cardiac arrest.
Lidocaine	*Lidocaine* has long been recommended for the treatment of ventricular arrhythmias in infants and children because it decreases automaticity and suppresses ventricular arrhythmias. Data from a study of shock-refractory VT in adults showed that lidocaine was inferior to amiodarone, so lidocaine has been recommended as a second-line drug in shock-refractory cardiac arrest when amiodarone is not available. Its indications in the treatment of other ventricular arrhythmias are uncertain. There have been no published studies on the use of lidocaine in pediatric cardiac arrest.
Magnesium sulfate	*Magnesium sulfate* should be administered for the treatment of torsades de pointes or hypomagnesemia. There is insufficient evidence to recommend for or against the routine use of magnesium in pediatric cardiac arrest.[48-57]
Other agents	
Atropine	*Atropine* is indicated for the treatment of bradyarrhythmias. There are no published studies suggesting its efficacy for treatment of cardiac arrest in pediatric patients. See Chapter 5 for a complete discussion.
Calcium	*Calcium* is indicated for the treatment of documented ionized hypocalcemia and hyperkalemia,[58] particularly in patients with hemodynamic compromise. Ionized hypocalcemia is relatively common in critically ill children, particularly those with sepsis[59,60] or after cardiopulmonary bypass. Calcium may also be considered for the treatment of hypermagnesemia[61] or calcium channel blocker overdose.[62] Routine use of calcium in cardiac arrest is not recommended because it does not improve survival.[63]
Sodium bicarbonate	*Sodium bicarbonate* is recommended for the treatment of symptomatic patients with hyperkalemia,[64] tricyclic antidepressant overdose, or an overdose of other sodium channel blocking agents.[65] Routine use of sodium bicarbonate in cardiac arrest is not recommended. After you have provided effective ventilation and chest compressions and administered epinephrine, you may consider sodium bicarbonate for prolonged cardiac arrest.

Advanced Airway Management

In managing the airway and ventilation in pediatric victims of cardiac arrest, consider the following important information:

- An advanced airway (eg, ET tube) may be placed during CPR. However, there was no proven advantage of ET intubation over effective bag-mask ventilation in a study of out-of-hospital cardiac arrest when EMS transport time was short.[45] This study does not address the utility or timing of ET intubation in the in-hospital setting but suggests that immediate intubation may not be necessary.
- Be careful to avoid excessive ventilation during resuscitation. Excessive ventilation can impede venous return and thus cardiac output.[66] Increased intrathoracic pressure also elevates right atrial pressure, thus reducing coronary perfusion pressure. When ventilation is provided through a mask (in "cycles" of 15 compressions and 2 breaths), minimize the time taken to provide breaths because this represents an interval without chest compressions. Excessive tidal volumes during bag-mask ventilation may also distend the stomach, thereby impeding ventilation and increasing the risk of aspiration.[67]
- Colorimetric exhaled CO_2 devices may produce false-negative readings (ie, the device color indicates no CO_2 detected despite correct placement of an ET tube in the trachea) during cardiac arrest. Use direct laryngoscopy to confirm tube placement if exhaled CO_2 is not detected and there is other evidence that the tube is in the trachea (eg, chest rise and bilateral breath sounds).
- Once an advanced airway is placed during CPR, provide 8 to 10 breaths/min (1 breath every 6 to 8 seconds) without pausing chest compressions.

Pediatric Pulseless Arrest Algorithm

Overview

The Pediatric Pulseless Arrest Algorithm (Figure 6) outlines the steps for assessment and management of the pulseless patient who does not respond to BLS interventions.

The algorithm consists of 2 pathways for a pulseless arrest:

- A shockable rhythm (VF/VT) pathway is displayed on the left side of the algorithm.
- A nonshockable rhythm (asystole/PEA) pathway is displayed on the right side of the algorithm.

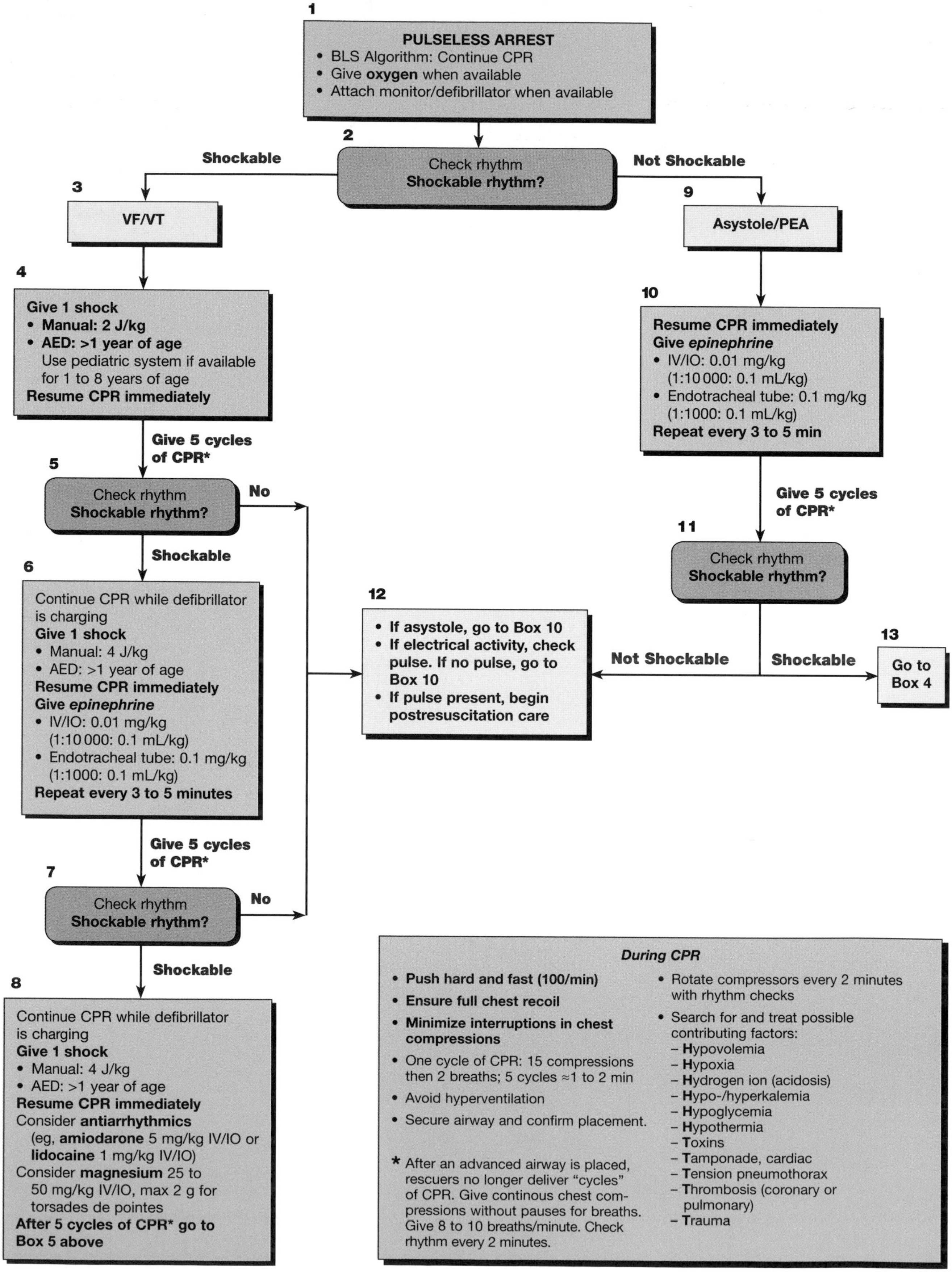

Figure 6. Pediatric Pulseless Arrest Algorithm.

Management of VF/Pulseless VT

The Pediatric Pulseless Arrest Algorithm is based on expert consensus. It is designed to maximize uninterrupted periods of CPR while enabling efficient delivery of electrical therapy, if appropriate, for victims of cardiac arrest. Although the actions are listed sequentially, when several rescuers are present, many actions will happen simultaneously.

Using the PALS algorithm, providers should structure assessments and interventions around 2-minute periods of uninterrupted, high-quality CPR. This requires organization so that every member of the team knows his or her responsibilities. About every 2 minutes, check the rhythm and deliver 1 shock if needed, rotate compressors, and prepare to deliver medications. Resume CPR, beginning with chest compressions, immediately after rhythm check or shock delivery. Administer drugs during compressions as soon as possible after a rhythm check has indicated persistent cardiac arrest. If an organized rhythm is observed during the rhythm check at 2 minutes, check for a pulse.

In the description of this sequence, we will refer to Box numbers 1 through 8. These are the numbers assigned to the boxes on the left side of the algorithm.

Basic Life Support (Boxes 1-2)

Box 1 prompts the rescuer to continue BLS management as reviewed in Table 1. Summary of BLS ABCD Maneuvers for Infants, Children, and Adults.

Administer oxygen if it is available and provide ventilations immediately to any child in pulseless arrest.

Once the monitor/defibrillator arrives and is attached, check the rhythm (Box 2) and determine whether the rhythm is shockable (VF/VT) or nonshockable (asystole/PEA). If the rhythm is shockable, proceed to the left side of the algorithm (Box 3).

For VF/VT, Deliver Shock (Boxes 3-4)

Box 4 directs you to deliver 1 unsynchronized shock. If the defibrillator requires more than 10 seconds to charge, perform CPR while the defibrillator is charging. The shorter the interval between the last compression and the shock delivery, the higher the predicted shock success. For this reason try to keep that interval as short as possible (ideally <10 seconds). Resume high-quality CPR, beginning with chest compressions, immediately after shock delivery. As noted previously, in a monitored setting this approach may be modified at the physician's discretion.

If during resuscitation from cardiac arrest, a child in a critical care setting has invasive hemodynamic monitoring in place, such as an intra-arterial catheter, the presence of a waveform with an adequate arterial pressure can be assessed during the rhythm check to determine if return of spontaneous circulation has occurred.

Defibrillation devices for children include the

- AED (able to recognize pediatric shockable rhythms and ideally equipped with a pediatric dose attenuator)
- manual defibrillator (enables administration of variable shock doses based on weight)

Institutions that care for children at risk for arrhythmias and cardiac arrest (eg, hospitals, emergency departments) ideally should have defibrillators available that are capable of energy adjustment appropriate for children.

AED

AEDs are programmed to evaluate the victim's ECG to determine if a shockable rhythm is present, charge to the appropriate dose, and prompt the rescuer to deliver a shock. The AED provides voice and visual prompts to assist the operator. Many, but not all, AED algorithms have been shown to be sensitive and specific for recognizing shockable arrhythmias in children.

Weight/Age	AED Energy Dose
≥25 kg (≥8 years old)	• Use a standard "adult" AED with adult pad-cable system
<25 kg (≥1 year old and <8 years old)	• Use attenuated dose if a pediatric system is available • Use adult system if pediatric system is not available
<1 year old	Currently insufficient evidence to recommend for or against the use of an AED

Manual Defibrillator

For manual defibrillation, an initial dose of 2 J/kg (biphasic or monophasic waveform) is recommended. If at the next rhythm check you find that VF or pulseless VT persists, deliver a dose of 4 J/kg for the second and any subsequent shocks.

You can use either paddles or electrode pads to deliver electrical therapy via a manual defibrillator. If paddles are used, you must use a conducting gel, cream, paste, or pad between the paddle and the patient's chest to reduce transthoracic impedance. Do not use saline-soaked gauze pads or sonographic gels. Do not use alcohol pads. They may pose a fire hazard and produce chest burns. Self-adhesive pads reduce the risk of current arcing, can be placed prior to arrest, and can be used for monitoring. You should routinely use self-adhesive pads when they are available instead of standard paddles.

See the student CD for the universal steps in operating a manual defibrillator.

Paddles/Pads

Use the largest paddles or self-adhering electrode pads that will fit on the chest wall without touching.[68-70] The recommended paddle size is described below.

Weight/Age	Paddle Size
>10 kg (>approximately 1 year old)	Large "adult" paddles (8 to 13 cm)
<10 kg (<1 year old)	Small "infant" paddles (4.5 cm)

Place the paddles/electrode pads so that the heart is between them. Place one paddle on the upper right side of the chest below the clavicle and the other to the left of the left nipple in the anterior axillary line directly over the heart. Make sure the paddles/electrode pads do not touch. Allow at least 3 cm between paddles.

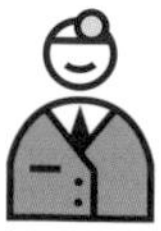

Alternatively, place paddles or self-adhesive electrode pads in an anterior-posterior position with one just to the left of the sternum and the other over the back. Anterior-posterior placement may be necessary in an infant, particularly if only large paddles/electrode pads are available.

Apply firm pressure to create good contact between the paddle/electrode pad and the skin. Placing paddles directly on the patient's bare skin decreases the delivered current. (See "Manual Defibrillator," above.)

Modifications to defibrillator use may be required in special situations.

Special Situation	Modifications
Standing water	Remove the victim from the water and wipe the chest. The chest does not need to be completely dry to deliver a shock using adhesive pads, but if there is water/liquid between the paddles or adhesive electrodes, current can arc between them and will not be delivered to the heart.
Implanted defibrillator or pacemaker	Do not place an electrode pad or paddle directly over implanted devices (eg, pacemaker or internal cardioverter/defibrillator) because the device may block current and reduce delivery of current to the heart. Place the paddle or electrode pad at least 1 inch (2.5 cm) to the side of the implanted device.
Transdermal medication patch	Do not place an electrode pad directly over a medication patch. If the patch is in the way, remove it and wipe the child's skin before attaching the electrode pad.
Oxygen	Several case reports have documented fires ignited by sparks from poorly attached defibrillator paddles in the presence of an oxygen-enriched atmosphere, such as oxygen delivered by ventilator tubing or even a simple face mask. The most severe fires were caused when ventilator tubing was disconnected from the ET tube and then left adjacent to the patient's head during attempted defibrillation. The oxygen-enriched atmosphere rarely extends >0.5 m (1.5 ft) in any direction from the oxygen outflow point. Rescuers should attempt to remove oxygen from the area immediately surrounding the child's chest during attempted defibrillation.

Clearing for Defibrillation

To ensure the safety of defibrillation, perform a visual check of the patient and the resuscitation team when you are about to deliver a shock. State a "warning" firmly and in a forceful voice before delivering each shock (this entire sequence should take less than 5 seconds):

- **"I am going to shock on three. One, I'm clear."** Check to make sure you are clear of contact with the patient, the stretcher, or other equipment.
- **"Two, you're clear."** Make a visual check to ensure that no one continues to touch the patient or stretcher. In particular, check the person providing ventilations. That person's hands should not be touching the ventilatory adjuncts, including the ET tube! Be sure oxygen is not flowing across the child's chest. Consider temporarily disconnecting the bag or the ventilation circuit from the ET tube during shock delivery.
- **"Three, everybody's clear."** Check yourself one more time before pressing the SHOCK button.

You need not use these exact words, but you must warn others that you are about to deliver shocks and that everyone must stand clear.

Deliver Shock and Resume CPR

Immediately after the shock, resume CPR beginning with chest compressions. Give about 2 minutes of CPR. (For 2 rescuers this will be about 10 cycles of 15 compressions followed by 2 ventilations.)

Check Rhythm (Box 5)

After 2 minutes of CPR, Box 5 directs you to check the rhythm. Try to minimize the time that chest compressions are interrupted. Before the rhythm check, the team leader should ensure that rescuers are prepared to rotate compressors, that the rescuer operating the defibrillator knows the shock dose to administer if VF/pulseless VT persists, that attempts have been made to establish IV/IO access, and that drugs are prepared for administration if indicated.

Try to limit interruptions in CPR to conduct a rhythm check to <10 seconds.

At this rhythm check, you may observe the following outcomes from the shock and CPR:

- Termination of VF/VT to a rhythm that is not treated with a shock (ie, a nonshockable rhythm); nonshockable rhythms include persistent pulseless arrest (ie, asystole or PEA) or an organized rhythm with a pulse
- Persistence of a shockable rhythm (VF/VT)

Termination of VF/VT (ie, Rhythm Is Nonshockable)

If a nonshockable rhythm is present, that rhythm may be an "organized" rhythm (ie, one with regular complexes [Figure 7]) with or without a pulse, or asystole. If the rhythm is organized, a team member should try to palpate a central pulse. If the rhythm is not organized, do not take the time to perform a pulse check; instead, immediately resume CPR.

Remember, rhythm and pulse checks should be brief (try to limit to <10 seconds). Pulse checks are unnecessary unless an organized rhythm (or other evidence of a perfusing rhythm, such as an arterial waveform) is present. Note that in specialized environments with intra-arterial or other hemodynamic monitoring in place (eg, an intensive care unit), physicians may alter this sequence.

If a pulse is present, begin postresuscitation care (Box 12).

If an organized rhythm is present but no pulse is palpable, PEA is present. If PEA or asystole is present, resume CPR beginning with compressions and proceed to the right side of the algorithm to Boxes 9-10.

If there is any doubt about the presence of a pulse, immediately resume CPR (Box 6). Chest compressions are unlikely to be harmful to a patient with a spontaneous rhythm but weak pulses. If there is no pulse, **do CPR.**

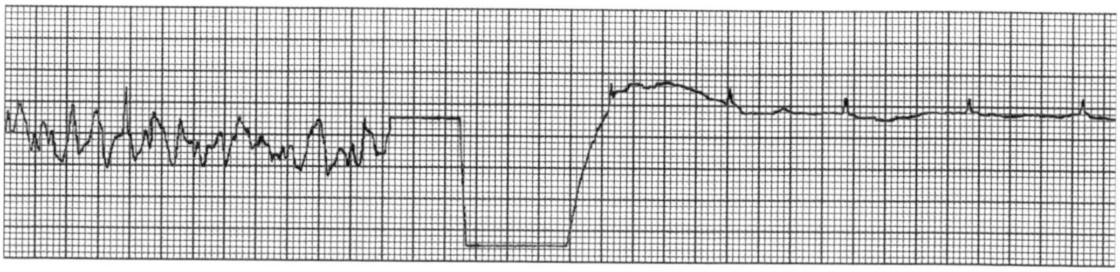

Figure 7. VF converted to organized rhythm after defibrillation (successful shock).

Persistence of VF/VT

If the rhythm check reveals a shockable rhythm (ie, persistent VF/VT), prepare to deliver a shock. If the defibrillator requires more than 10 seconds to charge, resume CPR (Box 6), beginning with immediate chest compressions while the defibrillator is charging. If IV/IO access is established, the rescuer delivering drugs should administer epinephrine during compressions as soon as possible after the rhythm check.

For Persistent VF/VT (Box 6)

Administer Shock

Give 1 shock by manual defibrillator (4 J/kg) or AED. Resume CPR immediately after the shock. A different compressor should be performing the compressions (ie, compressors should rotate every 2 minutes).

Immediately after the shock, resume CPR, beginning with chest compressions. Give about 2 minutes of CPR. (For 2 rescuers this will be about 10 cycles of 15 compressions followed by 2 ventilations.)

Give Epinephrine

If VF/VT persists despite delivery of 1 shock and 2 minutes of CPR, give epinephrine as soon as IV/IO access is available. Give the epinephrine during chest compressions either before (eg, if compressions are delivered while the defibrillator is charging) or after the second shock is delivered:

IV/IO	0.01 mg/kg (0.1 mL/kg) bolus (1:10 000)
ET tube	0.1 mg/kg (0.1 mL/kg) bolus (1:1000)
Repeat epinephrine administration about every 3 to 5 minutes if cardiac arrest persists. This will generally result in epinephrine delivery after every second (ie, every other) rhythm check.	

The algorithm and guidelines do not state a specific time when the first dose of epinephrine should be given because some patients will have early IV/IO access and hemodynamic monitoring and others will not. There is no published evidence to guide recommendations for timing of drug administration. By consensus epinephrine was not listed in Box 4 immediately after the *first* shock because epinephrine would not be needed if the first shock was successful.

In a monitored setting a physician may choose to administer epinephrine before or after the second shock. Where VF/VT is rapidly confirmed after the shock, administration of epinephrine with resumption of CPR is appropriate. Conversely, if an organized rhythm is seen after the shock in a monitored setting, it is reasonable to check for a pulse since epinephrine administration may produce adverse effects if not needed. For example, if the initial VF/VT was related to a cardiomyopathy, myocarditis, or drug toxicity, epinephrine administration immediately after elimination of VF/VT could induce recurrent VF/VT.

Drug Delivery During CPR

Ideally you should administer IV/IO drugs *during compressions* because blood flow generated by compressions circulates the drugs. By consensus the guidelines recommend drug delivery during the compressions immediately *before* (if compressions are delivered during charging of the defibrillator) or *after* shock delivery so that the drugs have time to circulate by the next rhythm check (and shock delivery if needed).

The rescuer(s) preparing the resuscitation drugs should refer to the algorithm and prepare the *next* drug dose that will be needed if cardiac arrest is present at the next rhythm check. Drug tables, charts, or other references should be readily available to expedite the preparation of drug doses. The use of a length-based, color-coded resuscitation tape facilitates rapid estimation of the appropriate drug dose.[71]

Administration of resuscitation drugs into the trachea results in lower blood concentrations than the same dose given intravascularly. Furthermore, recent animal studies suggest that the lower epinephrine concentrations achieved when the drug is delivered by the ET route may produce transient β-adrenergic effects. These effects can be detrimental, causing hypotension, lower coronary artery perfusion pressure and flow, and reduced potential for return of spontaneous circulation (ROSC). In addition, you will need to briefly interrupt chest compressions to deliver drugs by the ET route.

Thus, although ET administration of some resuscitation drugs is possible, IV or IO drug administration is preferred because it will provide a more predictable drug delivery and pharmacologic effect.[31,72-74] If the ET route is used, you should use a higher concentration of epinephrine (1:1000 solution) and give a dose that is 10 times the IV dose (ie, use 0.1 mg/kg).

Check Rhythm (Box 7)

Box 7 directs you to check the rhythm. Try to minimize the time that chest compressions are interrupted.

Try to limit interruptions in chest compressions for rhythm checks to <10 seconds.

If the rhythm check reveals	Then
Termination of VF/VT	Termination of VF/VT with a nonshockable arrest rhythm (asystole/PEA): go to Box 10 Termination of VF/VT with an organized rhythm and a pulse: begin postresuscitation care
Persistence of VF/VT	Go to Box 8

For Persistent VF/VT (Box 8)

Administer Shock

If VF/VT persists, give 1 shock by manual defibrillator (4 J/kg) or AED. If the defibrillator requires more than 10 seconds to charge, provide chest compressions while the defibrillator is charging. Resume CPR immediately after shock delivery.

Immediately after the shock, resume CPR, beginning with chest compressions. Give about 2 minutes of CPR. (For 2 rescuers this will be about 10 cycles of 15 compressions followed by 2 ventilations.)

Consider Antiarrhythmics or Magnesium Sulfate

Consider an antiarrhythmic agent (amiodarone or lidocaine) for VF/VT. Amiodarone is generally preferred to lidocaine. Use lidocaine if amiodarone is unavailable. Consider magnesium sulfate for torsades de pointes.

Dose antiarrhythmic agents as follows:

Drug	Dose
Amiodarone	5 mg/kg IV/IO (maximum single dose: 300 mg); may repeat dose to total of 15 mg/kg per 24 hours (maximum cumulative total of 2.2 g IV per 24 hours)
Lidocaine	1 mg/kg IV/IO
Magnesium sulfate	25 to 50 mg/kg IV/IO, maximum single dose: 2 g

Administer IV/IO drugs during chest compressions.

Check Rhythm (Box 5)

After about 2 minutes of CPR, check the rhythm (return to Box 5).

VF/Pulseless VT Treatment Sequences

Figure 8 summarizes the recommended sequence of CPR, rhythm checks, shocks, and delivery of drugs for VF/pulseless VT based on expert consensus.

Think of your management of pulseless arrest due to VF/VT as a nearly continuous stream of CPR, ideally interrupted only for rhythm checks and shock delivery. Drug preparation and administration should not require interruption of CPR and should not delay shock delivery.

Once an advanced airway (eg, ET tube) is in place, the CPR sequence changes from "cycles" to continuous chest compressions. One team member delivers chest compressions at a rate of about 100/min. Another team member delivers ventilations at a rate of about 8 to 10 breaths/min (one breath about every 6 to 8 seconds). Try to limit interruptions in CPR to those required for rhythm checks and shock delivery. This sequence may be modified in special settings (eg, an intensive care unit) with continuous ECG and hemodynamic monitoring in place.

The team leader will need to determine the appropriate time for inserting an advanced airway. Since insertion of an advanced airway is likely to require interruption of chest compressions, the team leader must weigh the priorities of securing the airway to ensure effective ventilations and minimizing interruptions in compressions. If an advanced airway is inserted, careful organization of supplies and personnel is needed to minimize the time that compressions are interrupted. Once the advanced airway is placed, confirm its correct position.

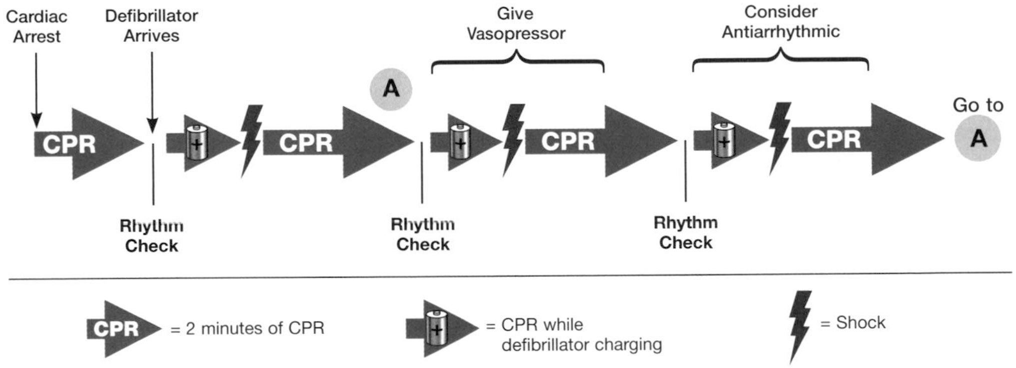

Figure 8. Pulseless arrest treatment sequences: ventricular fibrillation/pulseless VT. Prepare next drug prior to rhythm check. Administer drug during CPR, as soon as possible after the rhythm check confirms VF/pulseless VT. Do not delay shock. Continue CPR while drugs are prepared and administered and defibrillator is charging. Ideally, chest compressions should be interrupted only for ventilation (until advanced airway placed), rhythm check and actual shock delivery.

Management of PEA/Asystole

Management of children in pulseless cardiac arrest with PEA or asystole is outlined in the pathway on the right side of the Pediatric Pulseless Arrest Algorithm (Figure 6).

The most common ECG findings in infants and children in cardiac arrest are asystole and an organized rhythm without a pulse (ie, PEA). PEA is organized electrical activity—most commonly slow, wide QRS complexes—without palpable pulses. Less frequently there is a sudden impairment of cardiac output with an initially normal rhythm but with poor perfusion and no pulses. This subcategory of PEA (formerly known as electromechanical dissociation [EMD]) is more likely to be treatable.

You can recall potentially reversible causes of cardiac arrest or arrhythmias by using the H's and T's mnemonic. Causes of PEA that compromise venous return to the heart (eg, tension pneumothorax, cardiac tamponade, severe hypovolemia) may be particularly amenable to treatment. The outcome of PEA is poor unless there is a specific reversible cause that is identified and treated.

In addition to emergency measures such as needle decompression (ie, for tension pneumothorax) and pericardiocentesis (ie, for cardiac tamponade), children with PEA may need volume expansion and vasopressors or some combination of the 2 therapies.

During the treatment of cardiac arrest, including asystole or PEA, you will check the child's rhythm about every 2 minutes. Note that 25% of hospitalized children in the National Registry of CPR had a shockable rhythm at some point in their resuscitation; in many of these the VF was not present at the arrest but developed later.[6] If VF develops during resuscitation, return to the left side of the Pediatric Pulseless Arrest Algorithm (Box 4).

For treatment of asystole or PEA, resuscitation team members must provide high-quality CPR, deliver epinephrine as appropriate, and try to identify and treat potentially reversible causes of the arrest.

Give Epinephrine (Box 10)

If any rhythm check with pulse check (if appropriate) reveals a nonshockable rhythm of asystole or PEA (Box 9), resume CPR immediately and administer epinephrine (Box 10).

IV/IO	0.01 mg/kg (0.1 mL/kg) bolus 1:10 000
ET tube	0.1 mg/kg (0.1 mL/kg) bolus 1:1000
Repeat epinephrine administration about every 3 to 5 minutes if cardiac arrest persists. This will generally result in epinephrine delivery after every second (ie, every other) rhythm check.	

Administer the IV/IO epinephrine during chest compressions.

Check Rhythm (Box 11)

After about 2 minutes of CPR, check the rhythm (Box 11).

If Rhythm Is	Then
Shockable	Go to Box 4 and proceed through the steps on the left side of the algorithm
Nonshockable	Go to Box 12 Determine if the rhythm is organized: • If yes, check a pulse — If a pulse is present, begin postresuscitation care — If a pulse is not present, return to Box 10 • If not organized (asystole), return to Box 10

Asystole/PEA Treatment Sequence

Figure 9 summarizes the recommended sequence of CPR, rhythm checks, shocks, and delivery of drugs for asystole and PEA based on expert consensus.

Think of your management of pulseless arrest due to asystole and PEA as a nearly continuous stream of CPR, ideally interrupted only by rhythm checks. Do not interrupt CPR for drug preparation and administration. Administer IV/IO drugs during chest compressions.

Once an advanced airway (eg, ET tube) is in place, the CPR sequence changes from "cycles" to *continuous* chest compressions. One team member delivers chest compressions at a rate of about 100/min. Another team member delivers ventilations at a rate of about 8 to 10 breaths/min (one breath about every 6 to 8 seconds). Try to limit interruptions in chest compressions to those required for rhythm checks. This sequence may be modified in specialized settings (eg, intensive care units) with continuous ECG and hemodynamic monitoring in place.

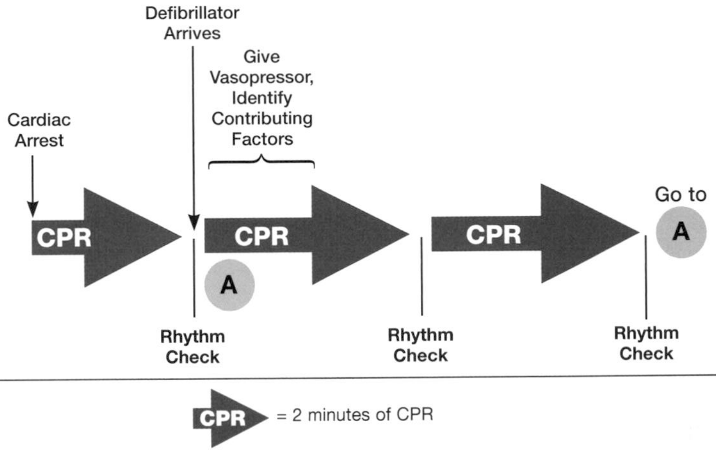

Figure 9. Pulseless arrest treatment sequences: asystole and PEA.

Identifying and Treating Underlying Causes

The outcome of pediatric cardiac arrest is generally poor. Rapid recognition, immediate high-quality CPR, and aggressive correction of contributing factors offer the best chance for successful resuscitation.

Ensure that high quality CPR is being provided:

- Monitor the rate and depth of chest compressions to be sure they are adequate and that the compressor allows full chest wall recoil after each compression.
- Consider palpating for a pulse during compressions. Although palpable "pulses" may represent venous pulsations, the absence of any palpable pulse should prompt rescuers to ensure that compressions are sufficiently deep with complete recoil after each compression and to determine if there is some factor limiting cardiac output.
- Deliver shocks as needed as soon as possible after the compressions are stopped.
- Consider exhaled CO_2 monitoring as an indicator of CPR quality; absence of detectable CO_2 may indicate inadequate cardiac output and pulmonary blood flow during CPR and is associated with poor outcome.

Some types of cardiac arrest may be associated with a reversible condition. If you can quickly identify the condition and treat it appropriately, your resuscitative efforts may be successful. It is important to identify and treat any reversible cause of arrest.

In the search for the reversible causes or contributing factors, do the following:

- Consider potentially reversible causes by recalling the H's and T's
- Review the ABCDs again to ensure that you are providing high-quality CPR and that the airway and ventilation are adequate.
- Be sure that the advanced airway is correctly placed and that ventilations produce visible chest rise without excessive volume or rate.
- Ensure that the manual resuscitation device is connected to a source of high-flow oxygen.

H's and T's

Cardiac arrest in children may be associated with a reversible condition. In addition, resuscitation efforts may be complicated by factors such as misplacement of an advanced airway or development of a tension pneumothorax. If you don't think about reversible causes or complicating factors, you are likely to miss them. Review the following H's and T's to help you identify potentially reversible causes of cardiac arrest or factors that may be complicating your resuscitative efforts.

H's	T's
Hypovolemia	**T**oxins
Hypoxia	**T**amponade (cardiac)
Hydrogen ion (acidosis)	**T**ension pneumothorax
Hyper-/Hypokalemia	**T**hrombosis (coronary or pulmonary)
Hypoglycemia	**T**rauma
Hypothermia	

Hypoglycemia

Hypoglycemia is commonly associated with poor outcome in critically ill children.[75] You should check blood glucose concentration during resuscitation with the goal of maintaining normoglycemia. Hypoglycemia is an important consideration in pediatric cardiac arrest and resuscitation for the following reasons:

- Critically ill infants and children have limited stores of glycogen that may be rapidly depleted during episodes of physiologic stress.
- Clinical signs of hypoglycemia may mimic those of hypoxemia and ischemia preceding cardiac arrest (ie, poor perfusion, diaphoresis, tachycardia, hypothermia, irritability or lethargy, and hypotension).
- Glucose is the major metabolic substrate for the neonatal myocardium, so hypoglycemia may especially depress neonatal myocardial function.
- Although fatty acids normally function as the major metabolic substrate for the myocardium of older infants and children, glucose provides a significant energy source during episodes of ischemia.

Hypovolemia

If hypovolemia is possible (eg, history consistent with dehydration) or occult bleeding may be present, consider administration of one or more fluid boluses during the attempted resuscitation.

Pediatric Cardiac Arrest: Special Circumstances

Introduction

The following special circumstances resulting in pediatric cardiac arrest require specific management:

- Trauma
- Drowning
- Anaphylaxis
- Toxins

Cardiac Arrest Due to Trauma

Cardiac arrest associated with trauma in children represents a significant subgroup of out-of-hospital pediatric cardiac arrests. In addition, improperly performed resuscitation is a major cause of preventable pediatric trauma deaths.[76] Despite rapid and effective out-of-hospital and trauma center response, children with out-of-hospital cardiac arrest due to trauma rarely survive.[77] In one study of out-of-hospital pediatric cardiac arrests, survival to hospital discharge was 1.1%.[8]

Factors associated with the best outcome from traumatic cardiac arrest are

- treatable penetrating injuries
- prompt transport (typically ≤10 minutes) to a trauma care facility.[78-81]

Traumatic cardiac arrest in children has multiple possible causes, including

- hypoxia secondary to respiratory arrest, airway obstruction, or tracheobronchial injury
- injury to vital structures (eg, heart, aorta, pulmonary arteries)
- severe head injury with secondary cardiovascular collapse
- upper cervical spinal cord injury with respiratory arrest progressing to cardiac arrest, which may be complicated by spinal shock
- diminished cardiac output or PEA from tension pneumothorax, cardiac tamponade, or massive hemorrhage

Basic and advanced life support techniques for the pediatric trauma victim in cardiac arrest are fundamentally the same as those for the child with nontraumatic cardiac arrest: support of airway, breathing, and circulation. The focus of resuscitation in the out-of-hospital setting is to

- anticipate airway obstruction by dental fragments, blood, or other debris (use a suction device if necessary)
- minimize motion of the cervical spine
- stop all external bleeding with pressure
- safely extricate the patient
- minimize interventions that will delay transport to definitive care
- transport the patient with multisystem trauma to a trauma center with pediatric expertise

Here is a summary of key management principles for the management of traumatic cardiac arrest in children.

Airway	• Open and maintain the airway using a jaw-thrust maneuver. • Restrict cervical spine motion by manual stabilization of the head and neck.
Breathing	• Ventilate with a bag-and-mask device using 100% oxygen; a 2-person technique is preferable in order to maintain immobilization of the head and neck. • If ET intubation is attempted, one rescuer should stabilize the head and neck in a neutral position. • Avoid routine hyperventilation; hyperventilate only if there are signs of impending brain herniation. • Consider empiric bilateral needle decompression for possible tension pneumothorax. • Seal any significant open pneumothorax and insert a thoracostomy tube.

(continued)

Circulation	• Perform high-quality CPR. • Attach a monitor-defibrillator. • Stop visible hemorrhage using direct compression. • Assume that the patient is hypovolemic and provide aggressive fluid resuscitation. • Consider empiric pericardiocentesis for possible cardiac tamponade. • Consider spinal shock (ie, loss of sympathetic innervation) resulting in fluid-refractory hypotension and bradycardia. Vasopressor therapy is indicated if spinal shock is suspected.
Disability	• Maintain spinal immobilization.
Exposure	• Maintain body temperature.

Cardiac Arrest Due to Drowning

For pediatric victims of cardiac arrest due to submersion, survival to hospital discharge (22.7%) and intact neurologic survival (6%) are better than overall survival from out-of-hospital pediatric cardiac arrest.[8]

Immediate CPR is the single most important factor influencing survival.

Chest compressions may be difficult to provide while the victim is still in the water, but you can initiate ventilations immediately. When possible, remove the child from the water on a backboard or other immobilization device. Start chest compressions as soon as you can do so safely and the child is lying face-up on a firm surface.

No modifications of standard Pediatric BLS (PBLS) sequencing are necessary for drowning victims other than consideration of cervical spine injury and the possibility of hypothermia as a contributing factor. Rescuers should remove drowning victims from the water by the fastest means available and should begin resuscitation as quickly as possible.

Airway	• Open the airway.
Breathing	• Ventilate with a bag-and-mask device using 100% oxygen. • If possible, another rescuer can provide cricoid pressure during bag-mask ventilation of the unresponsive victim to minimize the risk of vomiting and aspiration. • Be prepared to suction due to high likelihood of vomiting from swallowed water; decompress the stomach with a nasogastric or orogastric (NG/OG) tube after the airway is secured.
Circulation	• Perform high-quality CPR. • Attach a monitor/defibrillator. • If defibrillation is indicated, quickly wipe the patient's chest to minimize electrical arcing between the defibrillation pads or paddles. • Avoid pacing if the patient is hypothermic because this may induce VF.
Disability	Maintain immobilization of the cervical spine.
Exposure	Evaluate core body temperature and attempt rewarming if the patient is severely hypothermic (core temperature <30°C).

In hypothermic cardiac arrest patients, it is often difficult to know when to terminate resuscitative efforts. In victims of submersion in icy water, survival is possible after submersion times as long as 40 minutes and CPR times exceeding 2 hours. When drowning occurs in ice water, rewarming to at least 30°C is recommended before abandonment of CPR because the heart may be unresponsive to resuscitative efforts until this core temperature is achieved.

Conversely, if the patient drowns in cool water and is found hypothermic, this typically means the patient has been submerged for a prolonged period, and resuscitative efforts are unlikely to be effective.

For patients who are pulseless following ice water submersion with severe hypothermia, extracorporeal rewarming is the most rapid and effective technique. Avoid delays in the prehospital or community hospital setting for passive external rewarming or body cavity irrigation in favor of rapid transfer to a facility that is capable of pediatric extracorporeal membrane oxygenation (ECMO) or cardiopulmonary bypass.

Cardiac Arrest Due to Anaphylaxis

Near-fatal anaphylaxis produces profound vasodilation, which significantly increases intravascular capacity. Anaphylaxis is often accompanied by bronchoconstriction, which further impairs tissue oxygen delivery. If cardiac arrest develops, CPR, volume administration, and adrenergic drugs are the cornerstones of therapy. Patients with anaphylaxis are often young with healthy hearts and cardiovascular systems. They may respond to rapid correction of vasodilation and low intravascular volume. Effective CPR may maintain sufficient oxygen delivery until the catastrophic effects of the anaphylactic reaction resolve.

If cardiac arrest develops as a result of anaphylaxis, management may include the following critical therapies.

Airway	Open and maintain the airway using manual maneuvers.
Breathing	• Perform bag-mask ventilations using 100% oxygen. • If ET intubation is performed, be prepared for the possibility of airway edema and the need to use a smaller ET tube than predicted by age or length.
Circulation	• Perform effective chest compressions (may maintain sufficient oxygen delivery until the catastrophic effects of the anaphylactic reaction resolve). • Administer large volumes of isotonic crystalloid as quickly as possible using at least 2 large-bore IVs with pressure bags or IO access. • Administer epinephrine in standard doses (0.01 mg/kg IV/IO [0.1 mL/kg of 1:10 000]) or via the ET tube if no vascular access can be obtained (0.1 mg/kg [0.1 mL/kg of 1:1000]). • Titrate epinephrine infusion as needed.[82] • Manage according to the Pediatric Pulseless Arrest Algorithm if arrest rhythm is asystole or PEA (which is often the case).

There is little data about the value of antihistamines in anaphylactic cardiac arrest, but it is reasonable to assume that use of antihistamines would result in little harm. Although steroids given during cardiac arrest will have little effect, administer steroids (eg, methylprednisolone 1 mg/kg IV/IO) as soon as possible because of their potential value in the management of anaphylaxis during the early hours of the postresuscitation period.

Cardiac Arrest Associated With Poisoning

Drug overdose or poisoning may cause cardiac arrest as a result of direct cardiac toxicity or the secondary effects of respiratory depression, peripheral vasodilation, arrhythmias, and hypotension. The myocardium is often healthy, but temporary cardiac dysfunction may be present until the effects of the drug or toxin have been mediated or metabolized. This will require a variable amount of time, usually involving at least several hours, depending on the nature of the toxin, drug, or poison. Because the toxicity may be temporary, prolonged efforts and use of advanced support techniques such as extracorporeal cardiac life support may result in long-term good quality survival.

Initiate advanced life support measures according to the Pediatric Pulseless Arrest Algorithm. PALS treatments for victims of a suspected poisoning should include a search for and treatment of reversible causes. Early consultation with a poison control center or a toxicologist is recommended.

Social Issues and Ethics in Resuscitation

Special social and ethical issues during resuscitation of a child in cardiac arrest include

- family presence during resuscitation
- termination of resuscitative efforts

Family Presence During Resuscitation

Studies have shown that most family members would like to be present during the attempted resuscitation of a loved one.[83-88] Parents or family members may be reluctant to ask if they can be present, but healthcare providers should offer the opportunity whenever possible.[83-91] Family members may experience less anxiety, depression, and more constructive grief behaviors if they were present during resuscitative efforts.[92]

Planning for family-witnessed resuscitation includes the following:

- Discuss the plan in advance with the resuscitation team if possible.
- Assign one team member to remain with the family to answer questions, clarify information, and offer comfort.[93]
- Provide sufficient space to accommodate all family members who are present.
- Be sensitive to family presence during the resuscitative effort; team members must be mindful of the family members' presence while they communicate with each other.

In the out-of-hospital setting, family members are typically present during the attempted resuscitation of a loved one. Although out-of-hospital providers may be completely involved with the resuscitative effort, it may comfort family members if you offer brief explanations and the opportunity for them to remain with the loved one. Some EMS systems provide a follow-up visit to family members after an unsuccessful resuscitation attempt. See "Ethical and Legal Aspects of CPR in Children" on the student CD.

Terminating Resuscitative Efforts

There are no universally reliable predictors of when to stop resuscitative efforts in the setting of pediatric cardiac arrest. In the past children who underwent prolonged resuscitation with absence of ROSC after 2 doses of epinephrine were considered unlikely to survive.[1] However, intact survival after prolonged in-hospital resuscitation with more than 2 doses of epinephrine has been documented.[94-96]

The decision about when to stop resuscitative efforts is influenced by the likely cause of the arrest, available resources and location of the resuscitation attempt, and by the likelihood of any reversible or contributing conditions. Prolonged resuscitative efforts should be made for infants and children with

- recurring or refractory VF/VT
- drug toxicity (ie, until appropriate toxicologic management can be performed or the cardiovascular system can be supported until the drug effect resolves)
- primary hypothermic insult (ie, until appropriate warming measures have been undertaken)

If available, extracorporeal cardiac life support (eg, ECMO) may be beneficial for infants and children with acute, reversible conditions. Examples are cardiac or respiratory failure due to hypothermia or drug toxicity. It is currently used in a limited number of advanced pediatric centers, especially in children with primary cardiac conditions (eg, postcardiotomy patients) and in-hospital arrest, provided that high-quality CPR is performed until ECMO is available. One large pediatric study and several smaller studies showed that good outcome can be achieved when extracorporeal circulatory support is established after 30 to 90 minutes of refractory in-hospital arrest with standard CPR.[97]

Predictors of Outcome After Cardiac Arrest

Factors That Influence Outcome

The outcome after cardiac arrest in children may be influenced by

- interval from collapse to initiation of CPR
- quality of CPR provided
- duration of resuscitative efforts
- underlying conditions
- other factors

Initiation of prompt CPR is associated with improved outcomes. Witnessed events, bystander CPR, and a short interval from collapse to EMS personnel arrival are important prognostic factors associated with improved outcome in adult cardiac arrest, and it seems reasonable to extrapolate these factors to children. A pediatric study showed that the interval from collapse to initiation of CPR is a significant prognostic factor.[98] In out-of-hospital patients who have ROSC before arrival in the ED, chances for long-term survival are improved.[3,99,100]

The duration of resuscitative efforts is an indicator of outcome. In general, the likelihood of a good outcome declines with the length of the resuscitative efforts. Six pediatric studies show that prolonged resuscitation is associated with poor outcome in pediatric cardiac arrest.[98,101-104] Although the likelihood of a good outcome is greater with short duration of CPR, successful resuscitations have been documented with longer resuscitation efforts, particularly in the inpatient setting when the arrests were witnessed and prompt and presumably excellent CPR was provided.

Underlying conditions can significantly influence outcome. Some patients with PEA may have reversible causes of arrest that will respond to treatment. Patients with an initial rhythm of VF/pulseless VT arrest generally have a higher survival rate than patients with asystole or other nonperfusing rhythms.[4,35,99,105] This higher survival rate may not be observed in submersion victims with VF/pulseless VT, which has been associated with extremely poor prognosis.[106] Similarly, when VF/pulseless VT develops during the resuscitation of children with in-hospital cardiac arrest, the outcome is worse.[9] Children with out-of-hospital cardiac arrest caused by trauma[77] and in-hospital cardiac arrest caused by septic shock[94] rarely survive.

Other factors, however, can positively influence outcome despite prolonged resuscitative efforts. Examples include the following:

- Good outcomes for in-hospital pediatric cardiac arrest in patients with isolated heart disease (usually following surgical intervention) were achieved when ECMO was started after 30 to 90 minutes of refractory standard CPR. This demonstrates that 15 to 30 minutes of CPR do not define the limits of cardiac and cerebral viability.
- Good outcomes in an in-hospital witnessed arrest have been reported after 30 to 60 minutes of prompt (and presumably excellent) CPR.[94,107] Children with cardiac arrest due to environmental hypothermia or immersion in icy water can have excellent outcomes despite more than 30 minutes of CPR.[108,109]

Postresuscitation Management

Postresuscitation management begins with ROSC. See Chapter 8 for more information.

References

1. Young KD, Seidel JS. Pediatric cardiopulmonary resuscitation: a collective review. *Ann Emerg Med.* 1999;33(2):195-205.
2. Appleton GO, Cummins RO, Larson MP, et al. CPR and the single rescuer: at what age should you "call first" rather than "call fast"? *Ann Emerg Med.* 1995;25(4):492-494.
3. Hickey RW, Cohen DM, Strausbaugh S, et al. Pediatric patients requiring CPR in the prehospital setting. *Ann Emerg Med.* 1995;25(4):495-501.
4. Mogayzel C, Quan L, Graves JR, et al. Out-of-hospital ventricular fibrillation in children and adolescents: causes and outcomes. *Ann Emerg Med.* 1995;25(4):484-491.
5. Smith BT, Rea TD, Eisenberg MS. Ventricular fibrillation in pediatric cardiac arrest. *Acad Emerg Med.* 2006;13(5):525-529.
6. Nadkarni VM, Larkin GL, Peberdy MA, et al. First documented rhythm and clinical outcome from in-hospital cardiac arrest among children and adults. *JAMA.* 2006;295(1):50-57.
7. Sirbaugh PE, Pepe PE, Shook JE, et al. A prospective, population-based study of the demographics, epidemiology, management, and outcome of out-of-hospital pediatric cardiopulmonary arrest [published correction appears in *Ann Emerg Med.* 1999;33:358]. *Ann Emerg Med.* 1999;33(2):174-184.
8. Donoghue AJ, Nadkarni V, Berg RA, et al. Out-of-hospital pediatric cardiac arrest: an epidemiologic review and assessment of current knowledge. *Ann Emerg Med.* 2005;46(6):512-522.
9. Samson RA, Nadkarni VM, Meaney PA, et al. Outcomes of in-hospital ventricular fibrillation in children. *N Engl J Med.* 2006;354(22):2328-2339.
10. Eberle B, Dick WF, Schneider T, et al. Checking the carotid pulse check: diagnostic accuracy of first responders in patients with and without a pulse. *Resuscitation.* 1996;33(2):107-116.
11. Owen CJ, Wyllie JP. Determination of heart rate in the baby at birth. *Resuscitation.* 2004;60(2):213-217.
12. Graham CA, Lewis NF. Evaluation of a new method for the carotid pulse check in cardiopulmonary resuscitation. *Resuscitation.* 2002;53(1):37-40.
13. Ochoa FJ, Ramalle-Gomara E, Carpintero JM, et al. Competence of health professionals to check the carotid pulse. *Resuscitation.* 1998;37(3):173-175.
14. Mather C, O'Kelly S. The palpation of pulses. *Anaesthesia.* 1996;51(2):189-191.
15. Lapostolle F, Le Toumelin P, Agostinucci JM, et al. Basic cardiac life support providers checking the carotid pulse: performance, degree of conviction, and influencing factors. *Acad Emerg Med.* 2004;11(8):878-880.
16. Moule P. Checking the carotid pulse: diagnostic accuracy in students of the healthcare professions. *Resuscitation.* 2000;44(3):195-201.

17. Young KD, Gausche-Hill M, McClung CD, et al. A prospective, population-based study of the epidemiology and outcome of out-of-hospital pediatric cardiopulmonary arrest. *Pediatrics.* 2004;114(1):157-164.

18. Suominen P, Olkkola KT, Voipio V, et al. Utstein style reporting of in-hospital paediatric cardiopulmonary resuscitation. *Resuscitation.* Jun 2000;45(1):17-25.

19. Nadkarni V, Berg R, Kaye W, et al. Survival outcome for in-hospital pulseless cardiac arrest reported to the National Registry of CPR is better for children than adults. *Crit Care Med.* 2003;31:A14.

20. Ronco R, King W, Donley DK, et al. Outcome and cost at a children's hospital following resuscitation for out-of-hospital cardiopulmonary arrest. *Arch Pediatr Adolesc Med.* 1995;149(2):210-214.

21. Hedges JR, Barsan WB, Doan LA, et al. Central versus peripheral intravenous routes in cardiopulmonary resuscitation. *Am J Emerg Med.* Sep 1984;2(5):385-390.

22. Daga SR, Gosavi DV, Verma B. Intraosseous access using butterfly needle. *Trop Doct.* 1999;29(3):142-144.

23. Quinton DN, O'Byrne G, Aitkenhead AR. Comparison of endotracheal and peripheral intravenous adrenaline in cardiac arrest: is the endotracheal route reliable? *Lancet.* 1987;1(8537):828-829.

24. Ralston SH, Voorhees WD, Babbs CF. Intrapulmonary epinephrine during prolonged cardiopulmonary resuscitation: improved regional blood flow and resuscitation in dogs. *Ann Emerg Med.* 1984;13(2):79-86.

25. Kleinman ME, Oh W, Stonestreet BS. Comparison of intravenous and endotracheal epinephrine during cardiopulmonary resuscitation in newborn piglets. *Crit Care Med.* 1999;27(12):2748-2754.

26. Jasani MS, Nadkarni VM, Finkelstein MS, et al. Effects of different techniques of endotracheal epinephrine administration in pediatric porcine hypoxic-hypercarbic cardiopulmonary arrest. *Crit Care Med.* 1994;22(7):1174-1180.

27. Berg M, Clark LL, Valenzuela TD, et al. Post-shock chest compression delays with automated external defibrillator usage. *Resuscitation*. 2005;64:287-291.

28. Figa FH, Gow RM, Hamilton RM, et al. Clinical efficacy and safety of intravenous amiodarone in infants and children. *Am J Cardiol.* 1994;74(6):573-577.

29. Hoffman TM, Bush DM, Wernovsky G, et al. Postoperative junctional ectopic tachycardia in children: incidence, risk factors, and treatment. *Ann Thorac Surg.* 2002;74(5):1607-1611.

30. 2005 International Consensus on Cardiopulmonary Resuscitation and Emergency Cardiovascular Care Science with Treatment Recommendations, part 6: paediatric basic and advanced life support. *Resuscitation.* 2005;67(2-3):271-291.

31. Elizur A, Ben-Abraham R, Manisterski Y, et al. Tracheal epinephrine or norepinephrine preceded by beta blockade in a dog model. Can beta blockade bestow any benefits? *Resuscitation.* 2003;59(2):271-276.

32. Perondi MB, Reis AG, Paiva EF, et al. A comparison of high-dose and standard-dose epinephrine in children with cardiac arrest. *N Engl J Med.* 2004;350(17):1722-1730.

33. Patterson MD, Boenning DA, Klein BL, et al. The use of high-dose epinephrine for patients with out-of-hospital cardiopulmonary arrest refractory to prehospital interventions. *Pediatr Emerg Care.* 2005;21(4):227-237.

34. Carpenter TC, Stenmark KR. High-dose epinephrine is not superior to standard-dose epinephrine in pediatric in-hospital cardiopulmonary arrest. *Pediatrics.* 1997;99(3):403-408.

35. Dieckmann R, Vardis R. High-dose epinephrine in pediatric out-of-hospital cardiopulmonary arrest. *Pediatrics.* 1995;95(6):901-913.

36. Mann K, Berg RA, Nadkarni V. Beneficial effects of vasopressin in prolonged pediatric cardiac arrest: a case series. *Resuscitation.* 2002;52(2):149-156.

37. Voelckel WG, Lindner KH, Wenzel V, et al. Effects of vasopressin and epinephrine on splanchnic blood flow and renal function during and after cardiopulmonary resuscitation in pigs. *Crit Care Med.* 2000;28(4):1083-1088.

38. Voelckel WG, Lurie KG, McKnite S, et al. Effects of epinephrine and vasopressin in a piglet model of prolonged ventricular fibrillation and cardiopulmonary resuscitation. *Crit Care Med.* 2002;30(5):957-962.

39. Wenzel V, Krismer AC, Arntz HR, et al. A comparison of vasopressin and epinephrine for out-of-hospital cardiopulmonary resuscitation. *N Engl J Med.* 2004;350(2):105-113.

40. Stiell IG, Hebert PC, Wells GA, et al. Vasopressin versus epinephrine for inhospital cardiac arrest: a randomised controlled trial. *Lancet.* 2001;358(9276):105-109.

41. Lindner KH, Dirks B, Strohmenger HU, et al. Randomised comparison of epinephrine and vasopressin in patients with out-of-hospital ventricular fibrillation. *Lancet.* 1997;349(9051):535-537.

42. Guyette FX, Guimond GE, Hostler D, et al. Vasopressin administered with epinephrine is associated with a return of a pulse in out-of-hospital cardiac arrest. *Resuscitation.* 2004;63(3):277-282.

43. Fogel RI, Herre JM, Kopelman HA, et al. Long-term follow-up of patients requiring intravenous amiodarone to suppress hemodynamically destabilizing ventricular arrhythmias. *Am Heart J.* 2000;139(4):690-695.

44. Lee KL, Tai YT. Long-term low-dose amiodarone therapy in the management of ventricular and supraventricular tachyarrhythmias: efficacy and safety. *Clin Cardiol.* 1997;20(4):372-377.

45. Gausche M, Lewis RJ, Stratton SJ, et al. Effect of out-of-hospital pediatric endotracheal intubation on survival and neurological outcome: a controlled clinical trial. *JAMA.* 2000;283(6):783-790.

46. Perry JC, Fenrich AL, Hulse JE, et al. Pediatric use of intravenous amiodarone: efficacy and safety in critically ill patients from a multicenter protocol. *J Am Coll Cardiol.* 1996;27(5):1246-1250.

47. Soult JA, Munoz M, Lopez JD, et al. Efficacy and safety of intravenous amiodarone for short-term treatment of paroxysmal supraventricular tachycardia in children. *Pediatr Cardiol.* 1995;16(1):16-19.

48. Aung K, Htay T. Vasopressin for cardiac arrest: a systematic review and meta-analysis. *Arch Intern Med.* 2005;165(1):17-24.

49. Cannon LA, Heiselman DE, Dougherty JM, et al. Magnesium levels in cardiac arrest victims: relationship between magnesium levels and successful resuscitation. *Ann Emerg Med.* 1987;16(11):1195-1199.

50. Buylaert WA, Calle PA, Houbrechts HN. Serum electrolyte disturbances in the post-resuscitation period. *Resuscitation.* 1989;17(suppl):S189-S196.

51. Salerno DM, Elsperger KJ, Helseth P, et al. Serum potassium, calcium and magnesium after resuscitation from ventricular fibrillation: a canine study. *J Am Coll Cardiol.* 1987;10(1):178-185.

52. Allegra J, Lavery R, Cody R, et al. Magnesium sulfate in the treatment of refractory ventricular fibrillation in the prehospital setting. *Resuscitation.* 2001;49(3):245-249.

53. Fatovich DM, Prentice DA, Dobb GJ. Magnesium in cardiac arrest (the magic trial). *Resuscitation.* 1997;35(3):237-241.

54. Hassan TB, Jagger C, Barnett DB. A randomised trial to investigate the efficacy of magnesium sulphate for refractory ventricular fibrillation. *Emerg Med J.* 2002;19(1):57-62.

55. Longstreth WT Jr, Fahrenbruch CE, Olsufka M, et al. Randomized clinical trial of magnesium, diazepam, or both after out-of-hospital cardiac arrest. *Neurology.* 2002;59(4):506-514.

56. Thel MC, Armstrong AL, McNulty SE, et al. Randomised trial of magnesium in in-hospital cardiac arrest. Duke Internal Medicine Housestaff. *Lancet.* 1997;350(9087):1272-1276.

57. Miller B, Craddock L, Hoffenberg S, et al. Pilot study of intravenous magnesium sulfate in refractory cardiac arrest: safety data and recommendations for future studies. *Resuscitation.* 1995;30(1):3-14.

58. Bisogno JL, Langley A, Von Dreele MM. Effect of calcium to reverse the electrocardiographic effects of hyperkalemia in the isolated rat heart: a prospective, dose-response study. *Crit Care Med.* 1994;22(4):697-704.

59. Cardenas-Rivero N, Chernow B, Stoiko MA, et al. Hypocalcemia in critically ill children. *J Pediatr.* 1989;114(6):946-951.

60. Zaritsky A. Cardiopulmonary resuscitation in children. *Clin Chest Med.* 1987;8(4):561-571.

61. Bohman VR, Cotton DB. Supralethal magnesemia with patient survival. *Obstet Gynecol.* 1990;76(pt 2)(5):984-986.

62. Ramoska EA, Spiller HA, Winter M, et al. A one-year evaluation of calcium channel blocker overdoses: toxicity and treatment. *Ann Emerg Med.* 1993;22(2):196-200.

63. Stueven HA, Thompson B, Aprahamian C, et al. Lack of effectiveness of calcium chloride in refractory asystole. *Ann Emerg Med.* 1985;14(7):630-632.

64. Ettinger PO, Regan TJ, Oldewurtel HA. Hyperkalemia, cardiac conduction, and the electrocardiogram: a review. *Am Heart J.* 1974;88(3):360-371.

65. Hoffman JR, Votey SR, Bayer M, et al. Effect of hypertonic sodium bicarbonate in the treatment of moderate-to-severe cyclic antidepressant overdose. *Am J Emerg Med.* 1993;11(4):336-341.

66. Aufderheide TP, Sigurdsson G, Pirrallo RG, et al. Hyperventilation-induced hypotension during cardiopulmonary resuscitation. *Circulation.* 2004;109(16):1960-1965.

67. Becker LB, Berg RA, Pepe PE, et al. A reappraisal of mouth-to-mouth ventilation during bystander-initiated cardiopulmonary resuscitation. A statement for healthcare professionals from the Ventilation Working Group of the Basic Life Support and Pediatric Life Support Subcommittees, American Heart Association. *Resuscitation.* 1997;35(3):189-201.

68. Atkins DL, Sirna S, Kieso R, et al. Pediatric defibrillation: importance of paddle size in determining transthoracic impedance. *Pediatrics.* 1988;82(6):914-918.

69. Atkins DL, Kerber RE. Pediatric defibrillation: current flow is improved by using "adult" electrode paddles. *Pediatrics.* 1994;94(1):90-93.

70. Samson RA, Atkins DL, Kerber RE. Optimal size of self-adhesive preapplied electrode pads in pediatric defibrillation. *Am J Cardiol.* 1995;75(7):544-545.

71. Lubitz DS, Seidel JS, Chameides L, et al. A rapid method for estimating weight and resuscitation drug dosages from length in the pediatric age group. *Ann Emerg Med.* 1988;17(6):576-581.

72. Vaknin Z, Manisterski Y, Ben-Abraham R, et al. Is endotracheal adrenaline deleterious because of the beta adrenergic effect? *Anesth Analg.* 2001;92(6):1408-1412.

73. Manisterski Y, Vaknin Z, Ben-Abraham R, et al. Endotracheal epinephrine: a call for larger doses. *Anesth Analg.* 2002;95(4):1037-1041.

74. Efrati O, Ben-Abraham R, Barak A, et al. Endobronchial adrenaline: should it be reconsidered? Dose response and haemodynamic effect in dogs. *Resuscitation.* 2003;59(1):117-122.

75. Skrifvars MB, Pettila V, Rosenberg PH, et al. A multiple logistic regression analysis of in-hospital factors related to survival at six months in patients resuscitated from out-of-hospital ventricular fibrillation. *Resuscitation.* 2003;59(3):319-328.

76. Dykes EH, Spence LJ, Young JG, et al. Preventable pediatric trauma deaths in a metropolitan region. *J Pediatr Surg.* 1989;24(1):107-110.

77. Hazinski MF, Chahine AA, Holcomb GW 3rd, et al. Outcome of cardiovascular collapse in pediatric blunt trauma. *Ann Emerg Med.* 1994;23(6):1229-1235.

78. Copass MK, Oreskovich MR, Bladergroen MR, et al. Prehospital cardiopulmonary resuscitation of the critically injured patient. *Am J Surg.* 1984;148(1):20-26.

79. Durham LA III, Richardson RJ, Wall MJ Jr, et al. Emergency center thoracotomy: impact of prehospital resuscitation. *J Trauma.* 1992;32(6):775-779.

80. Kloeck W. Prehospital advanced CPR in the trauma patient. *Trauma Emerg Med.* 1993;10:772-776.

81. Schmidt U, Frame SB, Nerlich ML, et al. On-scene helicopter transport of patients with multiple injuries—comparison of a German and an American system. *J Trauma.* 1992;33(4):548-553.

82. Sampson HA, Munoz-Furlong A, Campbell RL, et al. Second symposium on the definition and management of anaphylaxis: summary report—Second National Institute of Allergy and Infectious Disease/Food Allergy and Anaphylaxis Network symposium. *J Allergy Clin Immunol.* 2006;117(2):391-397.

83. Barratt F, Wallis DN. Relatives in the resuscitation room: their point of view. *J Accid Emerg Med.* 1998;15(2):109-111.

84. Boie ET, Moore GP, Brummett C, et al. Do parents want to be present during invasive procedures performed on their children in the emergency department? A survey of 400 parents. *Ann Emerg Med.* 1999;34(1):70-74.

85. Doyle CJ, Post H, Burney RE, et al. Family participation during resuscitation: an option. *Ann Emerg Med.* 1987;16(6):673-675.

86. Hanson C, Strawser D. Family presence during cardiopulmonary resuscitation: Foote Hospital emergency department's nine-year perspective. *J Emerg Nurs.* 1992;18(2):104-106.

87. Meyers TA, Eichhorn DJ, Guzzetta CE. Do families want to be present during CPR? A retrospective survey. *J Emerg Nurs.* 1998;24(5):400-405.

88. Robinson SM, Mackenzie-Ross S, Campbell Hewson GL, et al. Psychological effect of witnessed resuscitation on bereaved relatives. *Lancet.* 1998;352(9128):614-617.

89. Boyd R. Witnessed resuscitation by relatives. *Resuscitation.* 2000;43(3):171-176.

90. Offord RJ. Should relatives of patients with cardiac arrest be invited to be present during cardiopulmonary resuscitation? *Intensive Crit Care Nurs.* 1998;14(6):288-293.

91. Shaner K, Eckle N. Implementing a program to support the option of family presence during resuscitation. *The Association for the Care of Children's Health (ACCH) Advocate.* 1997;3(1):3-7.

92. Boudreaux ED, Francis JL, Loyacano T. Family presence during invasive procedures and resuscitations in the emergency department: a critical review and suggestions for future research. *Ann Emerg Med.* 2002;40(2):193-205.

93. Eichhorn DJ, Meyers TA, Mitchell TG, et al. Opening the doors: family presence during resuscitation. *J Cardiovasc Nurs.* 1996;10(4):59-70.

94. Reis AG, Nadkarni V, Perondi MB, et al. A prospective investigation into the epidemiology of in-hospital pediatric cardiopulmonary resuscitation using the international Utstein reporting style. *Pediatrics.* 2002;109(2):200-209.

95. Lopez-Herce J, Garcia C, Rodriguez-Nunez A, et al. Long-term outcome of paediatric cardiorespiratory arrest in Spain. *Resuscitation.* 2005;64(1):79-85.

96. Parra DA, Totapally BR, Zahn E, et al. Outcome of cardiopulmonary resuscitation in a pediatric cardiac intensive care unit. *Crit Care Med.* 2000;28(9):3296-3300.

97. Morris MC, Wernovsky G, Nadkarni VM. Survival outcomes after extracorporeal cardiopulmonary resuscitation instituted during active chest compressions following refractory in-hospital pediatric cardiac arrest. Pediatr *Crit Care Med.* 2004;5(5):440-446.

98. Schindler MB, Bohn D, Cox PN, et al. Outcome of out-of-hospital cardiac or respiratory arrest in children. *N Engl J Med.* 1996;335(20):1473-1479.

99. Losek JD, Hennes H, Glaeser P, et al. Prehospital care of the pulseless, nonbreathing pediatric patient. *Am J Emerg Med.* 1987;5(5):370-374.

100. Kyriacou DN, Arcinue EL, Peek C, et al. Effect of immediate resuscitation on children with submersion injury. *Pediatrics.* 1994;94(pt 1)(2):137-142.

101. Mir NA, Faquih AM, Legnain M. Perinatal risk factors in birth asphyxia: relationship of obstetric and neonatal complications to neonatal mortality in 16,365 consecutive live births. *Asia Oceania J Obstet Gynaecol.* 1989;15(4):351-357.

102. Ondoa-Onama C, Tumwine JK. Immediate outcome of babies with low Apgar score in Mulago Hospital, Uganda. *East Afr Med J.* 2003;80(1):22-29.

103. Longstreth WT Jr, Diehr P, Cobb LA, et al. Neurologic outcome and blood glucose levels during out-of-hospital cardiopulmonary resuscitation. *Neurology.* 1986;36(9):1186-1191.

104. Gillis J, Dickson D, Rieder M, et al. Results of inpatient pediatric resuscitation. *Crit Care Med.* 1986;14(5):469-471.

105. Coffing CR, Quan L, Graves JR, et al. Etiologies and outcomes of the pulseless, nonbreathing pediatric patient presenting with ventricular fibrillation. *Ann Emerg Med.* 1992;21:1046.

106. Quan L, Gore EJ, Wentz K, et al. Ten-year study of pediatric drownings and near-drownings in King County, Washington: lessons in injury prevention. *Pediatrics.* 1989;83(6):1035-1040.

107. Lopez-Herce J, Garcia C, Dominguez P, et al. Characteristics and outcome of cardiorespiratory arrest in children. *Resuscitation.* 2004;63(3):311-320.

108. Kuisma M, Suominen P, Korpela R. Paediatric out-of-hospital cardiac arrests: epidemiology and outcome. *Resuscitation.* 1995;30(2):141-150.

109. Idris AH, Berg RA, Bierens J, et al. Recommended guidelines for uniform reporting of data from drowning: the "Utstein style." *Resuscitation.* 2003;59(1):45-57.

Chapter 8

Postresuscitation Management

Overview

Introduction

Following ROSC from cardiac arrest or resuscitation from severe shock or respiratory failure, a systematic approach to assessment and support of the respiratory, cardiovascular, and neurologic systems is critical. In addition, the PALS provider should evaluate and support other body systems (eg, renal, gastrointestinal) as needed. Although effective resuscitation is the main focus of the PALS course, ultimate patient outcome is often determined by the subsequent care of the patient, including transport of the child safely to a center with special expertise in caring for seriously ill or injured children.

One objective of optimal postresuscitation management is to avoid common causes of both early and late morbidity and mortality. Early mortality can be caused by hemodynamic instability and respiratory problems. Later morbidity and mortality can result from multi-organ failure or brain injury.[1,2]

Optimal postresuscitation management includes

- identifying and treating organ system dysfunction
- supporting tissue perfusion and cardiovascular function
- providing adequate oxygenation and ventilation
- correcting acid-base and electrolyte imbalances
- avoiding hyperthermia after cerebral insults
- maintaining adequate glucose concentrations
- ensuring adequate analgesia and sedation

The extent of postresuscitation evaluation and management will be influenced by the PALS provider's scope of practice and the available resources.

Learning Objectives

After completing this chapter you should be able to

- explain that postresuscitation management applies to care after cardiac arrest and care following resuscitation from severe shock or respiratory failure
- list the priorities for postresuscitation assessment and management
- differentiate between immediate and subsequent postresuscitation management
- discuss the systematic approach to postresuscitation management
- summarize how to prepare a child for transfer or transport and state the importance of using a transport checklist

Postresuscitation Management

Introduction

Postresuscitation management consists of 2 general phases to stabilize the child.

The first phase is immediate postresuscitation management. During this phase you continue to provide advanced life support for immediate life-threatening conditions and focus on the ABCs.

- **A**irway and **B**reathing. Assess and support oxygenation and ventilation. At this time you will typically use tertiary assessment tools, such as an arterial blood gas and chest x-ray, to further assess the adequacy of oxygenation, ventilation, and ET tube position.
- **C**irculation. Assess and maintain adequate blood pressure and perfusion. Treat arrhythmias. Tertiary assessment studies such as lactate concentration, venous oxygen saturation, and base deficit provide information on the adequacy of tissue perfusion. As you proceed through your assessment, identify and treat any reversible or contributing causes of the arrest or critical illness.

In the second phase of postresuscitation management, you provide broader multi-organ supportive care.

After stabilization coordinate the transfer or transport of the child to a tertiary care setting as appropriate.

Primary Goals

The primary goals of postresuscitation management are to

- optimize and stabilize cardiopulmonary function with emphasis on restoring and maintaining vital organ perfusion and function (especially of the brain)
- prevent secondary organ injury
- identify and treat the cause of acute illness
- minimize the risk of deterioration of the child during transport to the next level of care
- institute measures that may improve long-term, neurologically intact survival

Systematic Approach

Assess the patient using a systematic assessment approach. In addition to repeated primary assessments, your evaluation will often include secondary and tertiary assessments. The secondary assessment focuses on a review of patient history and a thorough physical examination. The tertiary assessment involves invasive and noninvasive monitoring and appropriate laboratory and nonlaboratory testing.

This chapter discusses assessment and management of the following systems during the postresuscitation period:

- Respiratory system
- Cardiovascular system
- Neurologic system
- Renal system
- Gastrointestinal system
- Hematologic system

Respiratory System

Management Priorities

Continue to monitor and support the patient's airway, oxygenation, and ventilation, looking for clinical signs and objective measurements of the adequacy of oxygenation and ventilation. (See Chapter 1 for more information on assessment of the respiratory system.) During resuscitation high-flow oxygen, inhaled medications, ET intubation, and mechanical ventilation may be required. In the postresuscitation phase elective intubation may be appropriate to achieve airway control and to perform diagnostic studies such as CT scanning. (See the student CD for more information about ET intubation and confirmation of ET tube placement.)

The goals of respiratory management in the immediate postresuscitation period are the following:

Goal	Considerations
Maintain adequate oxygenation (generally Pa_{O_2} >60 mm Hg, Sp_{O_2} >90%)	Determining the optimal Pa_{O_2} and oxygen saturation requires understanding that one important determinant of tissue oxygen delivery is the oxygen content. If the child is anemic, then tissue oxygen delivery may be better maintained by achieving a high Pa_{O_2}, whereas oxygen saturation of 90% is typically adequate in the child with a normal hemoglobin concentration and normal oxygen consumption.
Maintain adequate ventilation and acceptable Pa_{CO_2} levels	The acceptable Pa_{CO_2} level depends on the clinical circumstance. For example, in children with asthma and respiratory failure, rapid correction of the Pa_{CO_2} is not appropriate; efforts to achieve this with mechanical ventilation will likely result in increased morbidity. For patients with neurologic conditions, a normal Pa_{CO_2} is desirable and avoids hypocarbia.

General Recommendations

General recommendations for the assessment and management of the respiratory system may include those described in the table below.

Assessment and Management of the Respiratory System	
Assessment	
Monitoring	• Monitor the following parameters (at a minimum) continuously — SpO_2 and heart rate by pulse oximetry (compare pulse oximetry heart rate to ECG rate to ensure that pulse oximeter readings are accurate) — Heart rate and rhythm — Exhaled CO_2 by colorimetric device if patient is intubated; monitor end-tidal CO_2 by capnography if equipment and expertise are available • If the patient is already intubated, verify tube position, patency, and security using clinical assessment and a confirmation device • After proper tube position is confirmed, ensure that the tube is well-taped and that tube position at the lip or gum is documented *Providers must use both clinical assessment and confirmatory devices (such as monitoring of exhaled CO_2) to verify proper tube placement immediately after intubation, during transport, and when the patient is moved (eg, from gurney to bed). In the postresuscitation period, monitor exhaled CO_2, especially during transport and diagnostic procedures that require patient movement.*[3]
Physical examination	• Perform a clinical examination by observing chest rise and auscultating for abnormal or asymmetric breath sounds. • Evaluate for evidence of respiratory compromise (eg, tachypnea, increased work of breathing, agitation, decreased responsiveness, poor air exchange, cyanosis).
Laboratory tests	• Obtain an arterial blood gas (ABG) if possible in children following ROSC or treatment for respiratory failure or severe shock. If the patient is mechanically ventilated, obtain the ABG 10 to 15 minutes after establishing initial ventilatory settings; ideally correlate blood gases with capnographic end-tidal CO_2 concentration to enable noninvasive monitoring of ventilation.
Nonlaboratory tests	• Obtain a chest x-ray to identify pulmonary problems and depth of ET tube placement in the trachea.

Management	
Oxygenation	• If the child is not intubated, provide supplementary oxygen with a partial or a nonrebreathing mask until you confirm adequate SpO_2. • Adjust the inspired oxygen concentration to result in an $SpO_2 \geq 90\%$, keeping in mind the caveats noted previously. • If the patient has $SpO_2 < 90\%$ when receiving 100% inspired oxygen, consider additional invasive or noninvasive ventilatory support. • If the child has a cyanotic cardiac lesion, adjust the oxygen saturation goal with consideration of the patient's baseline SpO_2 and clinical status.
Ventilation	Assist ventilation as needed, targeting normal $PaCO_2$ levels (ie, 35 to 40 mm Hg) if the child had previously normal lung function. As noted previously, normalization of the $PaCO_2$ may not be appropriate in all situations. Avoid routine hyperventilation in patients with neurologic problems.
Respiratory failure	• Perform ET intubation if oxygen administration and other interventions are not successful in achieving adequate oxygenation or ventilation, or both, or if airway protection is needed because of depressed mental status. In some patients noninvasive positive-pressure ventilation (eg, bi-level positive airway pressure [BiPAP]) may be adequate). • Use appropriate ventilator settings (Table 1). • Verify ET tube position, patency, and security; retape if needed prior to transport. • Evaluate if the patient has a large glottic air leak. Consider reintubation with a cuffed tube or a larger uncuffed tube if the glottic air leak prevents adequate chest rise, oxygenation, or ventilation. Check the ET tube cuff pressure; maintain <20 cm H_2O. • Insert a gastric tube to relieve and help prevent gastric inflation. • Use the "DOPE" mnemonic to troubleshoot acute deterioration in a mechanically ventilated patient. (See Endotracheal Intubation on the student CD for more information on DOPE.)
Analgesia and sedation	• Control pain and discomfort with analgesics (eg, fentanyl or morphine) and sedatives (eg, lorazepam or midazolam). • Consider sedation and analgesia for all responsive intubated patients *Use lower doses of sedatives or analgesics if the child is hemodynamically unstable, and titrate dose while stabilizing hemodynamic function. Morphine is more likely than fentanyl to cause hypotension when used in equipotent doses because morphine causes histamine release.*
Neuromuscular blockade	• For the intubated patient consider neuromuscular blocking agents (eg, vecuronium, pancuronium) for any of the following indications after ruling out DOPE: — High peak or mean airway pressure due to high airway resistance or reduced lung compliance — Patient ventilator asynchrony — Difficult airway *Neuromuscular blockade may minimize the risk of ET tube displacement. Be aware that neuromuscular blockers do not provide sedation or analgesia and will mask seizures. When using neuromuscular blockers, always ensure that a patient is adequately sedated by evaluating for signs of stress, such as tachycardia, hypertension, pupil dilation, or tearing.* *It is also important to recall that peak airway pressure is affected by the inspiratory time and delivered tidal volume. Assess these parameters before assuming the child has high airway resistance or stiff lungs.*

Table 1. Initial Ventilator Settings*

Oxygen	100%
Tidal volume†	6 to 15 mL/kg
Inspiratory time†‡	0.6 to 1 second
Peak inspiratory pressure‡	20 to 35 cm H_2O (lowest level that results in adequate chest expansion)
Respiratory rate	Infants: 20 to 30 breaths/min Children: 16 to 20 breaths/min Adolescents: 8 to 12 breaths/min
PEEP	2 to 5 cm H_2O (adjust to optimize oxygen delivery)

PEEP indicates positive end-expiratory pressure.

*These settings should be adjusted based on clinical assessment and arterial blood gas analysis.

†For volume ventilators.

‡For time-cycled, pressure-limited ventilators.

Cardiovascular System

Management Priorities

The ischemia of cardiac arrest and effects of defibrillation and reperfusion can cause circulatory dysfunction that can last for hours after ROSC. Similarly, compromised tissue perfusion and oxygenation in shock and respiratory failure may result in secondary adverse effects on cardiovascular system function. The goals of circulatory management are to maintain adequate blood pressure and cardiac output to restore or maintain sufficient tissue oxygenation and delivery of metabolic substrates. Management priorities are to

- restore and maintain intravascular volume (preload)
- maintain normotension and adequate systemic perfusion
- maintain adequate Spo_2 and Pao_2
- maintain adequate hemoglobin concentration
- manage myocardial dysfunction
- control arrhythmias
- consider therapies to reduce metabolic demand (eg, support ventilation and reduce temperature)

This section includes

- general recommendations for advanced assessment and management of the cardiovascular system
- the PALS Postresuscitation Treatment of Shock Algorithm
- information about administration of maintenance fluids

Please review Chapters 4 and 5 for more information on the physiology of shock and use of drugs to maintain cardiac output.

General Recommendations

General recommendations for the assessment and management of the cardiovascular system may include those described in the table below.

Assessment and Management of the Cardiovascular System	
Assessment	
Monitoring	• Monitor the following parameters frequently or continuously — Heart rate and rhythm by cardiac monitor — Blood pressure and pulse pressure (noninvasively or invasively) — Spo_2 by pulse oximetry — Urine output by urinary catheter • In the critical care setting consider monitoring — CVP by central venous line — Svo_2 by central venous line (requires fiberoptic catheter) — Cardiac function (eg, echocardiogram) or continuous cardiac output from pulmonary artery catheter *Noninvasive blood pressure measurement (ie, by automated blood pressure devices) is often unreliable in patients who are poorly perfused or who have frequent arrhythmias. These patients will likely benefit from placement of an arterial line for invasive blood pressure measurement.* *The difference in oxygen saturation between the arterial and central venous circulations [$S(a\text{-}v)O_2$] gives an estimate of whether there is adequate oxygen delivery to meet tissue use. Assuming that oxygen consumption remains constant, it provides a physiologic assessment of the adequacy of cardiac output.*
Physical examination	• Repeat examination (eg, quality of central and peripheral pulses, heart rate, capillary refill, blood pressure, extremity temperature and color) frequently until the patient is stable. • Monitor end-organ function (eg, evidence of neurologic function, renal function, skin perfusion) to detect evidence of worsening circulatory compromise.
Laboratory tests	• Arterial blood gas • Hemoglobin and hematocrit • Serum glucose, electrolytes, BUN/creatinine, calcium • Consider lactate and central venous oxygen saturation (measured by co-oximetry) *In addition to the pH, note the magnitude of any metabolic acidosis (base deficit). A persistent metabolic (lactic) acidosis suggests inadequate cardiac output and oxygen delivery. Serum electrolytes can help identify if there is an anion gap with the acidosis, which may help identify the source of acidosis if the lactate is not increased in a patient with significant metabolic acidosis.*
Nonlaboratory tests	• Perform chest x-ray to evaluate ET tube depth of insertion and heart size and to identify pulmonary edema or other pathology. • Evaluate 12-lead ECG (if arrhythmias are present or there is concern for myocardial ischemia). • Consider echocardiogram if concern exists about pericardial tamponade or myocardial dysfunction.[2,4] *Radiographic evaluation of heart size may aid in the initial and subsequent assessment of intravascular volume. In the absence of heart disease, a small heart is consistent with hypovolemia and a large heart is consistent with volume overload. Pericardial effusion may also produce cardiomegaly on chest x-ray.*

Management	
Intravascular volume	• Establish secure vascular access (if possible 2 catheters; one can be an IO). • Administer fluid boluses (10 to 20 mL/kg of isotonic crystalloid, administered over 5 to 20 minutes) as needed to restore intravascular volume. Adjust the fluid administration rate to replace any fluid deficits and meet ongoing requirements. Once the patient is euvolemic, avoid excessive fluid administration in a patient with cardiac or respiratory failure. • Consider the need for colloid or blood administration. • Calculate maintenance fluid requirements and administer as appropriate. ***Do not use hypotonic or dextrose-containing fluids for volume resuscitation.*** *See "Administration of Maintenance Fluids" later in this chapter.*
Blood pressure	• **Treat hypotension aggressively,** titrating volume and vasoactive medications as appropriate. • If hypotension is due to an arrhythmia, treat the arrhythmia. • If hypotension is due to excessive vasodilation (eg, sepsis), early use of a vasopressor may be indicated. *Treatment of hypotension is crucial to avoid secondary multisystem injury. See the PALS Postresuscitation Treatment of Shock Algorithm in this chapter for more information on management of hypotensive and normotensive shock.*
Tissue oxygenation	• Provide supplementary oxygen in high concentration until you confirm adequate Spo_2, then titrate oxygen to maintain adequate Spo_2. • Support adequate perfusion. • Maintain adequate hemoglobin concentration.
Metabolic demand	• Control pain with appropriate analgesia (eg, morphine, fentanyl). • Control agitation with appropriate sedation (eg, lorazepam, midazolam); rule out hypoxemia, hypercarbia, or poor perfusion as potential causes of agitation. • Control fever with antipyretics. • Consider ET intubation and assisted ventilation to reduce work of breathing. *Caution: Sedatives or analgesics may cause hypotension.*
Arrhythmias	• Control tachyarrhythmias and bradyarrhythmias with appropriate medical therapy or cardioversion. • Seek expert consultation for arrhythmia management. *See Chapter 6 for more information.*
Postarrest myocardial dysfunction	• Anticipate postarrest myocardial dysfunction for 4 to 24 hours after ROSC. • Consider vasoactive agents to optimize hemodynamic function.[5-8] • Maintain adequate blood pressure and perfusion. *Myocardial dysfunction is common in children after resuscitation from cardiac arrest.[9,10] Postarrest myocardial dysfunction can produce hemodynamic instability and secondary organ injury and may precipitate another cardiac arrest.*

PALS Postresuscitation Treatment of Shock Algorithm

Introduction

After resuscitation from cardiac arrest or shock, hemodynamic compromise may result from a combination of

- inadequate intravascular volume
- decreased cardiac contractility
- increased systemic or pulmonary vascular resistance or very low systemic vascular resistance

Very low systemic vascular resistance is most common in children with septic shock. Recent data shows, however, that most children with fluid-refractory septic shock have high rather than low systemic vascular resistance and poor myocardial function.[8] Children with cardiogenic shock typically have poor myocardial function and a compensatory increase in systemic and pulmonary vascular resistance to attempt to maintain an adequate blood pressure.

Support of Systemic Perfusion

Four parameters can be manipulated to optimize systemic perfusion.

Parameter	Action (when needed)
Preload	Titrate volume administration.
Contractility	• Administer inotropes or inodilators. • Correct hypoxia, electrolyte and acid-base imbalances, and metabolic disorders. • Treat poisonings (eg, administer antidotes if available).
Afterload (systemic vascular resistance)	• Administer vasopressors or vasodilators as appropriate. • Correct hypoxia and acidosis.
Heart rate	• Administer chronotropes (eg, epinephrine). • Administer antiarrhythmics. • Correct hypoxia. • Consider pacing.

See "Physiology of Shock" in Chapter 4 for a discussion of preload, afterload, and contractility.

Overview of Algorithm

The PALS Postresuscitation Treatment of Shock Algorithm (Figure) outlines assessment and treatment steps for the management of shock during the postresuscitation period. In the description of this sequence, we will refer to Box numbers 1 through 6. These are the numbers assigned to the boxes on the algorithm.

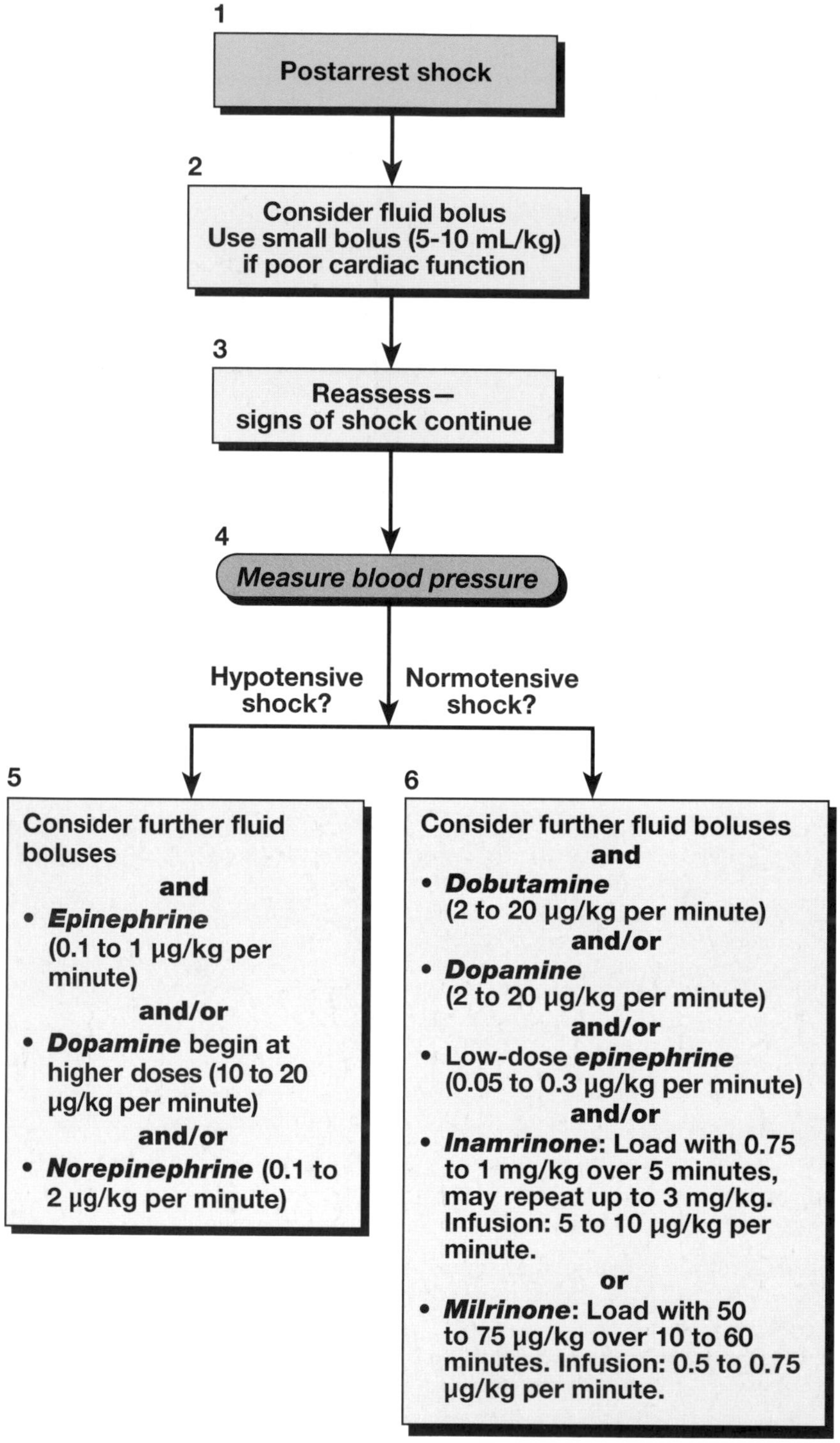

Figure 1. PALS Postresuscitation Treatment of Shock Algorithm

Estimation of Maintenance Fluid Requirements

- **Infants <10 kg:** Infusion of D_5 normal saline after initial stabilization at a rate of 4 mL/kg per hour. For example, the maintenance rate for an 8-kg baby is as follows:

  4 mL/kg per hour × 8 kg = 32 mL/h

- **Children 10 to 20 kg:** Infusion of 0.9% sodium chloride (normal saline) after initial stabilization at a rate of 40 mL/h plus 2 mL/kg per hour for each kilogram between 10 and 20 kg. For example, the maintenance rate for a 15-kg child is as follows:

  40 mL/h +
  (2 mL/kg per hour × 5 kg) =
  50 mL/h

- **Children >20 kg:** Infusion of 0.9% sodium chloride (normal saline) after initial stabilization at a rate of 60 mL/h plus 1 mL/kg per hour for each kilogram above 20 kg. For example, the maintenance rate for a 30-kg child is as follows:

  60 mL/h +
  (1 mL/kg per hour × 10 kg) =
  70 mL/h

- Shortcut for patients weighing >20 kg:

  weight in kg + 40 mL/h

Adjust rate and composition of fluids to child's clinical condition (eg, pulse, blood pressure, systemic perfusion) and level of hydration.

Postarrest Shock and Fluid Therapy (Boxes 1-3)

Since most children with ROSC after cardiac arrest have myocardial dysfunction, consider administering a small fluid bolus (5 to 10 mL/kg), then reassess. *If the child demonstrates signs of poor cardiac function (eg, large liver, pulmonary edema, jugular venous distension), carefully evaluate the need for fluid administration. Inappropriate fluid administration can potentially worsen cardiopulmonary function.*

Reassess the child to determine if signs of shock continue.

Blood Pressure Check (Box 4)

If you detect signs of shock, measure the blood pressure.

- If the patient is hypotensive, go to Box 5.
- If the patient is normotensive, go to Box 6.

If Hypotensive Shock (Box 5)

If the patient remains hypotensive (Box 5), consider additional fluid boluses (5 to 10 mL/kg) and infusion of one or a combination of the following drugs. Base your choice of drug on the cause of hypotension, whether from poor contractility or excessive vasodilation, or both, assuming that preload has been addressed.

Medication	Route	Dosage and Administration
Epinephrine	IV/IO	0.1 to 1 µg/kg per minute
and/or		
Dopamine	IV/IO	Begin at higher doses—10 to 20 µg/kg per minute
and/or		
Norepinephrine	IV/IO	0.1 to 2 µg/kg per minute

Epinephrine

Low-dose infusions (<0.3 µg/kg per minute) generally produce β-adrenergic action (potent inotropy and decreased systemic vascular resistance), and higher doses (>0.3 µg/kg per minute) generally produce α-adrenergic effects (vasoconstriction).[11] Because there is great interpatient variability,[12,13] titrate the drug to the desired effect. Epinephrine may be preferable to dopamine in patients (especially infants) with marked circulatory instability and hypotensive shock. It is a potent inotropic agent that can either lower or increase systemic vascular resistance, depending on the infusion dose.

Dopamine

Titrate dopamine to treat shock that is unresponsive to fluid and when systemic vascular resistance is low.[8,14] At higher doses (>5 µg/kg per minute), dopamine stimulates cardiac β-adrenergic receptors, but this effect may be reduced in infants and in chronic congestive heart failure. Doses of 10 to 20 µg/kg per minute increase systemic vascular resistance due to α-adrenergic effect.[11] Infusion rates >20 µg/kg per minute may result in excessive vasoconstriction.[11]

Norepinephrine

Norepinephrine is a potent inotropic and peripheral vasoconstricting agent. Titrate an infusion to treat shock with low systemic vascular resistance (septic, anaphylactic, or neurogenic) that is unresponsive to volume.

If Normotensive Shock (Box 6)

If the patient is normotensive (Box 6) but remains poorly perfused, consider further fluid boluses (10 to 20 mL/kg) and administration of one or a combination of the following drugs:

Medication	Route	Dosage and Administration
Dobutamine	IV/IO	2 to 20 μg/kg per minute
and/or		
Dopamine	IV/IO	2 to 20 μg/kg per minute
and/or		
Low-dose epinephrine	IV/IO	0.05 to 0.3 μg/kg per minute
and/or		
Milrinone	IV/IO	Load with 50 to 75 μg/kg over 10 to 60 minutes. Infusion: 0.5 to 0.75 μg/kg per minute
or		
Inamrinone	IV/IO	Load with 0.75 to 1 mg/kg over 5 minutes; may repeat up to 3 mg/kg. Infusion: 5 to 10 μg/kg per minute

Dobutamine

Dobutamine has a selective effect on β_1-adrenergic and β_2-adrenergic receptors and has intrinsic α-adrenergic blocking activity. It increases myocardial contractility and usually decreases peripheral vascular resistance. Titrate an infusion[12,15,16] to improve cardiac output and blood pressure, especially due to poor myocardial function.[16]

Dopamine

Typically dopamine is administered at an infusion rate of 2 to 20 μg/kg per minute. Although low-dose dopamine infusion has been frequently recommended to maintain renal blood flow or improve renal function, more recent data has failed to show a beneficial effect from such therapy. See "Dopamine" in Box 5 for more information on the use of this drug in the postresuscitation period.

Low-dose Epinephrine

See "Epinephrine" in Box 5.

Milrinone and Inamrinone

Milrinone and inamrinone are inodilators that augment cardiac output with little effect on heart rate and myocardial oxygen demand. Use an inodilator for treatment of myocardial dysfunction with increased systemic or pulmonary vascular resistance.[17-19] You may need to administer fluids because of the vasodilatory effects.

Compared with drugs like dopamine and norepinephrine, inodilators have a long half-life with a long delay in reaching a new steady-state hemodynamic effect after changing the infusion rate (4.5 hours with milrinone and 18 hours with inamrinone). In case of toxicity the adverse effects may persist for several hours after you stop the infusion.

Administration of Maintenance Fluids

Maintenance Fluid Composition

Consider administration of maintenance fluids once intravascular volume is restored and existing fluid deficits have been replaced. Account for the rate of vasoactive drug infusions when determining maintenance fluid rate.

In the first hours after resuscitation, an isotonic fluid with dextrose (D_5NS or D_5LR) is generally safe and effective for maintenance fluids.[20-22]

Specific components may be added to maintenance fluids based on the clinical condition:

- Dextrose should generally be included in all maintenance fluids, especially for infants and for patients who are hypoglycemic or who are at risk for hypoglycemia.
- Potassium chloride (KCl) 10 to 20 mEq/L is typically added once ongoing monitoring of potassium is available for children with adequate renal function and documented urine output. Avoid adding KCl to maintenance fluids in children with known hyperkalemia, renal failure, muscle injury, or severe acidosis.

Fluid Rate Calculation by 4-2-1 Method

A practical approach to estimating hourly maintenance fluid requirements is the 4-2-1 method (Table 2).

Table 2. Estimation of Maintenance Fluid Requirements

Weight (kg)	Fluid Rate	Example of Calculation
<10	4 mL/kg per hour	8 kg infant: 4 mL/kg per hour × 8 kg = 32 mL/h
10 to 20	40 mL/h + 2 mL/kg per hour per each kg between 10 and 20 kg	15 kg child: 40 mL/h + 2 mL/kg per hour × 5 kg = 50 mL/h
>20	60 mL/h + 1 mL/kg per hour per each kg above 20 kg	30 kg child: 60 mL/h + 1 mL/kg per hour × 10 kg = 70 mL/h

A shortcut calculation of maintenance hourly fluid rate for patients weighing >20 kg is weight in kg + 40 mL/h.

Once you have calculated the maintenance fluid requirements, adjust the actual rate of fluid administration to the child's clinical condition (eg, pulse, blood pressure, systemic perfusion, urine output) and level of hydration.

Neurologic System

Management Priorities

The goals of neurologic management during the postresuscitation period are to preserve brain function and prevent secondary neuronal injury. Management priorities are to

- maintain adequate brain perfusion
- maintain normoglycemia
- control temperature
- treat increased intracranial pressure (ICP)
- treat seizures aggressively; search for and treat their cause

General Recommendations

General recommendations for the assessment and management of the neurologic system may include those described in the table below.

Assessment and Management of the Neurologic System	
Assessment	
Monitoring	Monitor temperature. *In patients who are poorly perfused, reliable monitoring of core temperature requires advanced techniques (rectal, bladder).*
Physical examination	• Perform frequent, brief neurologic assessments (eg, GCS, pupillary responses, gag reflex, corneal reflexes, oculocephalic reflexes). • Identify signs of impending cerebral herniation. • Identify seizure activity, both convulsive and nonconvulsive. • Identify abnormal neurologic findings, including abnormal movements (posturing/myoclonus/hyperreflexia). *Signs of impending cerebral herniation include unequal or dilated unresponsive pupils, hypertension, bradycardia, respiratory irregularities or apnea, and reduced response to simulation. When ICP is measured, a sudden rise in ICP is often seen. Besides increased ICP, other causes of CNS dysfunction are hypoxic-ischemic brain injury, hypoglycemia, convulsive or nonconvulsive seizures, toxins/drugs, electrolyte abnormalities, hypothermia, traumatic brain injury, and central nervous system infection.* *See "Disability" in Chapter 1 for more information on neurologic assessment.*
Laboratory tests	• Evaluate glucose; repeat measurement following treatment of hyperglycemia or hypoglycemia. • Obtain serum electrolytes and calcium concentration if seizure activity is present; measure anticonvulsant concentrations if the child was receiving these agents. • Consider toxicologic studies if poisoning or overdose is suspected. • Consider cerebral spinal fluid studies if central nervous system (CNS) infection is suspected.
Nonlaboratory tests	• Consider CT scan if CNS dysfunction or neurologic deterioration is present. • Consider EEG if convulsive or nonconvulsive status epilepticus is suspected.

Management	
Brain perfusion	• Optimize brain perfusion by supporting cardiac output and systemic oxygen content. • Avoid hyperventilation unless there are signs of impending cerebral herniation. *Support cardiac output by optimizing preload, afterload, and contractility. See "Support of Systemic Perfusion" in this chapter for more information.*
Blood glucose	• Treat hypoglycemia. • Monitor glucose concentration. In general, try to avoid causing or worsening hyperglycemia. • Consider treating persistent hyperglycemia. *Although hyperglycemia is associated with poor outcome in critically ill children, the role of active treatment of hyperglycemia in critically ill children remains uncertain. In most animal studies hyperglycemia at the time of cerebral ischemia produces a worse outcome, but the effect of hyperglycemia occurring after ROSC is less clear.*[23]
Temperature control	Control hypothermia and hyperthermia. **Hypothermia** • Do not actively rewarm the patient who is hypothermic (ie, <37°C and >33°C) after ROSC following cardiac arrest. If the patient is hemodynamically unstable and you believe this is due at least in part to hypothermia, then rewarming is appropriate. • Consider initiating cooling in normothermic patients who remain comatose after resuscitation from cardiac arrest; you may need to treat or prevent shivering to achieve hypothermia. • Watch for and treat complications of hypothermia. *Cooling to a temperature of 32°C to 34°C for 12 to 24 hours or longer after resuscitation from a cardiac arrest may aid brain recovery. Complications of hypothermia include diminished cardiac output, arrhythmia, infection, pancreatitis, coagulopathy, thrombocytopenia, hypophosphatemia, and hypomagnesemia.* **Hyperthermia** • Avoid hyperthermia; adjust ambient temperature as needed. • Treat fever aggressively with antipyretics and cooling devices or procedures (eg, iced saline gastric lavage). *Fever adversely influences recovery from ischemic brain injury*[24-28] *and is associated with poor outcome following resuscitation from cardiac arrest.*[24, 25, 29-39] *Metabolic oxygen demand increases by 10% to 13% for each degree Celsius elevation of temperature above normal. Increased metabolic demand may worsen neurologic injury. Furthermore, fever increases the release of inflammatory mediators, cytotoxic enzymes, and neurotransmitters, all of which increase brain injury.*

(continued)

Management *(continued)*	
Increased ICP	• Elevate head of bed to 30° if blood pressure is adequate. • Keep head in midline. • Ventilate to maintain normocarbia. • Short periods of hyperventilation may be perfomed as a temporizing measure for the child with signs of impending cerebral herniation. • Consider steroids for CNS tumor or inflammatory process. • Use mannitol or hypertonic saline for acute herniation syndrome. • Consult a neurosurgical expert if — the GCS score is <13 (GCS <9 is generally an indication for ICP montioring in traumatic brain injury) — there is rapid neurologic deterioration *Prolonged hyperventilation is ineffective for treatment of increased ICP, and excessive hyperventilation may worsen neurologic outcome. Hypocarbia results in cerebral vasoconstriction, reducing cerebral blood flow. Hyperventilation also reduces venous return and cardiac output, contributing to cerebral ischemia.*
Seizures	• Treat seizures aggressively. Therapeutic options include a benzodiazepine (eg, lorazepam), fosphenytoin/phenytoin, or a barbiturate (eg, phenobarbital). Monitor blood pressure because phenytoin and phenobarbital may cause hypotension. • Search for a correctable metabolic cause, such as hypoglycemia or electrolyte imbalance (ie, hyponatremia or hypocalcemia). • Consider toxins or metabolic disease as the etiology. • Consult a neurologist if available.

Renal System

Management Priorities

Another goal of postresuscitation management is to minimize secondary injury to the kidneys, ensure there is adequate renal perfusion, and correct acid-base imbalance resulting from renal injury. Management priorities for support of the renal system are to

- optimize renal perfusion and function
- correct acid-base imbalance

General Recommendations

General recommendations for the assessment and management of the renal system may include those described in the table.

Assessment and Management of the Renal System	
Assessment	
Monitoring	• Monitor for decreased urine output (<1 mL/kg per hour in infants and children or <30 mL/h in adolescents) by urinary catheter. • Monitor for increased urine output as a result of glucosuria, diabetes insipidus, and osmotic and nonosmotic diuretics. *Insert a urinary catheter to enable accurate measurement of urine output. Consider use of a urinary catheter with a temperature probe that permits continuous core temperature monitoring.*
Physical examination	• Examine the abdomen for distended bladder or diffusely distended and tight abdomen, which may impair renal perfusion (abdominal compartment syndrome). • Examine for evidence of hypovolemia and circulatory dysfunction resulting in oliguria. • Ensure patency of the urinary catheter. *Causes of oliguria are prerenal conditions (eg, hypovolemia or inadequate systemic perfusion), intrinsic renal disease, or urinary tract obstruction.*
Laboratory tests	• Assess renal function — BUN/creatinine — Serum electrolytes • Obtain urinalysis if indicated by history or exam • Assess metabolic state — ABG (acid-base) — Serum glucose — Anion gap — Lactate concentration *Urine glucose measurement is important when evaluating urine output; glucosuria may indicate the cause of increased urine output (eg, diabetes mellitus).*
Management	
Renal function	• Augment renal perfusion by restoring intravascular volume and supporting systemic perfusion, as needed, with vasoactive drugs. • Treat with loop diuretics (eg, furosemide) in patients with volume overload/congestive heart failure and normal blood pressure. • When possible avoid nephrotoxic medications; adjust dose and timing of medications excreted by the kidneys if you know that renal function is impaired. • Add KCl to IV fluids cautiously if renal function is poor or if there is no urine output; potassium concentration should be measured when possible before adding potassium. • Consider that the oliguric patient may have intrinsic renal failure; if so, you may need to restrict fluid intake once intravascular volume is adequate. *Administration of fluid augments preload in volume-depleted patients. Vasoactive drugs may improve renal perfusion by improving cardiac output.*
Acid-base balance	• Correct lactic acidosis by improving tissue perfusion (ie, with fluid administration and vasoactive agents). • Consider correcting non-anion gap metabolic acidosis with sodium bicarbonate, particularly if the history or signs suggest bicarbonate loss in the stool from diarrhea. • Sodium bicarbonate is not indicated for the treatment of hyperchloremic metabolic acidosis (eg, associated with normal saline boluses).

Gastrointestinal System

Management Priorities

The major goals of gastrointestinal management during postresuscitation care are to restore and maintain gastrointestinal function, including liver and pancreatic function, and to minimize the risk of aspiration of gastric contents into the airway. Management priorities are to

- support systemic perfusion
- relieve gastric distention
- correct electrolyte abnormalities (eg, hypomagnesemia or hypokalemia) that may be contributing to ileus
- support hepatic function

General Recommendations

General recommendations for the assessment and management of the gastrointestinal system may include those described in the table below.

Assessment and Management of the Gastrointestinal System	
Assessment	
Monitoring	• Monitor type and quantity of nasogastric (NG) tube drainage.
Physical examination	• Perform a careful abdominal examination with attention to bowel sounds, abdominal girth, and abdominal tightness. *Critically ill or injured children may have delayed gastric emptying.* *A tight abdomen that is difficult to compress raises concern for an intra-abdominal catastrophe such as a perforated bowel or intra-abdominal bleeding. Additional studies (eg, abdominal ultrasound) and early surgical consultation are indicated as appropriate.*
Laboratory tests	Obtain laboratory tests of liver and pancreatic function based on the patient's condition and the etiology of the arrest. • Evaluate liver function — Transaminases (ALT/AST) — Biliary function (bilirubin, alkaline phosphatase, 5´-nucleotidase) — Synthetic function (albumin, PT/PTT) — Glucose — Ammonia (if concern about liver failure) • Evaluate for pancreatic injury — Amylase/lipase
Nonlaboratory tests	• Consider ultrasound to evaluate liver, gall bladder, pancreas, and bladder and to assess for intra-abdominal fluid. • Consider abdominal CT scan with intravenous and enteral contrast, particularly when evaluating abdominal trauma.

	Management
Gastric distention	• Insert orogastric (OG) or NG tube and aspirate stomach air and contents. Ideally use a sump tube rather than a single-lumen NG feeding tube to decompress the stomach.
Ileus	• Insert OG or NG tube and aspirate gastric contents. • Aspirate via NG tube at regular intervals or place NG tube on siphon drainage to provide bowel decompression. • Restore and maintain electrolyte and fluid balance.
Hepatic failure	• Infuse glucose at a rate to maintain normal glucose concentrations. • Correct clotting factor deficiency for clinical bleeding using fresh frozen plasma, cryoprecipitate, and activated factor VII when indicated.

Hematologic System

Management Priorities

The goals of hematologic management during the postresuscitation period are to optimize the oxygen-carrying capacity and coagulation function of the blood. Management priorities are to

- treat significant hemorrhage
- restore coagulation function
- restore adequate oxygen-carrying capacity

General Recommendations

General recommendations for the assessment and management of the hematologic system may include those described in the table below.

Assessment and Management of the Hematologic System	
	Assessment
Physical examination	• Identify external or internal hemorrhage. • Assess skin and mucous membranes for pallor, petechiae, or bruising.
Laboratory tests	• Hemoglobin and hematocrit • Platelet count • Prothrombin time, partial thromboplastin time, international normalized ratio (INR), fibrinogen, D-dimer, and fibrin split products

Management	
Blood component therapy	• Transfuse with packed red blood cells (PRBCs) 10 mL/kg if hemorrhagic shock is refractory to isotonic crystalloid (2 or 3 boluses of 20 mL/kg). *Type-specific blood is generally available within 5 minutes and is preferred over O-negative transfusions when time precludes complete crossmatching. Complications of massive transfusion include hypothermia, hyperkalemia, hypocalcemia, coagulopathies from dilution of platelets, and clotting factors.* • Platelet transfusion may be indicated: — If severe bleeding is present, transfuse with platelets if platelet count <50 000 to 100 000/mm^3 and severe bleeding is present. — If patient is at risk of bleeding (no bleeding is present) and platelet count <20 000/mm^3, consider platelet transfusion. — In general, 1 unit of random donor platelets/5 kg body weight will raise the platelet count by 50 000/mm^3. *Platelets should be ABO and Rh compatible; platelet crossmatching is not necessary.* • Administer fresh frozen plasma (10 to 15 mL/kg) if abnormal coagulation tests and patient is at risk for bleeding or is bleeding. • Consider vitamin K administration for depletion of vitamin K-dependent clotting factors. • Ensure that serum ionized calcium is normal since it is a cofactor in clotting. *Fresh frozen plasma contains all clotting factors but no platelets. Beware that fresh frozen plasma uses citrate as the anticoagulant—rapid infusions may acutely lower plasma ionized calcium concentrations, resulting in vasodilation and reduced cardiac contractility, causing hypotension despite the administration of a colloid solution.*

Postresuscitation Transport

Introduction

The PALS principles of postresuscitation assessment, monitoring, intervention, stabilization, communication, and documentation apply to the transport of the pediatric patient, whether the transport is interhospital or intrahospital. Important considerations of transport are

- coordination with receiving facility
- advance preparation for transport
- infectious disease considerations
- preparation immediately before transport
- communication between physicians
- communication between hospitals or other healthcare providers
- communication with family
- post-transport documentation and follow-up

Coordination With Receiving Facility

Coordinate transport and transfer with the receiving providers at the tertiary care center to ensure that the child is delivered safely in stable or improved condition.[40] Both the referring and receiving facilities should have well-defined protocols for specific clinical situations. Protocols, contracts, and agreements should be established *before* a seriously ill or injured child requires transport. In some areas of the country, transfer of uninsured patients may be restricted, especially if the nearest available pediatric center is across a state line. Advance preparation for transport should address such administrative matters in written, prearranged contracts between the referring and receiving hospitals. Advanced preparation should also include written protocols and agreements to initiate appropriate communication between administrators to avoid delays at the time of patient transport. Transport reimbursement arrangements should be discussed in advance.

Advance Preparation for Transport

Advance preparation for interhospital transport by the referring facility may include the following:

- List of pediatric tertiary care facilities and telephone numbers
- Identify nearest alternative hospital if there is only one pediatric tertiary care center in the area (even if it is in another state)
- List of pediatric transport systems and telephone numbers
- If transport is to be performed by personnel from the referring facility, maintain a list of pediatric equipment and supplies to include with standard EMS equipment. A more extensive list of equipment should be available if a physician accompanies the patient. Ideally pediatric transport packs, containing equipment of the correct size and medication doses for the particular emergency situation, should be prepared in advance.
- Personnel trained and experienced in pediatric care (see "Transport Team" later in this chapter)
- Periodic evaluation of transport vehicle equipment to ensure that it is appropriate for the entire range of ages and sizes of pediatric patients and to ensure that lost or missing equipment is immediately replaced
- Administrative protocols and use of a transport checklist to ensure that all appropriate interventions are provided and appropriate documents are sent with the patient

Infectious Disease Considerations

If the patient is suspected of having an infectious disease, obtain appropriate cultures (if not already obtained) before transport. Early antibiotic administration is critical when sepsis is suspected. If there is a possibility of a contagious disease, transport personnel should take appropriate precautions to avoid disease transmission (eg, masks).

Preparation Immediately Before Transport

For preparation immediately before transport consider the following:

- Obtain consent to transport
- Prepare the patient for transport
- Anticipate the requirements of the transport team

Obtain consent to transport

If the transport team is not from the referring or receiving hospital, the referring hospital must assist in the efficient transfer of the patient. Some transport teams operate on the basis of implied consent. Implied consent means that transport is considered part of the treatment for a life-threatening emergency, and formal consent is not required. Obtain written consent to transport from the child's legal guardian if possible. Many transport teams request that the parents remain at the referring hospital to give consent directly to the team.

Prepare the patient for transport

If airway patency or ventilatory status is questionable, secure the airway with an ET tube before transport and verify placement with clinical assessment and a confirmation device (eg, exhaled CO_2 detection). If radiology services are available in a timely manner or if there is uncertainty about the ET tube position, check depth of insertion with a chest x-ray. Tape intravascular lines and the ET tube securely in place. Vascular catheters and ET tubes may become dislodged during transport because they were inadequately secured for a moving environment.[41] The movement and vibrations that occur during transport make replacement of dislodged catheters or ET tubes difficult. In transporting trauma patients, stabilize the cervical spine and any fractured bones before transport.

Anticipate the requirements of the transport team

Transfer will be more efficient if the referring facility anticipates the requirements of the transport team and prepares to meet them. Copies of the patient's chart and x-rays should be made before the transport team arrives. If blood products may be required during transport, prepare a supply in advance to accompany the patient. Similarly, anticipate the need for specific vasoactive drug support.

Communication Between Physicians

Good communication is important prior to patient transfer. The initial call to transfer a patient should be made by one physician to another.[42] In general, the transport system should not be activated until the referring physician has discussed the patient's case with the physician who will accept the patient being transferred.

Other important components of this discussion and follow-up documentation may include the following:

- Consult the patient's chart at the time of the call to give specific details about estimated weight, vital signs, fluids administered, and timing of events.
- In a crisis give a brief history of the illness or accident, interventions, and the patient's current clinical status to facilitate decisions about treatment and method of transport.
- Document the names of the receiving physician and hospital.
- Document the advice provided by the receiving physician; the transport team may need additional specific information to select the proper equipment for transport.
- Discuss any potential need for isolation so that appropriate arrangements can be made at the receiving hospital.

Communication Between Hospitals or Other Healthcare Providers

Successful communication between the receiving and referring facilities is essential for successful transport. Important communications may include the following:

- Nurses from the receiving and referring facilities should respectively request and provide updates on the patient's status.
- When the transport team arrives, the referring physician should personally provide a current report about the patient directly to the transport team, transferring care of the patient.
- If the receiving hospital's transport team is not involved in the transport, the referring physician should telephone the receiving physician immediately before the patient's departure and report the patient's most recent vital signs, current clinical status, and estimated time of arrival at the receiving hospital.
- Include copies of all records, laboratory results, and x-rays with the patient. Note any laboratory results that are pending at the time of transport. Include the laboratory phone number with the patient's record so that the receiving physician can obtain the results.

The referring physician should notify the receiving facility if the patient's condition changes significantly at any time before arrival of the transport team.

Communication With the Family

Communication with the family is an essential part of postresuscitation care and transport care. Update the family about all interventions and diagnostic studies. Answer questions, clarify information, and offer comfort. See "Family Presence During Resuscitation" in Ethical and Legal Aspects of CPR in Children on the student CD.

Post-Transport Documentation and Follow-up

Post-transport follow-up provides important feedback that can improve the performance of the transport team and referring hospital.

Who	Action
Receiving physician	Contact the referring physician after the transport is complete to provide feedback about management, to advise of the patient's status, and to address transport issues.
Receiving hospital	Provide personnel at the referring hospital with subsequent follow-up information about the patient's condition, including the ultimate outcome. This may require written consent from the child's parent or guardian.
Referring physician	Ensure that laboratory results that become available after transport of the patient are communicated to the receiving hospital. If the receiving hospital does not provide communication about the patient's condition and ultimate outcome, contact the medical director of the transport system. Express any concerns about the transport. Such a discussion can often clarify misunderstandings, such as the necessity for interventions or timing of transport.

Mode of Transport and Transport Team Composition

Introduction

The mode of transport and composition of the transport team should be based on the care required by the individual pediatric patient and the logistics of the transfer.

Mode of Transport

Once the child has been stabilized, providers must determine the most appropriate method of transfer to a tertiary care facility. A child with significant respiratory or circulatory compromise requires constant medical supervision. Transport in the caregiver's vehicle is not an option. Interhospital transport can be provided by

- ground transportation by ambulance (eg, local EMS ambulance, advanced life support unit, or critical care transport vehicle)
- helicopter
- fixed-wing aircraft

Ground Transportation by Ambulance

Ambulances, whether a local ambulance or a critical care transport vehicle from the receiving hospital, provide readily available ground transportation. They are relatively inexpensive and spacious (compared with most transport aircraft). They are operable in most weather conditions and can stop easily if a procedure must be performed. One disadvantage of ground ambulance transport is increased transport time over long distances. Another disadvantage is the risk of traffic-related delays.

Helicopter

Helicopter transport is fast, allowing rapid transfer of care from the referring hospital to the receiving hospital, particularly when there is a long distance between the hospitals. This mode of transportation avoids traffic congestion. A disadvantage during helicopter transport is that it is difficult to monitor or evaluate the pediatric patient. Performing emergency procedures is usually impossible. Helicopters are not pressurized, and the patient compartment may experience extremes in temperature. Other disadvantages are the inability to fly due to weather conditions, increased safety concerns, and high cost.

Fixed-wing Aircraft

Fixed-wing aircraft are used only for long-distance transport or when it is necessary to reach a remote area, such as an island. These aircraft are pressurized and they land at controlled sites. It is easier to perform patient interventions and monitoring in a fixed-wing aircraft than in a helicopter. The disadvantages are long start-up times (usually offset by the speed of flight) and the need to transfer the patient from hospital to ambulance to aircraft with a reverse transfer sequence on landing.

Transport Team

Transport team members should have specific training and experience in pediatric evaluation, stabilization, and resuscitation. The members of the transport team may be

- local EMS personnel
- medical personnel from the referring hospital
- critical care teams
- pediatric critical care transport teams

Local EMS teams rarely have the training, experience, or equipment for long-distance transport of a critically ill or injured child after stabilization.[43,44] The use of local EMS personnel may also deprive the community of service in the event of other local emergencies.

Medical personnel from the referring hospital may be rapidly mobilized. But their involvement on the transport team may deprive their facility of necessary personnel unless they are specifically scheduled for transport. Personnel with limited experience in pediatric prehospital and critical care will find patient management especially difficult in a moving vehicle with limited or unfamiliar equipment (eg, portable monitors). Anticipated care during transfer should not exceed the level that the transport team is capable of providing.

Critical care teams who transport patients of all ages may have variable training, experience, and equipment for optimum care of a critically ill or injured child.[45] Evaluate the ability of transport teams to care for critically ill or injured children before this type of care is needed.[46]

Pediatric critical care transport teams provide optimum transport for critically ill children and often provide continuity of care from transport to the PICU. Unfortunately such teams are not available in all areas, and they may not have access to all types of transport vehicles. Use the most qualified team (as measured by existing pediatric transport guidelines) that is available within an acceptable time interval based on the child's condition.

It is often best to wait for the arrival of a team experienced in pediatric critical care for the transport of a critically ill or injured child even if this creates a delay. This type of transport team can initiate pediatric critical care at the referring hospital and maintain that level of care during transport.[47] An exception to this rule would be the child who requires immediate surgical intervention at the tertiary care center (eg, a craniotomy for epidural hematoma).[47]

Transport Triage

No specific criteria are available to reliably determine the need for a pediatric critical care transport team.[48-50] The following are broad criteria:

- Children who are expected to require PICU admission at the receiving hospital are likely to need that level of monitoring during transport
- Children with a respiratory, cardiovascular, or neurologic condition who have significant potential for deterioration during transport
- Children who have recently experienced a life-threatening event (even if they are stable at the time of transport) because the event may recur; examples are neonates and infants with a history of apnea and any child who has required aggressive stabilization (eg, after seizure with apnea or after resuscitation from severe shock)

Summary: Transport Checklist

Transport Checklist	
Coordination with receiving facility	
☐	Identify pediatric tertiary care center with appropriate receiving providers. Phone number:
Advance preparation for transport	
☐	Identify nearest alternative hospital if there is only one pediatric tertiary care center in the area. Phone number:
☐	Locate administrative protocol for interhospital patient transport.
Mode of transport	
☐	Determine appropriate mode of transport for patient and weather condition (ground ambulance, helicopter, fixed-wing aircraft).
Infectious disease considerations	
☐	Practice universal precautions.
☐	Obtain appropriate cultures if the patient is suspected of having an infectious disease.
☐	Administer antibiotics if sepsis is suspected.
☐	Consider need for patient isolation (ie, respiratory or contact).
Preparation immediately before transport	
☐	Obtain consent to transport.
☐	Prepare the patient for transport.
☐	Anticipate requirements of the transport team.
Communication between physicians	
☐	Identify and document the name of the receiving physician:
☐	Communicate appropriate details of the case to the receiving physician.
Communication between hospitals	
☐	Notify the receiving facility if the patient's condition changes significantly at any time before arrival of the transport team.
☐	Nurses from the referring facility should provide a report and updates as needed on the patient's status.
☐	The referring physician should provide a current report about the patient directly to the transport team, formally transferring the patient.
☐	The referring physician should contact the receiving physician immediately before departure to provide the most current update about the patient and estimated time of arrival if the receiving hospital's transport team is not involved in transport.
☐	Include copies of all records, laboratory results, and x-rays with the patient.
☐	Note laboratory results pending at the time of transport and include laboratory phone number with the patient's record so that the receiving physician can obtain the results.

Transport Checklist	
Communication with family	
☐	Communicate results of all interventions and diagnostic studies to the family. Answer questions, clarify information, and offer comfort.
Post-transport documentation and follow-up	
☐	Contact the medical director of the transport system if no communication is received from the receiving facility about the patient's condition and ultimate outcome.

References

1. Booth CM, Boone RH, Tomlinson G, et al. Is this patient dead, vegetative, or severely neurologically impaired? Assessing outcome for comatose survivors of cardiac arrest. *JAMA*. 2004;291(7):870-879.
2. Bunch TJ, White RD, Gersh BJ, et al. Long-term outcomes of out-of-hospital cardiac arrest after successful early defibrillation. *N Engl J Med.* 2003;348(26):2626-2633.
3. Tobias JD, Lynch A, Garrett J. Alterations of end-tidal carbon dioxide during the intrahospital transport of children. *Pediatr Emerg Care.* 1996;12(4):249-251.
4. Spaulding CM, Joly LM, Rosenberg A, et al. Immediate coronary angiography in survivors of out-of-hospital cardiac arrest. *N Engl J Med.* 1997;336(23):1629-1633.
5. Vasquez A, Kern KB, Hilwig RW, et al. Optimal dosing of dobutamine for treating post-resuscitation left ventricular dysfunction. *Resuscitation*. 2004;61(2):199-207.
6. Kern KB, Hilwig RW, Berg RA, et al. Postresuscitation left ventricular systolic and diastolic dysfunction: treatment with dobutamine. *Circulation*. 1997;95(12):2610-2613.
7. Meyer RJ, Kern KB, Berg RA, et al. Post-resuscitation right ventricular dysfunction: delineation and treatment with dobutamine. *Resuscitation*. 2002;55(2):187-191.
8. Ceneviva G, Paschall JA, Maffei F, et al. Hemodynamic support in fluid-refractory pediatric septic shock. *Pediatrics*. 1998;102(2):e19.
9. Hildebrand CA, Hartmann AG, Arcinue EL, et al. Cardiac performance in pediatric near-drowning. *Crit Care Med.* 1988;16(4):331-335.
10. Checchia PA, Sehra R, Moynihan J, et al. Myocardial injury in children following resuscitation after cardiac arrest. *Resuscitation*. 2003;57(2):131-137.
11. Zaritsky AL. Catecholamines, inotropic medications, and vasopressor agents. In: Chernow B, ed. *The Pharmacologic Approach to the Critically Ill Patient.* 3rd ed. Baltimore, Md: Williams & Wilkins; 1994:387-404.
12. Berg RA, Padbury JF. Sulfoconjugation and renal excretion contribute to the interpatient variation of exogenous catecholamine clearance in critically ill children. *Crit Care Med.* 1997;25(7):1247-1251.
13. Fisher DG, Schwartz PH, Davis AL. Pharmacokinetics of exogenous epinephrine in critically ill children. *Crit Care Med.* 1993;21(1):111-117.
14. Ushay HM, Notterman DA. Pharmacology of pediatric resuscitation. *Pediatr Clin North Am.* 1997;44(1):207-233.
15. Habib DM, Padbury JF, Anas NG, et al. Dobutamine pharmacokinetics and pharmacodynamics in pediatric intensive care patients. *Crit Care Med.* 1992;20(5):601-608.
16. Martinez AM, Padbury JF, Thio S. Dobutamine pharmacokinetics and cardiovascular responses in critically ill neonates. *Pediatrics*. 1992;89(1):47-51.

17. Barton P, Garcia J, Kouatli A, et al. Hemodynamic effects of i.v. milrinone lactate in pediatric patients with septic shock: a prospective, double-blinded, randomized, placebo-controlled, interventional study. *Chest*. 1996;109(5):1302-1312.

18. Bailey JM, Miller BE, Lu W, et al. The pharmacokinetics of milrinone in pediatric patients after cardiac surgery. *Anesthesiology*. 1999;90(4):1012-1018.

19. Abdallah I, Shawky H. A randomised controlled trial comparing milrinone and epinephrine as inotropes in paediatric patients undergoing total correction of Tetralogy of Fallot. *Egyptian J Anaesthesia.* 2003;19(4):323-329.

20. Moritz ML, Ayus JC. Prevention of hospital-acquired hyponatremia: a case for using isotonic saline. *Pediatrics*. 2003;111(2):227-230.

21. Choong K, Kho ME, Menon K, et al. Hypotonic versus isotonic saline in hospitalized children: a systematic review. *Arch Dis Child.* 2006; 91:828-835.

22. Hoorn EJ, Geary D, Robb M, et al. Acute hyponatremia related to intravenous fluid administration in hospitalized children: an observational study. *Pediatrics*. 2004;113(5):1279-1284.

23. Srinivasan V, Spinella PC, Drott HR, et al. Association of timing, duration, and intensity of hyperglycemia with intensive care unit mortality in critically ill children. *Pediatr Crit Care Med.* 2004;5(4):329-336.

24. Zeiner A, Holzer M, Sterz F, et al. Hyperthermia after cardiac arrest is associated with an unfavorable neurologic outcome. *Arch Intern Med.* 2001;161(16):2007-2012.

25. Takasu A, Saitoh D, Kaneko N, et al. Hyperthermia: is it an ominous sign after cardiac arrest? *Resuscitation*. 2001;49(3):273-277.

26. Ginsberg MD, Busto R. Combating hyperthermia in acute stroke: a significant clinical concern. *Stroke*. 1998;29(2):529-534.

27. Hickey RW, Kochanek PM, Ferimer H, et al. Induced hyperthermia exacerbates neurologic neuronal histologic damage after asphyxial cardiac arrest in rats. *Crit Care Med.* 2003;31(2):531-535.

28. Shum-Tim D, Nagashima M, Shinoka T, et al. Postischemic hyperthermia exacerbates neurologic injury after deep hypothermic circulatory arrest. *J Thorac Cardiovasc Surg.* 1998;116(5):780-792.

29. Obrist WD, Langfitt TW, Jaggi JL, et al. Cerebral blood flow and metabolism in comatose patients with acute head injury. Relationship to intracranial hypertension. *J Neurosurg.* 1984;61(2):241-253.

30. Hickey RW, Kochanek PM, Ferimer H, et al. Hypothermia and hyperthermia in children after resuscitation from cardiac arrest. *Pediatrics*. 2000;106(pt 1)(1):118-122.

31. Hypothermia After Cardiac Arrest Study Group. Mild therapeutic hypothermia to improve the neurologic outcome after cardiac arrest. *N Engl J Med.* 2002;346(8):549-556.

32. Bernard SA, Gray TW, Buist MD, et al. Treatment of comatose survivors of out-of-hospital cardiac arrest with induced hypothermia. *N Engl J Med.* 2002;346(8):557-563.

33. Gluckman PD, Wyatt JS, Azzopardi D, et al. Selective head cooling with mild systemic hypothermia after neonatal encephalopathy: multicentre randomised trial. *Lancet*. 2005;365(9460):663-670.

34. Battin MR, Penrice J, Gunn TR, et al. Treatment of term infants with head cooling and mild systemic hypothermia (35.0 degrees C and 34.5 degrees C) after perinatal asphyxia. *Pediatrics*. 2003;111(2):244-251.

35. Compagnoni G, Pogliani L, Lista G, et al. Hypothermia reduces neurological damage in asphyxiated newborn infants. *Biol Neonate.* 2002;82(4):222-227.

36. Debillon T, Daoud P, Durand P, et al. Whole-body cooling after perinatal asphyxia: a pilot study in term neonates. *Dev Med Child Neurol.* 2003;45(1):17-23.

37. Gunn AJ, Gluckman PD, Gunn TR. Selective head cooling in newborn infants after perinatal asphyxia: a safety study. *Pediatrics*. 1998;102(4 Pt 1):885-892.

38. Albrecht RF 2nd, Wass CT, Lanier WL. Occurrence of potentially detrimental temperature alterations in hospitalized patients at risk for brain injury. *Mayo Clin Proc.* 1998;73(7):629-635.

39. Takino M, Okada Y. Hyperthermia following cardiopulmonary resuscitation. *Intensive Care Med.* 1991;17(7):419-420.

40. Henning R. Emergency transport of critically ill children: stabilisation before departure. *Med J Aust.* 1992;156(2):117-124.

41. Gausche M, Lewis RJ, Stratton SJ, et al. Effect of out-of-hospital pediatric endotracheal intubation on survival and neurological outcome: a controlled clinical trial. *JAMA*. 2000;283(6):783-790.

42. Seidel JS, Knapp JF, eds. *Childhood Emergencies in the Office, Hospital, and Community.* Elk Grove Village, Ill: American Academy of Pediatrics; 2000.

43. Seidel JS. Emergency medical services and the pediatric patient: are the needs being met? II: training and equipping emergency medical services providers for pediatric emergencies. *Pediatrics*. 1986;78(5):808-812.

44. Seidel JS, Hornbein M, Yoshiyama K, et al. Emergency medical services and the pediatric patient: are the needs being met? *Pediatrics*. 1984;73(6):769-772.

45. McCloskey KA, Faries G, King WD, et al. Variables predicting the need for a pediatric critical care transport team. *Pediatr Emerg Care.* 1992;8(1):1-3.

46. American Academy of Pediatrics Task Force on Interhospital Transport. *Guidelines for Air and Ground Transport of Neonatal and Pediatric Patients.* Elk Grove Village, Ill: American Academy of Pediatrics; 1993.

47. Aoki BY, McCloskey K. *Evaluation, Stabilization, and Transport of the Critically Ill Child.* St. Louis, Mo: Mosby Year Book; 1992.

48. Orr RA, Venkataraman ST, Cinoman MI, et al. Pretransport Pediatric Risk of Mortality (PRISM) score underestimates the requirement for intensive care or major interventions during interhospital transport. *Crit Care Med.* 1994;22(1):101-107.

49. Kissoon N, Frewen TC, Kronick JB, et al. The child requiring transport: lessons and implications for the pediatric emergency physician. *Pediatr Emerg Care.* 1988;4(1):1-4.

50. Orr R, Venkataraman S, McCloskey K, et al. Predicting the need for major interventions during pediatric interhospital transport using pretransport variables. *Pediatr Emerg Care.* 1992;8:371.

Chapter 9

Pharmacology

Overview

Introduction	This chapter contains information on drugs referenced in the *PALS Provider Manual.* A summary of indications and doses of the drugs outlined in this chapter may be found in the *PALS Course Guide* (Part 10: Pharmacology).
Drug Doses	The scientific basis for the pharmacologic treatment of seriously ill or injured infants and children is dynamic. Advances in management options and drug therapies occur rapidly. Readers are advised to check for changes in recommended doses, indications, and contraindications in the following sources: *Currents in Emergency Cardiovascular Care,* which is available at http://www.americanheart.org/cpr, the ECC Handbook, and the package insert product information sheet for each drug and medical device.
Note	This chapter contains selected pharmacology information. The focus of this information is the pharmacology of these agents when used for the treatment of seriously ill or injured children. The chapter contents should not be considered complete information on the pharmacology of these drugs.

Adenosine

Classification: Antiarrhythmic
Indications: SVT
Available Forms: Injection: 3 mg/mL
Dose and Administration:

SVT		
IV/IO	First dose	0.1 mg/kg IV/IO *rapid* push (maximum dose 6 mg)
	Second dose	0.2 mg/kg IV/IO *rapid* push (maximum dose 12 mg)

Actions:

- Stimulates adenosine receptors in heart and vascular smooth muscle
- Briefly blocks conduction through AV node
  - Interrupts reentry pathways through AV node
  - Allows return of normal sinus rhythm in patients with SVT, including SVT associated with Wolff-Parkinson-White (WPW) Syndrome
- Depresses sinus node automaticity

Pharmacokinetics:

Absorption	(not applicable with IV/IO route of administration)
Distribution	erythrocytes, vascular endothelium
Metabolism	erythrocytes, endothelium rapidly take up and metabolize adenosine
Excretion	urine
Half-life	≤10 seconds

Pharmacodynamics:

IV/IO

- Onset—rapid if given by rapid bolus
- Peak—unknown
- Duration—usually <1 minute

Monitoring: Monitor blood pressure frequently and ECG continuously.
Adverse Effects:

CNS	lightheadedness, dizziness, arm tingling, numbness, apprehension, blurred vision, headache
EENT	metallic taste, throat tightness
RESP	dyspnea, hyperventilation, bronchospasm
CV	hypotension, transient bradycardia or asystole, atrial tachyarrhythmias, angina, palpitations
GI	nausea
SKIN	facial flushing, sweating

Special Considerations:

- If possible record rhythm strip during administration.
- Administer via central venous access if present, otherwise by IV/IO site most proximal in extremity.
- Push adenosine rapidly IV/IO followed immediately by NS flush (5 to 10 mL).
- Theophylline is an adenosine receptor antagonist and reduces adenosine effectiveness.

Albumin

Classification: Blood product derivative (plasma volume expander)
Indications:

- Shock
- Trauma
- Burns

Available Forms: Injection: 5% (5 g/100 mL), 25% (25 g/100 mL)
Dose and Administration:

Shock, Trauma, Burns	
IV/IO	0.5 to 1 g/kg IV/IO by *rapid* infusion (10 to 20 mL/kg of 5% solution)

Actions:

- Expands intravascular volume through colloid oncotic effect. As a large molecule, albumin is more likely to remain in the intravascular space for a longer time than administered crystalloid. Oncotic effect may help expand the intravascular space by pulling water from the extravascular compartment.
- Supports preload and cardiac output.

Pharmacokinetics:

Absorption	(not applicable with IV/IO route of administration)
Distribution	initially to intravascular space, then throughout extracellular space at a rate affected by capillary permeability
Metabolism	liver
Excretion	unknown
Half-life	variable (affected by clinical setting); usually <24 hours

Pharmacodynamics:

IV/IO

- Onset—15 to 30 minutes
- Peak—unknown
- Duration—unknown

Monitoring: Monitor cardiorespiratory function and systemic perfusion.
Adverse effects:

RESP	pulmonary edema, increased respiratory rate, bronchospasm
CV	fluid overload, hypotension, tachycardia, hypertension (if fluid overload)
SKIN	rash, urticaria, flushing
MISC	fever

Precautions:

- Monitor for signs of pulmonary edema. Albumin binds calcium, so rapid infusions may decrease ionized calcium concentration, leading to hypotension.
- Albumin also binds many drugs, such as phenytoin, which may reduce free drug concentration and therapeutic effect. Albumin infusion may lead to increase in serum sodium concentration because it is prepared in NS.

Special Considerations:

- Blood product—transfusion-like reactions rarely occur.
- For IV administration, use within 4 hours of opening vial.
- The 5% albumin is generally used undiluted. The 25% albumin may be given undiluted or diluted in NS.

Albuterol

Classification: Bronchodilator, β_2-adrenergic agent
Indications:

- Asthma
- Anaphylaxis (bronchospasm)
- Hyperkalemia

Available Forms:

- Nebulized solution: 0.5% (5 mg/mL)
- Prediluted nebulized solution: 0.63 mg/3 mL NS, 1.25 mg/3 mL NS, 2.5 mg/3 mL NS (0.083%)
- Metered-dose inhaler (MDI): 90 µg/puff

Dose and Administration:

Asthma, Anaphylaxis (mild to moderate), Hyperkalemia		
MDI		4 to 8 puffs (inhalation) q 20 minutes PRN with spacer
Nebulizer	weight <20 kg	2.5 mg/dose (inhalation) q 20 minutes
	weight >20 kg	5 mg/dose (inhalation) q 20 minutes
Asthma, Anaphylaxis (severe)		
Continuous nebulizer		0.5 mg/kg per hour continuous inhalation (maximum dose 20 mg/h)
MDI (recommended if intubated)		4 to 8 puffs (inhalation) via ETT q 20 minutes PRN or with spacer if not intubated

Action: Stimulates β_2-adrenergic receptors, causing bronchodilation, tachycardia, vasodilation, movement of potassium from extracellular to intracellular space (serum potassium will fall).
Pharmacokinetics:

Absorption	well absorbed
Distribution	unknown
Metabolism	liver (extensive), tissues
Excretion	urine
Half-life	3 to 8 hours

Pharmacodynamics:

Inhalation

- Onset—5 to 15 minutes
- Peak—1 to 1½ hours
- Duration—4 to 6 hours

Monitoring:

- Monitor SpO_2, blood pressure, breath sounds, and ECG continuously.
- Consider checking potassium concentration, especially if low prior to administration or if high doses of albuterol used.

Adverse Effects:

CNS	tremors, anxiety, insomnia, headache, dizziness, hallucinations, altered smell
EENT	dry nose and throat, irritation of nose and throat, bad taste
RESP	cough, wheezing, dyspnea, bronchospasm (these side effects are rare)
CV	palpitations, tachycardia, hypertension, angina, hypotension, arrhythmias
GI	heartburn, nausea, vomiting, diarrhea
SKIN	flushing, sweating, angioedema

Contraindications: Tachyarrhythmias, severe cardiac disease, or hypersensitivity to albuterol or adrenergic amines

Special Considerations:

- May be combined in same nebulizer with ipratropium bromide
- Increased risk of tachyarrhythmias when combined with theophylline or simultaneous use of other adrenergic agents (eg, terbulatine, dopamine)

Alprostadil (PGE_1)

Classification: Vasodilator, prostaglandin
Indications: Ductal-dependent congenital heart disease (to maintain patency of ductus arteriosus)

- Cyanotic lesions (eg, transposition of great vessels, tricuspid atresia, tetralogy of Fallot)
- Left heart or ascending aortic obstructive lesions (eg, hypoplastic left heart syndrome, critical aortic stenosis, coarctation of aorta, interrupted aortic arch)

Available Forms: Injection: 500 µg/mL
Dose and Administration:

Ductal-Dependent Congenital Heart Disease (all forms)		
IV/IO	Initial	0.05 to 0.1 µg/kg per minute IV/IO infusion
	Maintenance	0.01 to 0.05 µg/kg per minute IV/IO infusion

Actions:

- Acts through PGE_1 receptors to cause vasodilation of *all* arteries and arterioles (including ductus arteriosus)
- Inhibits platelet aggregation
- Stimulates uterine and intestinal smooth muscle

Pharmacokinetics:

Absorption	(not applicable with IV/IO route of administration)
Distribution	wide
Metabolism	endothelium in the lung (90% metabolized in one passage)
Excretion	urine
Half-life	5 to 10 minutes

Pharmacodynamics:

IV/IO

- Onset—within seconds
- Peak—<1 hour (cyanotic lesions); several hours (acyanotic lesions)

Monitoring: Monitor SpO_2, respiratory rate, blood pressure, ECG, and temperature continuously.

Adverse Effects:

CNS	seizures
RESP	apnea (common complication), bronchospasm
CV	vasodilation (common), hypotension, bradycardia, tachycardia, cardiac arrest
GI	gastric outlet obstruction, diarrhea
GU	renal failure
MS	cortical proliferation of long bones (after prolonged treatment, seen as periosteal new bone formation on x-ray)
SKIN	flushing, edema, urticaria
ENDO	hypoglycemia
HEME	disseminated intravascular coagulation, leukocytosis, hemorrhage, thrombocytopenia
ELECT	hypocalcemia
MISC	fever (common)

Precautions:

- Higher dose is associated with increased risk of adverse effects.
- Extravasation may cause tissue sloughing and necrosis.

Special Considerations:

- Drug may also be given via umbilical arterial catheter (UAC) positioned near ductus arteriosus.
- Prostaglandin E_1 should be refrigerated until administered.
- One method for infusion preparation is to multiply 0.3 by the infant's weight in kilograms. The result is the number of milligrams of prostaglandin to add to sufficient diluent (D_5W or NS) to create a solution totaling 50 mL. An infusion rate of 0.5 mL/h controlled by an infusion pump will deliver 0.05 µg/kg per minute.

Amiodarone

Classification: Antiarrhythmic (Class III)

- SVT
- VT (with pulses)
- Pulseless arrest (VF/pulseless VT)

Available Forms: Injection: 50 mg/mL, 15 mg/mL (aqueous solution without benzyl alcohol and polysorbate 80)

Dose and Administration:

SVT, VT (with pulses)	
IV/IO	5 mg/kg IV/IO *load* over 20 to 60 minutes (maximum dose 300 mg), repeat to maximum daily dose 15 mg/kg (2.2 g in adolescents)
Pulseless Arrest (VF/pulseless VT)	
IV/IO	5 mg/kg IV/IO *bolus* (maximum dose 300 mg), can repeat to maximum daily dose 15 mg/kg (2.2 g in adolescents)

Actions:

- Prolongs action potential duration and effective refractory period
- Slows sinus rate
- Prolongs PR and QT intervals
- Noncompetitively inhibits α-adrenergic and β-adrenergic receptors

Pharmacokinetics:

Absorption	(not applicable with IV/IO route of administration)
Distribution	wide
Metabolism	liver
Excretion	bile/feces, urine (minimal)
Half-life	15 to 50 days (oral doses have very long half-life)

Pharmacodynamics:

IV/IO

- Onset—within hours
- Peak—2 to 3 days
- Duration—2 weeks to months after stopping drug

Monitoring: Monitor blood pressure and ECG continuously.

Adverse Effects:

CNS	headache, dizziness, involuntary movement, tremors, peripheral neuropathy, malaise, fatigue, ataxia, paresthesias, syncope
RESP	pulmonary fibrosis, pulmonary inflammation, ARDS (Note: Gasping was reported in neonates as a complication of the benzyl alcohol preservative in non–water soluble form of the drug; water soluble product is not associated with this problem)
CV	*main toxicity:* hypotension, bradycardia, SA node dysfunction, sinus arrest, CHF, prolonged QT interval, torsades de pointes
GI	nausea, vomiting, diarrhea, abdominal pain
SKIN	rash, photosensitivity, blue-gray skin discoloration, alopecia, ecchymosis, toxic epidermal necrolysis, flushing
ENDO	hyperthyroidism, hypothyroidism (common with chronic use)
HEME	coagulation abnormalities

Precautions:

- Routine administration in combination with procainamide (or other agents that prolong QT interval) is *not* recommended without expert consultation.
- Use with caution if hepatic failure is present.
- Amiodarone inhibits cytochrome P450 system and therefore can increase drug concentration and risk of toxicity of a number of agents (eg, diltiazem).

Contraindications: Sinus node dysfunction, 2nd degree or 3rd degree AV block

Special Considerations: Because of its long half-life and potential drug interactions, consultation with a cardiologist is encouraged before using amiodarone outside of the cardiac arrest setting.

Atropine

Classification: Anticholinergic
Indications:

- Symptomatic bradycardia (usually secondary to vagal stimulation)
- Toxins/overdose (eg, organophosphate, carbamate)
- Rapid sequence intubation (RSI): (ie, age <1 year, age 1 to 5 years receiving succinylcholine, age >5 years receiving second dose of succinylcholine)

Available Forms: Injection: 0.05, 0.1, 0.3, 0.4, 0.5, 0.8, 1 mg/mL
Dose and Administration:

Bradycardia (symptomatic)		
IV/IO	0.02 mg/kg IV/IO (minimum dose 0.1 mg, maximum single dose for child is 0.5 mg, maximum single dose for adolescent is 1 mg). May repeat dose once (maximum total dose for child is 1 mg, maximum total dose for adolescent is 2 mg). Larger doses may be needed for treatment of organophosphate poisoning.	
ET	0.04 to 0.06 mg/kg ET	
Toxins/Overdose (eg, organophosphate, carbamate)		
IV/IO	<12 years	0.02 to 0.05 mg/kg IV/IO initially, then repeated IV/IO q 20 to 30 min until muscarinic symptoms reverse
	>12 years	0.05 mg/kg IV/IO initially, then 1 to 2 mg IV/IO q 20 to 30 min until muscarinic symptoms reverse
RSI		
IV/IO	0.01 to 0.02 mg/kg IV/IO (minimum dose 0.1 mg, maximum dose 1 mg)	
IM	0.02 mg/kg IM	

Action:

- Blocks acetylcholine and other muscarinic agonists at parasympathetic neuroeffector sites
- Increases heart rate and cardiac output by blocking vagal stimulation
- Reduces saliva production and increases saliva viscosity
- Causes mydriasis

Pharmacokinetics:

Absorption	(not applicable with IV/IO route of administration)
Distribution	crosses blood-brain barrier
Metabolism	liver
Excretion	urine, unchanged (70% to 90%)
Half-life	2 to 4 hours (longer if age <2 years)

Pharmacodynamics:

IV/IO

- Onset—2 to 4 minutes
- Peak—2 to 4 minutes
- Duration—2 to 6 hours

Monitoring: Monitor SpO_2, blood pressure, and ECG continuously.
Adverse Effects:

CNS	headache, dizziness, involuntary movement, confusion, psychosis, anxiety, coma, flushing, drowsiness, weakness
EENT	blurred vision, photophobia, glaucoma, eye pain, pupil dilation, nasal congestion, dry mouth, altered taste
CV	tachycardia, hypotension, paradoxical bradycardia, angina, premature ventricular contractions, hypertension
GI	nausea, vomiting, abdominal pain, constipation, paralytic ileus, abdominal distention
GU	urinary retention, dysuria
SKIN	rash, urticaria, contact dermatitis, dry skin, flushing, decreased sweating

Precautions:

- To avoid paradoxical bradycardia, do not use less than the minimum dose (ie, 0.1 mg).
- Document clearly if used for patients with head injury, because atropine will distort pupillary exam (causing pupil dilation).

Contraindications: Angle closure glaucoma, tachyarrhythmias, thyrotoxicosis
Special Considerations:

- Drug blocks bradycardic response to hypoxia. Monitor SpO_2 with pulse oximetry.
- Use drug in any child with bradycardia at time of endotracheal intubation.
- Consider using drug to prevent increased oral secretions if ketamine is used.
- Consider using drug to prevent bradycardia when succinylcholine is used in an infant or young child, especially in the presence of hypoxia and acidosis.

Calcium Chloride

Classification: Electrolyte
Indications:

- Hypocalcemia
- Hyperkalemia
- Consider for treatment of hypermagnesemia
- Consider for treatment of calcium channel blocker overdose

Available Forms: Injection: 100 mg/mL (10%)
Dose and Administration:

Hypocalcemia, Hyperkalemia, Hypermagnesemia, Calcium Channel Blocker Overdose	
IV/IO	20 mg/kg (0.2 mL/kg) IV/IO *slow* push during cardiac arrest (if hypocalcemia known or suspected); may repeat if documented or suspected clinical indication persists. Infuse over 30 to 60 minutes for other indications.

Actions:

- Needed for maintenance of nervous, muscular, skeletal systems, enzyme reactions, normal cardiac contractility, blood coagulation
- Affects secretory activity of endocrine and exocrine glands

Pharmacokinetics:

Absorption	(not applicable with IV/IO route of administration)
Distribution	extracellular
Metabolism	liver, bone uptake
Excretion	feces (80%), urine (20%)
Half-life	unknown

Pharmacodynamics:

IV/IO

- Onset—immediate
- Peak—rapid
- Duration—variable

Monitoring: Monitor blood pressure and ECG.

Adverse Effects (note that overdose can produce hypercalcemia and its signs):

CV	hypotension, bradycardia, asystole, shortened QT interval, heart block, cardiac arrest, arrhythmias
SKIN	sclerosis of peripheral veins, venous thrombosis, burn/necrosis (occurs with infiltration of surrounding tissue)
ELECT	hypercalcemia (with overdose)

Precautions:

- Do not use routinely during resuscitation (may contribute to cellular injury).
- Drug is not recommended for routine treatment of asystole or PEA unless hypocalcemia is suspected or documented.
- Avoid rapid administration (may cause adverse cardiovascular effects—eg, bradycardia—particularly if patient is receiving digoxin).

Contraindications: Hypercalcemia, digitalis toxicity, VF (except in the setting of suspected hyperkalemia)

Special Considerations:

- A dose of 20 mg/kg of calcium chloride 10% (0.2 mL/kg) IV or IO is equivalent to 5.4 mg/kg of elemental calcium.
- Central venous administration is preferred if available.
- When infusing calcium and sodium bicarbonate emergently, flush the tubing with NS before and after infusion of each drug to avoid formation of an insoluble precipitate in the catheter lumen.

Dexamethasone

Classification: Corticosteroid

Indications:

- Croup (mild to severe)
- Asthma (mild to moderate)
- Vasogenic cerebral edema (eg, from brain tumor or abscess)

Available Forms:

- Injection: 4, 10 mg/mL
- Elixir: 0.5 mg/5 mL
- Oral solution: 0.1, 1 mg/mL

Dose and Administration:

Croup	
Moderate to severe	0.6 mg/kg PO/IM/IV × 1 dose (maximum dose 16 mg)
Impending respiratory failure	0.6 mg/kg IV (maximum dose 16 mg)
Asthma	
Mild to moderate	0.6 mg/kg PO/IM/IV q 24 hours × 2 doses (maximum dose 16 mg)
Vasogenic Cerebral Edema	
	1 to 2 mg/kg IV/IO *load,* then 1 to 1.5 mg/kg per day divided every 4 to 6 hours (maximum daily dose 16 mg)

Actions:

- Reduces the number and activation of lymphocytes, eosinophils, mast cells, and macrophages and downregulates production and release of proinflammatory cytokines
- Inhibits vascular leak induced by proinflammatory mediators
- Restores disrupted endothelium tight junctions
- Increases expression of β-adrenergic receptors on cell surface, helping to restore responsiveness to catecholamines

Pharmacokinetics:

Absorption	rapid absorption through oral and IM routes (not applicable with IV/IO route of administration)
Distribution	wide distribution; acts at intracellular receptor
Metabolism	liver
Excretion	urine, bile/feces
Half-life	3 to 4½ hours for clearance; pharmacologic effect is much longer

Pharmacodynamics:

	PO	**IM**
Onset	1 hour	<1 hour
Peak	1 to 2 hours	8 hours
Duration	2½ days	6 days

Monitoring: Monitor SpO_2, blood pressure, and ECG.

Adverse Effects:

CNS	depression, headache, irritability, insomnia, euphoria, seizures, psychosis, hallucinations, weakness
EENT	fungal infections, increased intraocular pressure, blurred vision
CV	hypertension, thrombophlebitis, embolism, tachycardia, edema
GI	diarrhea, nausea, abdominal distention, pancreatitis
MS	fractures, osteoporosis
SKIN	flushing, sweating, acne, poor wound healing, ecchymosis, petechiae, hirsutism
ENDO	hypothalamic-pituitary-adrenal axis suppression, hyperglycemia, sodium and fluid retention
HEME	hemorrhage, thrombocytopenia
ELECT	hypokalemia

Special Considerations: Use for more than a few days can cause hypertension and hyperglycemia and increased risk of gastric bleeding.

Dextrose (Glucose)

Classification: Carbohydrate
Indications: Hypoglycemia
Available Forms: Injection: D_5W (0.05 g/mL), $D_{10}W$ (0.1 g/mL), $D_{50}W$ (0.5 g/mL)
Dose and Administration:

Hypoglycemia	
IV/IO	0.5 to 1 g/kg IV/IO

Concentration	*Dose*
$D_{50}W$	1 to 2 mL/kg
$D_{25}W$	2 to 4 mL/kg
$D_{10}W$	5 to 10 mL/kg
D_5W	10 to 20 mL/kg

Action: Essential for cellular respiration, the process by which chemical energy of "food" molecules is metabolized to produce ATP
Monitoring: Use rapid glucose test to rapidly confirm suspicion of hypoglycemia and monitor response to therapy.
Adverse Effects:

SKIN	sclerosis of veins (with hypertonic glucose concentrations)
ENDO	hyperglycemia, hyperosmolarity

Precautions: Do not administer drug routinely during resuscitation unless hypoglycemia is documented.
Special Considerations:

- Bolus glucose therapy for treatment of documented hypoglycemia should generally be followed by a continuous glucose infusion.
- Maximum recommended concentration for bolus administration is $D_{25}W$ (can be prepared by mixing $D_{50}W$ 1:1 with sterile water).
- Maximum concentration for newborn administration is $D_{12.5}W$ (0.125 g/mL).

Diphenhydramine

Classification: Antihistamine
Indications: Anaphylactic shock (after administration of epinephrine)
Available Forms: Injection: 10, 50 mg/mL
Dose and Administration:

Anaphylactic Shock	
IV/IO/IM	1 to 2 mg/kg IV/IO/IM q 4 to 6 hours (maximum dose 50 mg)

Actions:

- Competes with histamine for H_1-receptor sites
- Decreases allergic response by blocking histamine

Pharmacokinetics:

Absorption	(not applicable with IV/IO route of administration)
Distribution	wide
Metabolism	liver (95%)
Excretion	urine
Half-life	2 to 8 hours

Pharmacodynamics:

	IM	IV/IO
Onset	30 minutes	immediate
Peak	1 to 4 hours	unknown
Duration	4 to 8 hours	4 to 8 hours

Monitoring: Monitor Spo_2 and blood pressure continuously.

Adverse Effects:

CNS	dizziness, drowsiness, poor coordination, fatigue, anxiety, euphoria, confusion, paresthesia, neuritis, seizures, dystonic reaction, hallucinations, sedation (can cause paradoxical excitation in children)
EENT	blurred vision, pupil dilation, tinnitus, nasal stuffiness, dry nose/mouth/throat
CV	hypotension, palpitations, tachycardia
RESP	chest tightness
GI	nausea, vomiting, diarrhea
GU	urinary retention, dysuria, frequency
SKIN	photosensitivity, rash
HEME	thrombocytopenia, agranulocytosis, hemolytic anemia
MISC	anaphylaxis

Precautions: Drug may exacerbate angle closure glaucoma, hyperthyroidism, peptic ulcer, and urinary tract obstruction.

Dobutamine

Classification: Catecholamine, β-adrenergic agent

Indications:

- Congestive heart failure
- Cardiogenic shock

Available Forms:

- Injection: 12.5 mg/mL
- Premixed dilutions: 1 mg/mL, 2 mg/mL, 4 mg/mL

Dose and Administration:

Congestive Heart Failure, Cardiogenic Shock	
IV/IO	2 to 20 μg/kg per minute IV/IO infusion (titrated to desired effect)

Actions:

- Stimulates β_1-receptors (predominant effect)
  - Increases heart rate (SA node effect)
  - Increases myocardial contractility, automaticity, and conduction velocity (ventricular effect)
- Stimulates β_2-receptors, which increases heart rate and causes vasodilation
- Stimulates and inhibits α-receptors, which tend to cancel out vasoconstriction, but dobutamine has intrinsic α-adrenergic blocking effects, increasing the risk of hypotension from vasodilation

Pharmacokinetics:

Absorption	(not applicable with IV/IO route of administration)
Distribution	extracellular fluid
Metabolism	liver, kidney
Excretion	urine
Half-life	2 minutes

Pharmacodynamics:

IV/IO

- Onset—1 to 2 minutes
- Peak—10 minutes
- Duration—<10 minutes when infusion stopped

Monitoring: Monitor blood pressure and ECG continuously.
Adverse Effects:

CNS	anxiety, headache, dizziness
CV	hypotension, hypertension, palpitations, tachyarrhythmias, premature ventricular contractions, angina
GI	nausea, vomiting, mucositis
HEME	myelosuppression, neutropenia, thrombocytopenia, anemia

Precautions:

- Extravasation of dobutamine may produce tissue ischemia and necrosis.
- Do not mix with sodium bicarbonate.

Special Considerations:

- Drug is inactivated in alkaline solutions.
- Consider carefully in vasodilated septic shock because drug tends to further lower systemic vascular resistance.

Dopamine

Classification: Catecholamine, vasopressor, inotrope
Indications:

- Cardiogenic shock
- Distributive shock

Available Forms:

- Injection: 40, 80, 160 mg/mL
- Prediluted in D_5W: 0.8, 1.6, 3.2 mg/mL

Dose and Administration:

Cardiogenic Shock, Distributive Shock	
IV/IO	2 to 20 μg/kg per minute IV/IO infusion (titrate to desired effect)

Actions:

- Stimulates α-adrenergic receptors
  - Increases SVR (via constriction of arterioles)
- Stimulates β_1-adrenergic receptors
  - Increases heart rate (SA node effect)
  - Increases myocardial contractility, automaticity, and conduction velocity (ventricular effect)
- Stimulates β_2-adrenergic receptors
  - Increases heart rate
  - Lowers systemic vascular resistance
- Stimulates dopaminergic receptors
  - Causes renal and splanchnic vasodilation
  - Increases renal sodium and water loss by direct renal tubular action

Pharmacokinetics:

Absorption	(not applicable with IV/IO route of administration)
Distribution	extracellular space
Metabolism	liver, kidney
Excretion	urine
Half-life	2 minutes

Pharmacodynamics:

IV/IO

- Onset—1 to 2 minutes
- Peak—10 minutes
- Duration—<10 minutes when infusion stopped

Monitoring: Monitor blood pressure and ECG.

Adverse Effects:

CNS	headache
RESP	dyspnea
CV	palpitations, premature ventricular contractions, SVT, VT, hypertension, peripheral vasoconstriction
GI	nausea, vomiting, diarrhea
GU	acute renal failure
SKIN	local necrosis (with infiltration), gangrene

Precautions:

- High infusion rates (>20 μg/kg per minute) may produce peripheral, renal, and splanchnic vasoconstriction and ischemia.
- Do not mix with sodium bicarbonate.
- Thyroid function may be affected with prolonged use because dopamine may inhibit TSH release.

Special Considerations:

- High concentrations and large-volume infusions should be administered via a central venous catheter.
- Drug is inactivated in alkaline solutions.
- Effects are dose dependent: low infusions (1 to 5 μg/kg per minute) usually stimulate dopaminergic and β-adrenergic receptors; α-adrenergic effects become more prominent as infusion rate is increased.

Epinephrine

Classification: Catecholamine, vasopressor, inotrope

Indications:

- Anaphylaxis
- Asthma
- Bradycardia (symptomatic)
- Croup
- Pulseless arrest
- Shock (hypotensive)
- Toxins/overdose (eg, β-adrenergic blocker, calcium channel blocker)

Available Forms:

- Injection: 1:1000 aqueous (1 mg/mL), 1:10 000 aqueous (0.1 mg/mL)
- IM auto-injector: 0.3 mg (0.3 mL 1:1000 solution)
- Child IM junior auto-injector (for patient weight 10 to 30 kg): 0.15 mg (0.3 mL 1:2000 solution)
- Racemic solution: 2.25%

Dose and Administration:

Anaphylaxis	
IM	0.01 mg/kg (0.01 mL/kg) 1:1000 IM in thigh q 15 minutes PRN (maximum dose 0.5 mg) or
	IM auto-injector 0.3 mg (for patient weight ≥30 kg) or child IM junior auto-injector 0.15 mg (for patient weight 10 to 30 kg)
IV/IO	• 0.01 mg/kg (0.1 mL/kg) 1:10 000 IV/IO q 3 to 5 minutes (maximum dose 1 mg) if hypotension • If hypotension persists despite fluid administration and IV/IO injection, consider continuous IV/IO infusion of 0.1 to 1 μg/kg per minute
Asthma	
SQ	0.01 mg/kg (0.01 mL/kg) 1:1000 SQ q 15 minutes (maximum dose 0.5 mg; 0.5 mL)
Bradycardia (symptomatic)	
IV/IO	0.01 mg/kg (0.1 mL/kg) 1:10 000 IV/IO q 3 to 5 minutes (maximum dose 1 mg; 1 mL)
Croup	
Nebulizer	• 0.25 mL racemic solution (2.25%) mixed in 3 mL NS by inhaled nebulizer if moderate to severe illness (ie, stridor at rest) in infants or young children; up to 0.5 mL mixed in 3 mL NS for older children *or* • 3 mL 1:1000 by inhaled nebulizer (can mix in 3 mL NS)
Pulseless Arrest	
IV/IO	0.01 mg/kg (0.1 mL/kg) 1:10 000 IV/IO q 3 to 5 minutes (maximum IV/IO dose 1 mg)
ET	0.1 mg/kg (0.1 mL/kg) 1:1000 ET q 3 to 5 minutes

Shock (hypotensive)	
IV/IO infusion	0.1 to 1 μg/kg per minute IV/IO infusion (consider higher doses if needed)
Toxins/Overdose (eg, β-adrenergic blocker, calcium channel blocker)	
IV/IO	0.01 mg/kg (0.1 mL/kg) 1:10 000 IV/IO (maximum IV/IO dose 1 mg); if no response, consider higher doses up to 0.1 mg/kg (0.1 mL/kg) 1:1000 IV/IO
IV/IO infusion	0.1 to 1 μg/kg per minute IV/IO infusion (consider higher doses if hypotension refractory to this dose)

Actions:

- Stimulates α-adrenergic receptors at higher infusion rates, usually >0.3 μg/kg per minute *in infants and young children.* Older children need lower infusion rates to achieve vasoconstriction (response is dose-dependent but difficult to predict in individual patients).
  - Increases SVR (via constriction of arterioles, recognized by increase in diastolic blood pressure)
- Stimulates β_1-adrenergic receptors
  - Increases heart rate (SA node effect)
  - Increases myocardial contractility, automaticity, and conduction velocity (SA node, AV node, and ventricular effect)
- Stimulates β_2-adrenergic receptors (predominates at lower infusion rates, usually ≤0.3 μg/kg per minute)
  - Increases heart rate (SA node effect)
  - Causes bronchodilation
  - Causes vasodilation of arterioles; recognize fall in SVR by decrease in diastolic blood pressure. Data suggests that vasodilation preferentially occurs in the skeletal muscle vascular beds and infusion may result in a relative decrease in splanchnic perfusion when used in shock.

Pharmacokinetics:

Absorption	IM absorption is affected by perfusion (not applicable with IV/IO route of administration)
Distribution	unknown
Metabolism	liver, kidney, endothelium
Excretion	unknown
Half-life	2 to 4 minutes

Pharmacodynamics:

	IM	IV/IO	(Inhalation)
Onset	5 to 10 minutes	immediate	1 minute
Peak	unknown	within 1 minute	unknown

Monitoring: Monitor SpO_2, blood pressure, and ECG continuously.

Adverse Effects:

CNS	tremors, anxiety, insomnia, headache, dizziness, weakness, drowsiness, confusion, hallucinations, intracranial hemorrhage (from severe hypertension)
RESP	dyspnea
CV	arrhythmias (especially tachyarrhythmias, eg, SVT and VT), palpitations, tachycardia, hypertension, ST-segment elevation, postresuscitation myocardial dysfunction
GI	nausea, vomiting
GU	renal vascular ischemia
ENDO	hyperglycemia, postresuscitation hyperadrenergic state

ELECT	hypokalemia (direct effect to move potassium intracellularly resulting from β_2-adrenergic stimulation; may be used to treat hyperkalemia)
MISC	increased lactate (ie, independent of any change in organ perfusion as part of the gluconeogenesis response, making use of lactate as a marker of ischemia more difficult)

Precautions:

- High doses produce vasoconstriction and may compromise organ perfusion.
- Low doses may increase cardiac output with redirection of blood flow to skeletal muscles and decrease renal and splanchnic blood flow.
- Myocardial oxygen requirements are increased (due to increased heart rate, myocardial contractility, and with higher doses, increased SVR).
- Tissue ischemia and necrosis may result if IV infiltration occurs.
- Central venous access is preferred for administration.
- Catecholamines are inactivated in alkaline solutions.
- Observe at least 2 hours post croup treatment for "rebound" (ie, recurrence of stridor).

Contraindications: Cocaine-induced VT

Special Considerations: When given IM in anaphylaxis, data shows that best absorption occurs from thigh rather than deltoid muscle injection. Subcutaneous administration is not recommended for treatment of anaphylaxis because absorption is delayed when compared with IM route.

Furosemide

Classification: Loop diuretic

Indications:

- Pulmonary edema
- Fluid overload

Available Forms: Injection: 10 mg/mL

Dose and Administration:

Pulmonary Edema, Fluid Overload	
IV/IM	1 mg/kg IV/IM (usual maximum dose 20 mg for patient not chronically on loop diuretics)

Actions:

- Acts on ascending limb of loop of Henle inhibiting reabsorption of sodium and chloride, causing excretion of sodium, chloride, calcium, magnesium, and water; increased potassium excretion occurs in distal tubule in exchange for sodium
- Increases excretion of potassium in distal tubule as indirect effect

Pharmacokinetics:

Absorption	IM absorption not documented (not applicable with IV/IO route of administration)
Distribution	unknown
Metabolism	liver (30% to 40%); most excreted unchanged
Excretion	urine, feces
Half-life	½ to 1 hour

Pharmacodynamics:

	PO	IM	IV
Onset	½ to 1 hour	½ hour	5 minutes
Peak	1 to 2 hours	Unknown	½ hour
Duration	6 to 8 hours	4 to 8 hours	2 hours

Monitoring:

- Monitor blood pressure and ECG.
- Monitor blood glucose, BUN, uric acid, CBC, ABG.
- Monitor electrolytes: potassium, sodium, chloride, calcium, magnesium, and total CO_2.

Adverse Effects:

CNS	headache, fatigue, weakness, vertigo, paresthesias
EENT	hearing loss, ear pain, tinnitus, blurred vision, dry mouth, oral irritation
CV	orthostatic hypotension, angina, ECG changes (from electrolyte abnormalities), circulatory collapse
GI	nausea, vomiting, diarrhea, abdominal cramps, gastric irritation, pancreatitis
GU	polyuria, renal failure, glycosuria
MS	muscle cramps, stiffness
SKIN	pruritus, purpura, Stevens-Johnson syndrome, sweating, photosensitivity, urticaria
ENDO	hyperglycemia
HEME	thrombocytopenia, agranulocytosis, leucopenia, anemia, neutropenia
ELECT	hypokalemia, hypochloremia, hypomagnesemia, hyperuricemia, hypocalcemia, hyponatremia
MISC	metabolic alkalosis

Special Considerations: Hypokalemia may be significant and requires close monitoring and replacement therapy.

Hydrocortisone

Classification: Corticosteroid
Indications: Adrenal insufficiency (may be associated with septic shock)
Available Forms: Sodium succinate injectable in 100, 250, 500, 1000 mg/vial
Dose and Administration:

Adrenal Insufficiency	
IV/IO	2 mg/kg IV/IO bolus (maximum dose 100 mg)

Actions:

- Reduces the number and activation of lymphocytes, eosinophils, mast cells, and macrophages, which downregulates the production and release of proinflammatory cytokines
- Inhibits vascular leak induced by proinflammatory mediators
- Restores disrupted endothelial tight junctions
- Decreases mucus secretion
- Increases expression of β-adrenergic receptors on cell surface, helping to restore responsiveness to catecholamines

Pharmacokinetics:

Absorption	(not applicable with IV/IO route of administration)
Distribution	widely distributed; acts at intracellular receptor
Metabolism	liver (extensive)
Excretion	urine
Half-life	3 to 5 hours

Pharmacodynamics:

IV/IO

- Onset—rapid
- Peak—unknown
- Duration—8 to 24 hours

Adverse Effects:

CNS	depression, headache, mood changes
EENT	fungal infections, increased intraocular pressure, blurred vision
CV	hypertension
GI	diarrhea, nausea, abdominal distention, peptic ulcer
MS	fractures, osteoporosis, weakness
SKIN	flushing, sweating, thrombophlebitis, edema, acne, poor wound healing, ecchymosis, petechiae, pruritis
ENDO	hyperglycemia, suppression of hypothalamic-pituitary axis
HEME	hemorrhage, thrombocytopenia, hypercoagulability
MISC	increased risk of infection

Special Considerations: Consider measuring cortisol concentration before use in children with shock. Some centers perform a cosyntropin stimulation test before hydrocortisone administration.

Inamrinone

Classification: Phosphodiesterase inhibitor, inodilator
Indications: Myocardial dysfunction and increased SVR/PVR (eg, cardiogenic shock with high SVR, postcardiac surgery CHF)
Available Forms: Injection: 5 mg/mL
Dose and Administration:

Myocardial Dysfunction and Increased SVR/PVR	
IV/IO	loading dose of 0.75 to 1 mg/kg IV/IO slow bolus over 5 minutes (give over longer period if patient is unstable), may repeat twice (maximum total loading dose 3 mg/kg)
	5 to 10 μg/kg per minute IV/IO infusion

Actions:

- Increases myocardial contractility
- Reduces preload and afterload by relaxation of vascular smooth muscle

Pharmacokinetics:

Absorption	(not applicable with IV/IO route of administration)
Distribution	unknown
Metabolism	liver (50%)
Excretion	urine (10% to 40% unchanged), metabolites (60% to 90%)
Half-life	2 to 10 hours

Pharmacodynamics:

IV/IO

- Onset—2 to 5 minutes
- Peak—10 minutes
- Duration—variable

Monitoring: Monitor SpO_2, blood pressure, and ECG continuously.

Adverse Effects:

RESP	hypoxemia (from increased V/Q mismatch)
CV	hypotension, arrhythmias, angina
GI	nausea, vomiting, abdominal pain, hepatotoxicity, ascites, jaundice
SKIN	allergic reactions, irritation to veins
HEME	thrombocytopenia

Precautions:

- Hypovolemia may worsen hypotensive effects of drug.
- Drug may increase platelet destruction. Thrombocytopenia is more frequent and severe with inamrinone than with milrinone.
- Drug may accumulate in renal failure and in patients with low cardiac output.
- Drug can be co-infused with dextrose solutions but should not be primarily diluted in a dextrose solution.

Special Considerations: Loading dose may cause significant hypotension. If patient is hemodynamically unstable, give the loading dose slowly and monitor blood pressure closely. Be prepared to administer isotonic crystalloid (and possible vasopressors) as needed to treat hypotension.

Ipratropium Bromide

Classification: Anticholinergic, bronchodilator

Indications: Asthma

Available Forms:

- Nebulized solution: 0.02% (500 μg/2.5 mL)
- MDI: 18 μg/puff

Dose and Administration:

Asthma	
Nebulizer	250 to 500 μg (inhaled) q 20 minutes × 3 doses

Actions:

- Blocks action of acetylcholine at parasympathetic sites in bronchial smooth muscle, resulting in bronchodilation
- Inhibits secretions from serous and seromucous glands lining the nasal mucosa

Pharmacokinetics:

Absorption	minimal
Distribution	does not cross blood-brain barrier
Metabolism	liver (minimal)
Excretion	unknown
Half-life	2 hours

Pharmacodynamics:

Inhaled (INH)

- Onset—1 to 15 minutes
- Peak—1 to 2 hours
- Duration—3 to 6 hours

Monitoring: Monitor Spo_2 continuously.

Adverse Effects:

CNS	anxiety, dizziness, headache, nervousness
EENT	dry mouth, blurred vision (pupillary dilation)
RESP	cough, worsening bronchospasm
CV	palpitations
GI	nausea, vomiting, abdominal cramps
SKIN	rash

Special Considerations:

- Ipratropium is not absorbed into the bloodstream; its cardiovascular side effects are minimal.
- Inhaled ipratropium may cause pupillary dilation due to inadvertent deposition of nebulized solution in the eyes.

Lidocaine

Classification: Antiarrhythmic (Class IB)

Indications:

- VF/pulseless VT
- Wide-complex tachycardia (with pulses)
- Rapid sequence intubation (RSI) (ie, ICP protection)

Available Forms: Injection and infusion prepared in D_5W: 0.2% (2 mg/mL), 0.4% (4 mg/mL), 0.8% (8 mg/mL)

Dose and Administration:

VF/Pulseless VT, Wide-Complex Tachycardia (with pulses)		
IV/IO	Initial	1 mg/kg IV/IO loading bolus
	Maintenance	20 to 50 µg/kg per minute IV/IO infusion (repeat bolus dose if infusion initiated >15 minutes after initial bolus therapy)
ET		2 to 3 mg/kg ET
RSI		
IV/IO	1 to 2 mg/kg IV/IO	

Actions:

- Increases electrical stimulation threshold of ventricle and His-Purkinje system (stabilizing cardiac membrane and decreasing automaticity)
- Reduces intracranial pressure through inhibition of sodium channels in neurons, which reduces metabolic activity

Pharmacokinetics:

Absorption	(not applicable with IV/IO administration)
Distribution	erythrocytes, vascular endothelium
Metabolism	liver, active metabolites
Excretion	urine
Half-life	biphasic (8 minutes, 1 to 3 hours)

Pharmacodynamics:

IV/IO

- Onset—1 to 2 minutes
- Peak—unknown
- Duration—10 to 20 minutes because of rapid redistribution; terminal elimination 1½ to 2 hours

Monitoring: Monitor blood pressure and ECG continuously.

Adverse Effects:

CNS	seizures (high concentrations), headache, dizziness, involuntary movement, confusion, tremor, drowsiness, euphoria
EENT	tinnitus, blurred vision
CV	hypotension, myocardial depression, bradycardia, heart block, arrhythmias, cardiac arrest
RESP	dyspnea, respiratory depression or arrest
GI	nausea, vomiting
SKIN	rash, urticaria, edema, swelling, phlebitis at IV site

Precautions: High plasma concentration may cause myocardial and circulatory depression.

Contraindication: Wide-complex ventricular escape beats associated with bradycardia, high-degree heart block

Special Considerations:

- Reduce infusion dose if severe CHF or low cardiac output is compromising hepatic and renal blood flow.
- Drug may decrease ICP response during laryngoscopy for RSI.
- Drug attenuates intraocular pressure response during laryngoscopy for RSI.

Magnesium Sulfate

Classification: Electrolyte, bronchodilator
Indications:

- Asthma (refractory status asthmaticus)
- Torsades de pointes
- Hypomagnesemia

Available Forms: Injection: 100 mg/mL (0.8 mEq/mL), 125 mg/mL (1 mEq/mL), 250 mg/mL (2 mEq/mL), 500 mg/mL (4 mEq/mL)
Dose and Administration:

Asthma (refractory status asthmaticus), **Torsades de Pointes, Hypomagnesemia**	
IV/IO	• 25 to 50 mg/kg IV/IO bolus in pulseless VT with torsades • 25 to 50 mg/kg IV/IO over 10 to 20 minutes for VT with pulses associated with torsades or hypomagnesemia • 25 to 50 mg/kg IV/IO by slower infusion (15 to 30 minutes) for treatment of status asthmaticus • maximum dose 2 g

Actions:

- Inhibits calcium uptake, thereby causing smooth muscle relaxation
- Exerts antiarrhythmic action

Pharmacokinetics:

Absorption	(not applicable with IV/IO route of administration)
Distribution	wide
Metabolism	taken up by cells and bone
Excretion	urine
Half-life	unknown

Pharmacodynamics:

IV/IO

- Onset—immediate
- Peak—depends on duration of infusion
- Duration—30 minutes

Monitoring: Monitor ECG continuously and SpO_2 and blood pressure frequently.
Adverse Effects (most are related to hypermagnesemia):

CNS	confusion, sedation, depressed reflexes, flaccid paralysis, weakness
RESP	respiratory depression
CV	hypotension, bradycardia, heart block, cardiac arrest (may develop with rapid administration)
GI	nausea, vomiting
MS	cramps
SKIN	flushing, sweating
ELECT	hypermagnesemia

Precautions: Rapid bolus may cause severe hypotension and bradycardia.
Contraindication: Renal failure
Special Considerations: Have calcium chloride (or calcium gluconate) available if needed to reverse magnesium toxicity.

Methylprednisolone

Classification: Corticosteroid
Indications:

- Asthma (status asthmaticus)
- Anaphylactic shock

Available Forms: Injection: 40, 125, 500, 1000, 2000 mg
Dose and Administration:

Asthma (status asthmaticus), **Anaphylactic Shock**		
IV/IO/IM	Load	2 mg/kg IV/IO/IM (maximum 80 mg) Note: must use acetate salt IM
IV	Maintenance	0.5 mg/kg IV q 6 hours or 1 mg/kg q 12 hours up to 120 mg/day

Actions:

- Reduces the number and activation of lymphocytes, eosinophils, mast cells, and macrophages, resulting in downregulation of the production and release of proinflammatory cytokines
- Inhibits vascular leak induced by proinflammatory mediators
- Restores disrupted endothelial tight junctions
- Decreases mucus secretion
- Increases expression of β-adrenergic receptors on cell surface, helping to restore responsiveness to catecholamines

Pharmacokinetics:

Absorption	(not applicable with IV/IO route of administration)
Distribution	wide distribution; binds to intracellular steroid receptor
Metabolism	liver (extensive)
Excretion	urine
Half-life	3 to 5 hours for clearance; duration of effect is longer

Pharmacodynamics:

IV/IO

- Onset: rapid
- Peak: unknown
- Duration: 1 to 2 days

Adverse Effects:

CNS	depression, headache, mood changes, weakness
CV	hypertension, embolism
GI	hemorrhage, diarrhea, nausea, abdominal distention, pancreatitis, peptic ulcer
MS	fractures, osteoporosis, arthralgia
ENDO	hyperglycemia
HEME	hemorrhage, thrombocytopenia, transient leukocytosis
MISC	anaphylaxis (rare)

Special Considerations: Acetate salt is recommended for IM use.

Milrinone

Classification: Phosphodiesterase inhibitor, inodilator

Indications: Myocardial dysfunction and increased SVR/PVR (eg, cardiogenic shock with high SVR, postcardiac surgery, CHF)

Available Forms:

- Injection: 1 mg/mL
- Premixed injection in D_5W: 200 μg/mL

Dose and Administration:

Myocardial Dysfunction and Increased SVR/PVR	
IV/IO	• Loading dose of 50 to 75 μg/kg IV/IO over 10 to 60 minutes • Infusion of 0.5 to 0.75 μg/kg per minute IV/IO

Actions:

- Increases myocardial contractility
- Reduces preload and afterload by relaxation of vascular smooth muscle

Pharmacokinetics:

Absorption	(not applicable with IV/IO route of administration)
Distribution	unknown
Metabolism	liver (12%)
Excretion	urine, unchanged (83%), metabolites (12%)
Half-life	2.4 hours

Pharmacodynamics:

IV/IO

- Onset—2 to 5 minutes
- Peak—10 minutes
- Duration—variable (1½ to 5 hours)

Monitoring:

- Monitor blood pressure and ECG continuously.
- Routinely monitor platelet count.

Adverse Effects:

CNS	headache, tremor
CV	hypotension, ventricular arrhythmias, angina
GI	nausea, vomiting, abdominal pain, hepatotoxicity, jaundice
HEME	thrombocytopenia
ELECT	hypokalemia

Precautions:

- Hypovolemia may worsen hypotensive effects of drug.
- Drug has shorter half-life and less effect on platelets compared with inamrinone.
- Drug may accumulate in patients with renal failure or low cardiac output.

Special Considerations: Longer infusion times reduce risk of hypotension.

Naloxone

Classification: Opioid receptor antagonist
Indications: Narcotic (opiate) reversal
Available Forms: Injection: 0.4, 1 mg/mL
Dose and Administration:

Narcotic (opiate) Reversal Note: Total reversal is indicated for narcotic toxicity secondary to overdose; significantly smaller doses are required for patients with respiratory depression associated with therapeutic narcotic use.
• Total reversal: 0.1 mg/kg IV/IO/IM/SQ bolus q 2 minutes PRN (maximum dose 2 mg) • Total reversal *not* required: 1 to 5 μg/kg IV/IO/IM/SQ (titrated to effect) • 0.002 to 0.16 mg/kg per hour IV/IO infusion

Action: Competes with opiates at opioid receptor sites (reversing opioid effects)
Pharmacokinetics:

Absorption	rapid absorption after IM, SQ administration (not applicable with IV/IO route of administration)
Distribution	rapid
Metabolism	liver
Excretion	urine
Half-life	1 hour (up to 3 hours in neonates)

Pharmacodynamics:

IV/IO
- Onset—1 minute
- Peak—unknown
- Duration—20 to 60 minutes (variable and dose dependent)

Monitoring: Monitor SpO_2, blood pressure, and ECG continuously.
Adverse Effects:

CNS	seizures, drowsiness, nervousness
RESP	hyperpnea, pulmonary edema
CV	VF/VT, tachycardia, hypertension, asystole (especially if total reversal dose administered)
GI	nausea, vomiting

Precautions:

- Repeat dosing is often required because half-life of naloxone is often shorter than half-life of opioid being reversed.
- Administration to infants of addicted mothers may precipitate seizures or other withdrawal symptoms.
- In overdose patients, establish effective assisted ventilation before naloxone administration to avoid excessive sympathetic reaction.
- Drug reverses effects of narcotic analgesics; consider administration of nonopioid analgesics for treatment of pain.

Special Considerations: Drug exerts some analgesic effects.

Nitroglycerin

Classification: Vasodilator, antihypertensive
Indications:

- Congestive heart failure
- Cardiogenic shock

Available Forms:

- Injection: 0.5, 5, 10 mg/mL
- Prediluted injection in D_5W: 100 μg/mL, 200 μg/mL, 400 μg/mL

Dose and Administration:

Congestive Heart Failure, Cardiogenic Shock	
IV/IO	0.25 to 0.5 μg/kg per minute IV/IO infusion, may increase by 0.5 to 1 μg/kg per minute q 3 to 5 minutes PRN to 1 to 5 μg/kg per minute (maximum dose 10 μg/kg per minute in children) In adolescents start with 10 to 20 μg *per minute* (Note: This dose is *not* per kg per minute) and increase by 5 to 10 μg per minute every 5 to 10 minutes to maximum of 200 μg *per minute*

Action: Releases nitric oxide, which stimulates cGMP production; cGMP is an intracellular messenger that results in vascular smooth muscle relaxation. Action is greatest in venous system and pulmonary vascular bed, with relatively less effect on systemic arterial resistance.

Pharmacokinetics:

Absorption	(not applicable with IV/IO route of administration)
Distribution	unknown
Metabolism	liver (extensive); no active metabolites
Excretion	urine
Half-life	1 to 4 minutes

Pharmacodynamics:

IV/IO

- Onset—1 to 2 minutes
- Peak—unknown
- Duration—3 to 5 minutes

Monitoring: Monitor blood pressure and ECG continuously.
Adverse Effects:

CNS	headache, dizziness
RESP	hypoxemia (due to increased V/Q mismatch)
CV	postural hypotension, tachycardia, cardiac arrest, syncope, paradoxical bradycardia
SKIN	flushing, pallor, sweating

Norepinephrine

Classification: Inotrope, vasopressor, catecholamine
Indications: Hypotensive (usually distributive) shock (ie, associated with low systemic vascular resistance and unresponsive to fluid resuscitation)
Available Forms: Injection: 1 mg/mL
Dose and Administration:

Hypotensive Shock	
IV/IO	0.1 to 2 μg/kg per minute IV/IO infusion (titrate to desired effect)

Actions:

- Activates α-adrenergic receptors (increased smooth muscle tone)
- Activates myocardial β_1-adrenergic receptors (increased contractility and heart rate). The heart rate effect is blunted by baroreceptor stimulation that results from the vasoconstrictive effects.

Pharmacokinetics:

Absorption	(not applicable with IV/IO route of administration)
Distribution	extracellular space
Metabolism	liver, kidney, sympathetic nerves
Excretion	urine
Half-life	2 to 4 minutes

Pharmacodynamics:

IV/IO
- Onset—<30 seconds
- Peak—5 to 10 minutes
- Duration—≤10 minutes after stopping infusion

Monitoring: Monitor blood pressure and ECG continuously.
Adverse Effects:

CNS	headache, anxiety
RESP	respiratory distress
CV	hypertension, tachycardia, bradycardia, arrhythmias
GU	renal failure
SKIN	local necrosis (infiltration)

Precautions:

- If IV infiltration occurs, may produce severe tissue ischemia and necrosis due to prominent vasoconstrictive effects.
- Do not mix with sodium bicarbonate.

Special Considerations:

- Ideally should be administered via a central venous catheter.
- Drug is inactivated in alkaline solutions.

Oxygen

Classification: Element, gas

Indications:

- Hypoxia/hypoxemia
- Respiratory distress/respiratory failure
- Shock
- Trauma
- Cardiopulmonary failure
- Cardiac arrest
- Rapid sequence intubation (RSI) (ie, preoxygenation)

Available Forms: 100%

Dose and Administration:

Hypoxia/Hypoxemia, Respiratory Distress/Respiratory Failure, Shock, Trauma, Cardiopulmonary Failure, Cardiac Arrest
Administer 100% O_2 initially via high-flow O_2 delivery system; titrate to desired effect
RSI (preoxygenation)
Administer 100% O_2 via well-fitted face mask for at least 3 minutes (if spontaneous ventilations)

Delivery System	Oxygen (%)	Flow Rate (L/minute)
Low-flow System		
Nasal cannula	22 to 60 (depending on patient size and flow rate)	0.25 to 4
Oxygen mask	35 to 60	6 to 10
High-flow System		
Face tent	<40	10 to 15
Oxygen hood	80 to 90	10 to 15
Oxygen tent	>50	>10
Partial rebreathing mask with reservoir	50 to 60	10 to 12
Nonrebreathing mask with reservoir	95	10 to 15
Venturi mask	25 to 60 (mask specific)	variable

Actions:

- Increases arterial oxygen saturation
- Increases arterial oxygen content
- May improve tissue oxygen delivery if cardiac output is adequate

Monitoring: Monitor SpO_2 continuously.

Adverse Effects:

CNS	headache (high-flow rates)
EENT	dry mucous membranes (high-flow rates)
RESP	airway obstruction (due to drying of secretions)
GI	gastric distention (high-flow rates)

Precautions:

- Insufficient flow rates delivered via oxygen mask, oxygen hood, and oxygen tent may cause CO_2 retention.
- Oxygen delivery systems can cause obstruction of the small airways due to drying of secretions.

Special Considerations:

- Titrate therapy based on SpO_2 once adequate oxygen delivery has been achieved.
- Tight mask seal and high flow rates delivered via rebreathing systems are required to deliver maximum oxygen concentration.
- Collapsed reservoir bag on nonrebreathing system indicates air leak or inadequate flow rate.
- Add humidification to oxygen delivery systems as soon as feasible.
- In children with some cyanotic heart conditions with single ventricle physiology (eg, following surgical palliation before correction of hypoplastic left heart syndrome), use oxygen with caution. In these children the balance of systemic versus pulmonary blood flow can be substantially altered by effects of oxygen administration on pulmonary vascular resistance. Seek expert advice before use if you are unsure.

Procainamide

Classification: Antiarrhythmic (class IA)

- SVT
- Atrial flutter
- VT (with pulses)

Available Forms: Injection: 100, 500 mg/mL

Dose and Administration:

SVT, Atrial Flutter, VT (with pulses)	
IV/IO	15 mg/kg IV/IO load over 30 to 60 minutes

Actions:

- Depresses excitability of cardiac muscle
- Slows conduction in atrium, bundle of His, and ventricle
- Increases refractory period

Pharmacokinetics:

Absorption	(not applicable with IV/IO route of administration)
Distribution	rapid
Metabolism	liver to active metabolite (NAPA)
Excretion	urine, unchanged (50% to 70%)
Half-life	2.5 to 4.5 hours (procainamide); approximately 6 to 8 hours (NAPA)

Pharmacodynamics:

IV/IO

- Onset—rapid
- Peak—15 to 60 minutes
- Duration—3 to 6 hours

Monitoring: Monitor blood pressure and ECG continuously with focus on QT interval.
Adverse Effects:

CNS	headache, dizziness, confusion, psychosis, restlessness, irritability, weakness
CV	hypotension, negative inotropic effects, prolonged QT interval, torsades de pointes, heart block, cardiac arrest
GI	nausea, vomiting, diarrhea, hepatomegaly
SKIN	rash, urticaria, edema, swelling, pruritus, flushing
HEME	systemic lupus erythematosus syndrome, agranulocytosis, thrombocytopenia, neutropenia, hemolytic anemia

Precautions:

- Seek expert consultation when using this agent.
- Routine use in combination with amiodarone (or other drugs that prolong QT interval) is not recommended without expert consultation.
- Risk of hypotension and negative inotropic effects increases with rapid administration. Therefore, this drug is not an appropriate agent for treatment of VF or pulseless VT.
- Reduce dose for patients with poor renal or cardiac function.

Special Considerations: Monitor procainamide and NAPA concentrations.

Sodium Bicarbonate

Classification: Alkalinizing agent, electrolyte
Indications:

- Metabolic acidosis (severe)
- Hyperkalemia
- Sodium channel blocker overdose (eg, tricyclic antidepressant)

Available Forms:

- Injection: 4% (0.48 mEq/mL), 4.2% (0.5 mEq/mL), 7.5% (0.89 mEq/mL), 8.4% (1 mEq/mL)
- Injection (premixed): 5% (0.6 mEq/mL)

Dose and Administration:

Metabolic Acidosis (severe), Hyperkalemia	
IV/IO	1 mEq/kg IV/IO *slow* bolus
Sodium Channel Blocker Overdose (eg, tricyclic antidepressant)	
IV/IO	1 to 2 mEq/kg IV/IO bolus until serum pH is >7.45 (7.50 to 7.55 for severe poisoning) followed by IV/IO infusion of 150 mEq $NaHCO_3$/L solution to maintain alkalosis

Action: Increases plasma bicarbonate, which buffers H^+ ion (reversing metabolic acidosis) forming carbon dioxide; elimination of carbon dioxide via the respiratory tract increases pH

Pharmacokinetics:

Absorption	(not applicable with IV/IO route of administration)
Distribution	wide (extracellular fluid)
Metabolism	combines with protons; taken up by cells
Excretion	urine, exhalation as CO_2
Half-life	unknown

Pharmacodynamics:

IV/IO

- Onset—rapid
- Peak—rapid
- Duration—unknown

Monitoring:

- Monitor SpO_2 and ECG continuously.
- Monitor ABG with attention to pH as appropriate.

Adverse Effects:

CNS	irritability, headache, confusion, stimulation, tremors, hyperreflexia, tetany, seizures, weakness
RESP	respiratory depression, apnea
CV	arrhythmia, hypotension, cardiac arrest
GI	abdominal distention, paralytic ileus
GU	calculi
SKIN	cyanosis, edema, sclerosis/necrosis (infiltration), vasodilation
ELECT	hypernatremia, hyperosmolarity
MISC	metabolic alkalosis, weight gain, water retention

Precautions:

- Ensure adequate ventilation because buffering action produces CO_2, which crosses blood-brain barrier and cell membranes more rapidly than (HCO_3^-). If ventilation is inadequate, increased CO_2 may result in transient paradoxical CSF and intracellular acidosis.
- Drug may inactivate catecholamines.
- When combined with calcium salts, precipitates into insoluble calcium carbonate crystals that may obstruct the IV catheter or tubing.

Special Considerations:

- Drug should not be administered via the endotracheal route.
- Irrigate IV/IO tubing with NS before and after infusions.

Sodium Nitroprusside

Classification: Vasodilator, antihypertensive

Indications:

- Cardiogenic shock (ie, associated with high SVR)
- Hypertension (severe)

Available Forms: Injection: 50 mg

Dose and Administration:

Cardiogenic Shock (high SVR), Hypertension (severe)		
IV/IO	<40 kg	1 to 8 μg/kg per minute IV/IO infusion
	>40 kg	0.1 to 5 μg/kg per minute IV/IO infusion

Action: Relaxes tone in all vascular beds (arteriolar and venous) through release of nitric oxide. This vasodilation results in reduced cardiac filling pressures and right and left ventricular afterload.

Pharmacokinetics:

Absorption	(not applicable with IV/IO route of administration)
Distribution	extracellular fluid
Metabolism	endothelial cells and RBCs (to cyanide), then liver (to thiocyanate)
Excretion	urine (thiocyanate)
Half-life	3 to 7 days (thiocyanate)

Pharmacodynamics:

IV/IO

- Onset—1 to 2 minutes
- Peak—Rapid
- Duration—1 to 10 minutes after stopping infusion

Monitoring:

- Monitor blood pressure and ECG continuously.
- Monitor thiocyanate (should be <50 mg/L) and cyanide (toxic is >2 μg/mL) levels in patients receiving prolonged infusion, particularly if rate is >2 μg/kg per minute or in patient with hepatic or renal dysfunction.

Adverse Effects:

CNS	seizures (thiocyanate toxicity), dizziness, headache, agitation, decreased reflexes, restlessness
CV	hypotension, bradycardia, tachycardia
GI	nausea/vomiting/abdominal cramps (thiocyanate toxicity)
ENDO	hypothyroidism
MISC	cyanide and thiocyanate toxicity

Precautions:

- Hypovolemia may worsen hypotensive effects of drug.
- Cyanide and thiocyanate toxicity may result if administered at high rates, for >48 hours, or to patients with decreased hepatic or renal function (drug is metabolized by endothelial cells to cyanide, then metabolized in the liver to thiocyanate).

Special Considerations:

- Drug is routinely mixed in D_5W. Drug may be administered into solutions containing saline.
- Use special administration tubing or wrap drug reservoir in aluminum foil or another opaque material to protect it from deterioration on exposure to light.
- Use solution immediately once prepared.
- Freshly prepared solution may have a very faint brownish tint without any change in drug potency.
- Drug may react with a variety of substances to form highly colored reaction products.

Terbutaline

Classification: Selective β_2-adrenergic agonist, bronchodilator
Indications: Asthma (status asthmaticus), hyperkalemia
Available Forms: Injection: 1 mg/mL
Dose and Administration:

Asthma (status asthmaticus), Hyperkalemia	
IV/IO	0.1 to 10 μg/kg per minute IV/IO infusion; consider 10 μg/kg load over 5 minutes
SQ	10 μg/kg SQ q 10 to 15 minutes until IV/IO infusion is initiated (maximum dose 0.4 mg)

Action: Stimulates β_2-adrenergic receptors

- Causes bronchodilation
- Causes vasodilation of arterioles
- Causes potassium to move intracellularly (will reduce serum potassium)

Pharmacokinetics:

Absorption	(not applicable with IV/IO route of administration)
Distribution	extracellular fluid
Metabolism	liver (partial)
Excretion	primarily unchanged in urine
Half-life	3 to 16 hours

Pharmacodynamics:

IV/IO

- Onset—rapid
- Peak—unknown
- Duration—2 to 6 hours

Monitoring: Monitor SpO_2, blood pressure, and ECG continuously.
Adverse Effects:

CNS	tremors, anxiety, headache, dizziness, stimulation
CV	palpitations, tachycardia, hypertension, hypotension, arrhythmias, myocardial ischemia
GI	nausea, vomiting

Special Considerations: Like other β_2-adrenergic agonists, terbutaline can lower potassium concentrations, which may be helpful therapeutically. The drug should be used cautiously in children with hypokalemia.

Index

A

ABCDE assessment, 4, 7–25
- of airways, 7–8, 25
- of breathing, 8–14, 25
- in cardiac arrest, 157
  - in submersion and drowning accidents, 180
  - in trauma, 179–180
- in cardiogenic shock, 77
- in cardiopulmonary failure, 156–157
- of circulation, 15–21, 25
- of disability, 21–24, 25
- exposure for examination in, 24, 25
- in hypovolemic shock, 70
- in supraventricular tachycardia, 130

Abdominal (seesaw) breathing, 11–12

Accessory muscles of respiration, 39

Accessory pathway reentry, 128

Acid-base balance, 27, 28, 30
- in hypovolemic shock, 101
- postresuscitation, 207

Acidosis
- arterial blood gas analysis in, 27, 30
- bicarbonate therapy in, 252–253
- bradycardia with pulse in, 123
- carbon dioxide serum levels in, 30
- cardiac arrest in, 168, 178
- diabetic ketoacidosis, 69, 94, 98
- lactate levels in, 30, 84
- postresuscitation, 197, 207
- respiratory, 36, 37
- in shock, 84
  - hypovolemic, 101
- tachycardia with pulse and poor perfusion in, 145, 147

Acrocyanosis, 21

ACTH stimulation test in septic shock and adrenal insufficiency, 103, 105

Adenosine, 222
- in tachyarrhythmias, 137, 222
  - with adequate perfusion, 141, 143
  - with poor perfusion, 145, 146

Adrenal disorders in septic shock, 74, 102, 103, 105
- hydrocortisone in, 103, 105, 239–240

Adrenocorticotropic hormone stimulation test in septic shock and adrenal insufficiency, 103, 105

Advanced life support, pediatric, 163–167

AED use, 162, 168, 169–170

Afterload, cardiac, 64, 65
- in cardiogenic shock, 76, 107
- postresuscitation, 199

Age-related differences
- in basic life support, 161–162
- in blood pressure, 17
- in Glasgow Coma Scale, 23
- in glucose levels, 96
- in heart rate, 16
- in pulse rate, 52
- in respiratory rate, 9
- in urine output, 21

Air movement
- auscultation of, 12, 13–14
- laminar, 38
- turbulent, 38

Aircraft transport, postresuscitation, 214

Airway assessment and management
- in bradycardia with pulse, 122
- in cardiac arrest
  - advanced airway in, 162, 167
  - in anaphylaxis, 181
  - in basic life support, 161
  - in submersion and drowning accidents, 180
  - in trauma, 179
- in cardiopulmonary failure, 156
- postresuscitation, 192
  - in transport, 212
- primary assessment in, 7–8, 25
- in respiratory distress and failure, 46

Airway obstruction, 5, 42, 47–53
- assessment of, 7–8
- auscultation of air movement in, 12
- hypoxemic hypoxia in, 63
- lower, 5, 42, 50–53

in asthma, 51–53
in bronchiolitis, 51
lung and airway sounds in, 13
management of, 47–53
advanced interventions in, 8
simple measures in, 8
signs of, 8, 42
upper, 5, 7–8, 42, 47–50
in anaphylaxis, 49, 75, 106
in croup, 47, 48–49
respiratory effort in, 11
Airway resistance, 38
Albumin, 223–224
Albuterol, 224–225
in anaphylaxis, 106, 224
in asthma, 53, 224
Algorithms
on bradycardia with pulse, 122–126
on postresuscitation treatment of shock, 199–202
on pulseless arrest, 167–178
on septic shock, 102, 103
on tachycardia with pulse, 141–147
and adequate perfusion, 141–144
and poor perfusion, 144–147
Alkalosis, respiratory, in hypovolemic shock, 101
Allergies, 26
anaphylaxis in. *See* Anaphylaxis
lung tissue disease in, 43, 53
Alprostadil, 225–226
Altitude, high, hypoxemia in, 20, 36, 63
Ambulance transport, postresuscitation, 214
Amiodarone, 226–227
in cardiac arrest, 166, 168, 174, 226–227
in tachyarrhythmias, 138, 226–227
with adequate perfusion, 141, 143
with poor perfusion, 145, 147
Analgesia, postresuscitation, 195
Anaphylaxis
albuterol in, 106, 224
cardiac arrest in, 181
diphenhydramine in, 106, 232–233
epinephrine in, 106, 181, 236
methylprednisolone in, 106, 245
shock in, 70, 75, 83, 106
upper airway obstruction in, 49, 75, 106
Anemia
hypoxia in, 35, 63
pulse oximetry in, 14
Angioedema in anaphylactic shock, 75, 106
Antiarrhythmic drugs in cardiac arrest, 166, 174
Anticoagulant therapy in pulmonary embolism, 111
Antihistamines in anaphylactic shock, 106, 232–233
Apnea, 10
Appearance, general assessment of, 6
Arrhythmias, 16, 115–147
bradyarrhythmias, 116–126. *See also* Bradyarrhythmias
cardiac arrest in, 153, 154–155
postresuscitation, 198
tachyarrhythmias, 126–147. *See also* Tachyarrhythmias
Arterial blood gas analysis
in circulatory assessment, 30
postresuscitation, 194
in respiratory assessment, 27
in shock, 88
Asphyxia, cardiac arrest in, 154
Aspiration pneumonitis, 55
Assess-categorize-decide-act model, 4–5
Assessment, pediatric, 1–31
ABCDE approach in. *See* ABCDE assessment
in advanced life support, 163
assess-categorize-decide-act model on, 4–5
in bradycardia with pulse, 122, 124
in cardiac arrest, 157
in submersion and drowning accidents, 180
in trauma, 179–180
in cardiopulmonary failure, 156–157
circulatory, 6, 15–21, 25, 29–31
general, 4, 6
heart rate and rhythm in, 115
in hypercarbia, 37
in hypoxemia, 34
learning objectives on, 3
ongoing reassessments in, 5
in shock, 86–87, 90, 95
pediatric assessment triangle on, 4, 6
postresuscitation
cardiovascular, 197
gastrointestinal, 208
hematologic, 209
neurologic, 204
renal, 207
respiratory, 194
primary, 4, 7–25
respiratory. *See* Respiratory assessment
SAMPLE mnemonic on, 25–26
secondary, 4, 25–26
in shock, 86–88

advanced measures in, 91–92
ancillary studies in, 87–88, 90
cardiogenic, 77–78, 108
and fluid therapy, 95
glucose levels in, 96
hypovolemic, 69–70, 98, 99, 100
ongoing monitoring in, 86–87, 90, 95
standardized approach to, 1
in supraventricular tachycardia, 130
tertiary, 4, 26–31
and timely intervention for prevention of cardiac arrest, 3, 33
and transition of care, 5
Asthma, 42, 51–53
albuterol in, 53, 224
dexamethasone in, 230–231
epinephrine in, 236
ipratropium bromide in, 53, 241–242
lung and airway sounds in, 13, 52
magnesium sulfate in, 53, 244
methylprednisolone in, 53, 245
peak expiratory flow rate in, 29, 52
pulse in, 18, 52
respiratory effort in, 10, 11
severity of, 52–53
terbutaline in, 53, 255
Asystole, 158
algorithm on management of, 168, 175–177
Atrial escape rhythm, 118
Atrial fibrillation, 139
Atrial flutter, 132
cardioversion in, 136, 140
drug therapy in, 139
procainamide, 251–252
Atrial tachycardia
ectopic, 129
paroxysmal, 128
Atrioventricular block, 118–119, 121
causes of, 119
first degree, 118, 119, 121
management of, 123, 125
second degree Mobitz types, 118, 119, 121
symptoms in, 119
third degree, 118, 119, 121
Atrioventricular nodal reentry, 129
Atropine, 228–229
in bradycardia, 123, 124–125, 166, 228, 229
in cardiac arrest, 166
Automated external defibrillator use, 162, 168, 169–170
AVPU (Alert-Voice-Painful-Unresponsive) Pediatric Response Scale, 19, 22

B
Basic life support, 161–162, 168, 169
age-related differences in, 161–162
Bicarbonate
serum levels, 30
therapy, 84, 252–253
in cardiac arrest, 166
in hypovolemic shock, 101
Blood count, complete, in shock, 87
Blood gas analysis
arterial. *See* Arterial blood gas analysis
venous. *See* Venous blood gas analysis
Blood pressure, 16–18, 66
age-related changes in, 17
arterial monitoring, 31
in shock, 91
and cardiac output, 66
central venous, 31
as measure of preload, 65, 91
in shock, 65, 91
in compensated shock, 67
in distributive shock, 71, 72
in hypotension, 17–18, 67–68. *See also* Hypotension
in hypovolemic shock, 100
measurement of, 16
invasive monitoring, 31, 91
in shock, 66, 91
in neurogenic shock, 107
normal systolic and diastolic values, 17
in normotensive shock, 200, 202
septic, 103, 105
postresuscitation, 197, 198, 200, 201–202
in septic shock, 103, 104–105
and severity of shock, 66–68
and systemic vascular resistance, 66
Blood products, 95, 198, 210. *See also* Transfusion therapy
Blood volume
in hypovolemic shock, 69, 98
hemorrhagic, 99, 100
and preload, 65
Bradyarrhythmias, 116–126. *See also specific arrhythmias*
atrioventricular block, 118–119
bradycardia, 116, 117
management of, 122–126
recognition of, 117–121
sinus node arrest, 118, 120

symptoms of, 117
Bradycardia, 16, 116
atropine in, 123, 124–125, 166, 228, 229
causes of, 116, 117, 123, 126
electrocardiography in, 117, 120, 122
epinephrine in, 123, 124, 236
primary, 116
with pulse, algorithm on management of, 122–126
relative, 116
secondary, 116
sinus, 117, 120
Bradypnea, 10
Brain perfusion, 19
postresuscitation management of, 205
signs of, 19
Breath sounds, 12, 13–14
Breathing
airway resistance in, 38
assessment of, 8–14, 25. *See also* Respiratory assessment
in cardiac arrest, 161
in anaphylaxis, 181
compression-to-ventilation ratio in, 162, 175, 177
in trauma, 179
central nervous system control of, 40
disordered control of, 5, 43, 57–58
causes of, 43, 57
management of, 57–58
signs of, 43
lung compliance in, 39
muscles in, 39–40
physiology in respiratory problems, 37–40
postresuscitation, 192
rate of, 9–10
in airway obstruction, 42
in asthma, 52
voluntary control of, 40
work of, 6, 10–12
airway resistance affecting, 38
lung compliance affecting, 39
Bronchiolitis, 42
lung and airway sounds in, 13, 51
management of, 51
respiratory effort in, 10, 11
Bronchopulmonary dysplasia, 27
Bundle branch block, 131
Burns
albumin therapy in, 223
hypovolemic shock in, 69, 98

C
Calcium
serum levels in shock, 84, 88
blood products affecting, 95
septic, 102
therapy, 229–230
in cardiac arrest, 166
Capillary refill time, 19
in shock, 67, 72
Capnography, 29
Carbon dioxide
arterial, 27, 36–37
in hypercarbia, 27, 30, 34, 36–37, 56
postresuscitation, 193, 195
end-tidal, 29
exhaled, 28
in advanced airway, 167
postresuscitation, 194
total serum levels, 30
venous, 28
Carbon monoxide poisoning, 27
histotoxic hypoxia in, 63
pulse oximetry in, 14
Cardiac arrest, 153–184
advanced life support in, 163–167
algorithm on, 167–178
in anaphylaxis, 181
basic life support in, 161–162, 168, 169
causes of, 153, 155–156
reversible, 168, 176, 177–178
definition of, 153
drug therapy in, 165–166, 168, 174, 176
amiodarone, 166, 168, 174, 226–227
in anaphylaxis, 181
in asystole/PEA, 168, 176
and cardiopulmonary resuscitation, 173–174
endotracheal administration of, 164, 174
and persistent VF/VT, 173
routes of administration, 163–164
family presence during resuscitation in, 182
heart rhythms in, 157–160
hypoxic or asphyxial, 154
in-hospital, 155–156
initial management in, 161
outcome in, 183, 184
learning objectives on, 154
management of, 160–178
out-of-hospital, 155–156
lone rescuer in, 160–161

outcome in, 183
outcome in, 153–154, 183–184
oxygen therapy in, 250–251
in poisoning, 182
prevention of, 3, 33, 154
recognition of, 157–160
in shock, 62, 68
in submersion and drowning accidents, 180–181
sudden, 153, 154–155
survival rates in, 153, 183
termination of resuscitation in, 182–183
in trauma, 155, 168, 178, 179–180
Cardiac output, 64–66
and blood pressure, 66
in cardiogenic shock, 76, 78, 83, 107, 109
in distributive shock, 71
septic, 72–73
in hypovolemic shock, 69
measures improving, 82–83
in obstructive shock, 110
Cardiogenic shock, 5, 62, 76–78, 107–109
causes of, 76
differentiated from hypovolemic shock, 77, 107
drug therapy in, 78, 88, 109
dobutamine, 233–234
dopamine, 234–236
nitroglycerin, 248
nitroprusside, 253–254
fluid therapy in, 78, 86, 94, 107, 108, 109
physiology of, 76–77
pulse in, 77, 91
signs of, 77–78, 83
stroke volume in, 65
Cardiopulmonary failure
definition of, 156
oxygen therapy in, 250–251
recognition of, 156–157
Cardiopulmonary resuscitation, 160–178
in advanced airway, 162, 167
in bradycardia with pulse, 122, 123, 124
chest compressions in. *See* Chest compressions
and defibrillation, 169, 172, 174
drug delivery during, 173–174
duration of efforts in, 183
family presence during, 182
interval from collapse to initiation of, 183
by lone rescuer, 160–161, 162
and postresuscitation management, 191–217
pulse checks in, 172, 177
in pulseless electrical activity/asystole, 168, 175–177
push hard and fast recommendation on, 123, 124
sequence of, 175, 176–177
termination of, 182–183
in ventricular fibrillation/ventricular tachycardia, 168–175
Cardiovascular system
in hemorrhage and shock, 100
postresuscitation, 196–203
signs in assessment of, 15–19
Cardioversion in tachyarrhythmias, 135–136, 140
energy dose in, 136, 144, 146
indications for, 136
pharmacologic, 141, 143
potential problems in, 136
with pulse and adequate perfusion, 141, 143–144
with pulse and poor perfusion, 145, 146
synchronized shocks in, 136, 144, 146
Catheterization
arterial, for blood pressure monitoring, 31, 91
central venous, for blood pressure monitoring, 31, 91
intraosseous
in cardiac arrest advanced life support, 164
in shock, 86, 90
peripheral venous
in cardiac arrest advanced life support, 163–164
in shock, 86, 90
of pulmonary artery in shock, 92, 108
Central nervous system
in control of breathing, 40
infections affecting, 43, 57
postresuscitation assessment and management of, 204–206
and signs of brain perfusion, 19
Central venous oxygen saturation, 30
in shock, 92
Central venous pressure, 31
as measure of preload, 65, 91
in shock, 65, 91
Chemical pneumonitis, 55
Chemoreceptors in respiratory regulation, 40
Chest compressions, 161–162
in advanced airway, 162, 167, 175, 177
in bradycardia with pulse, 122, 123, 124
and defibrillation, 169, 172, 174
minimizing interruptions in, 162, 172, 174
push hard and fast recommendation on, 123, 124
ratio to ventilation, 162, 175, 177
Chest retractions and respiratory effort, 11
Chest tube placement in tension pneumothorax, 110

Chest wall
compliance of, 39
expansion of, in tidal volume assessment, 12
Chest x-rays
in cardiogenic shock, 108
in circulatory assessment, 31, 197
postresuscitation, 194, 197
in respiratory assessment, 29, 194
in sinus tachycardia, 131
in supraventricular tachycardia, 131
Circulation
in bradycardia with pulse, 122
in cardiac arrest, 157, 161
in anaphylaxis, 181
in submersion and drowning accidents, 180
in trauma, 180
in cardiopulmonary failure, 156
cardiovascular function signs of, 15–19
end-organ perfusion signs of, 19–21
general assessment of, 6
postresuscitation, 192, 196–203
primary assessment of, 15–21, 25
in respiratory distress and failure, 46
in shock, 67
in supraventricular tachycardia, 130
tertiary assessment of, 29–31
type and severity problems in, 5
Clothing removed for physical examination, 24
Cold shock, 71, 103, 105
Colloid solutions
postresuscitation, 198
in shock, 93, 98
Color and temperature of skin. *See* Skin color and temperature
Communication issues in postresuscitation transport, 211, 212–213, 216–217
with family, 213, 217
between hospitals, 211, 213, 216
between physicians, 212, 216
Compensatory mechanisms in shock, 65–66, 67
cardiogenic, 76
distributive, 71
hypovolemic, 67, 69
warning signs in failure of, 82
Compliance, pulmonary, 39
Congenital heart disease, ductal-dependent
obstructive shock in, 78, 79, 111
prostaglandin E_1 therapy in, 111, 225
Consciousness levels, assessment of, 21–24
Consent issues in postresuscitation transport, 212, 216
Consultations in shock management, 89, 90
Contractility of heart, 64, 65
in compensatory mechanisms, 65, 66
postresuscitation, 199
Contusions, pulmonary, 43, 53
Corticosteroid therapy, 230–231, 239–240, 245
in anaphylactic shock, 106, 245
in septic shock and adrenal insufficiency, 103, 105, 239–240
Cortisol levels in septic shock and adrenal insufficiency, 105
Crackles (rales), 14
Croup, 47, 48–49
dexamethasone in, 48, 49, 230–231
epinephrine in, 48, 236
Crystalloid solutions, isotonic. *See* Isotonic crystalloid solutions
Cushing's triad in intracranial pressure increase, 57
Cyanide poisoning, 63
Cyanosis, 20–21
in cardiogenic shock, 77
in ductal-dependent congenital heart disease, 79
Cytotoxic hypoxia, 35, 63

D
Defibrillation, 168, 169–173, 174
in advanced life support, 165
with automated external defibrillator, 162, 168, 169–170
in basic life support, 162
clearing for, 171
implanted defibrillator affecting, 171
with manual defibrillator, 168, 169, 170
paddles/pads in, 170
in persistent VF/VT, 173, 174
special situations affecting, 171
treatment sequence in, 169, 172, 174, 175, 177
Dehydration, hypovolemic shock in, 98, 99
Dexamethasone, 230–231
in croup, 48, 49, 230–231
Dextrose, 232
in postresuscitation therapy, 203
Diabetic ketoacidosis, 69, 94, 98
Diaphragm as respiratory muscle, 39, 40
Diarrhea, hypovolemic shock in, 69, 98
Diffusion defect, hypoxemia in, 20, 36
Diphenhydramine, 232–233
in anaphylactic shock, 106, 232–233
Disability
in cardiac arrest, 157
in submersion and drowning accidents, 180
in trauma, 180
in cardiopulmonary failure, 157

primary assessment of, 21–24, 25
in supraventricular tachycardia, 130
Distributive shock, 5, 62, 70–75, 101–107
anaphylactic, 70, 75, 83, 106
fluid therapy in, 94
management of, 83, 101–107
dopamine in, 234–236
neurogenic, 70, 75, 83, 107
physiology of, 71
septic, 72–74, 102–106. *See also* Septic shock
signs of, 71–72, 83
Diuretics, 238–239
in pulmonary edema, 109, 238–239
Dobutamine, 89, 233–234
postresuscitation, 200, 202
in septic shock, 103, 105
Documentation in postresuscitation transport and follow-up, 213, 217
Dopamine, 89, 234–236
postresuscitation, 200, 201, 202
in septic shock, 103, 105
Drowning and submersion accidents, cardiac arrest in, 180–181
Drug overdose and toxicity
bicarbonate therapy in, 166, 252–253
bradycardia with pulse in, 126
calcium therapy in, 166, 229–230
cardiac arrest in, 182
disordered control of breathing in, 57, 58
fluid therapy in, 94
tachycardia in, 133
with pulse and poor perfusion, 145, 147
Drug therapy, 221–255
in bradycardia with pulse, 123, 124–125
in cardiac arrest. *See* Cardiac arrest, drug therapy in
postresuscitation, 195, 200, 201–202
in shock, 88–89, 90
anaphylactic, 106
cardiogenic. *See* Cardiogenic shock, drug therapy in
classes of agents in, 89
hypotensive, 200, 201
hypovolemic, 100
normotensive, 200, 202
obstructive, 111
septic, 74, 88, 103, 104–105
vascular access for, 86
in tachyarrhythmias, 137–140
with pulse and adequate perfusion, 141, 143
with pulse and poor perfusion, 145, 146, 147
with transdermal patch, defibrillation in, 171
Ductal-dependent congenital heart disease
obstructive shock in, 78, 79, 111
prostaglandin E_1 therapy in, 111, 225

E
Echocardiography, 31
in cardiogenic shock, 108
postresuscitation, 197
Ectopic atrial focus, 129
Ectopic tachycardia
atrial, 129
junctional, 129
Edema
angioedema in anaphylactic shock, 75, 106
cerebral, dexamethasone in, 230–231
pulmonary, 43, 53, 55–56
airway resistance in, 38
in cardiogenic shock, 76, 77, 78
diuretics in, 109, 238–239
lung and airway sounds in, 13
respiratory effort in, 10
in septic shock, 74, 102
Electrocardiography
in asystole, 158
in atrial flutter, 132
in atrioventricular blocks, 118, 119, 121
in bradycardia, 117, 120, 122
in cardiogenic shock, 108
postresuscitation, 197
in pulseless electrical activity, 158
in sinus node arrest, 118, 120
in sinus tachycardia, 127, 128, 131
in supraventricular tachycardia, 130, 131, 140
in ventricular fibrillation, 159
in ventricular tachycardia, 132–133, 160
Embolism, pulmonary, 80, 111
central venous pressure in, 91
obstructive shock in, 78, 80, 111
Emergency response system, activation of, 161
End-organ perfusion, 19–21
Endotracheal intubation. *See* Tracheal intubation
Epinephrine, 89, 236–238
in anaphylaxis, 106, 181, 236
in bradycardia, 123, 124, 236
in cardiac arrest, 166, 168
in anaphylaxis, 181
in asystole/PEA, 168, 176
and cardiopulmonary resuscitation, 174
and persistent VF/VT, 173

in croup, 48, 236
postresuscitation, 200, 201, 202
in septic shock, 103, 105
Escape rhythms
atrial, 118
idioventricular, 118, 120
junctional, 118, 120
Ethical issues in termination of resuscitation, 182–183
Expiration
grunting sounds in, 13
muscles in, 39
as passive process, 39
peak expiratory flow rate in, 29
signs of airway obstruction in, 42
Exposure for physical examination in primary assessment, 24, 25
Extracorporeal cardiac life support, 183, 184
Eye opening in Glasgow Coma Scale, 22, 23

F
Family
communication with, postresuscitation, 213, 217
present during resuscitation, 182
Fever, postresuscitation management of, 205
Fibrillation
atrial, 139
ventricular. *See* Ventricular fibrillation
Fluid therapy
albumin in, 223
in cardiac arrest, routes of, 163–164
postresuscitation, 198, 200, 201, 203
algorithm on, 200, 201
composition of, 203
rate of delivery, 203
in shock, 86, 90, 92–95
cardiogenic, 78, 86, 94, 107, 108, 109
composition of, 93
hypovolemic, 83, 94, 97, 98–100, 101
monitoring and reassessment during, 95
obstructive, 110
rate of delivery, 94
septic, 94, 102, 103, 104
vascular access for, 86
volume of, 94
Flutter, atrial, 132
Food intake in last meal, assessment of, 26
Foreign-body airway obstruction, 8, 42
management of, 47, 49–50
Furosemide, 238–239

G
Gases
arterial blood. *See* Arterial blood gas analysis
venous blood. *See* Venous blood gas analysis
Gastric distention, postresuscitation management of, 209
Gastrointestinal disorders
hypovolemic shock in, 69, 98
postresuscitation, 208–209
General assessment, 4, 6
Glasgow Coma Scale, 22–24
Glucose blood levels
in cardiac arrest, 168, 178
and dextrose administration, 232
and lactate levels, 30
postresuscitation, 203, 204, 205
in shock, 84, 87, 96–97
septic, 102
in tachycardia with pulse, 145, 147
and urine output, 21
Grunting sounds, 13
and chest retractions, 11
Gurgling sounds, 13

H
Head bobbing and respiratory effort, 11
Head injury
disordered control of breathing in, 43, 57
Glasgow Coma Scale in, 22, 24
neurogenic shock in, 75
Head tilt–chin lift maneuver, 8
Healthcare providers
basic life support maneuvers, 161–162
in postresuscitation transport, 213
Heart failure
dobutamine in, 233–234
nitroglycerin in, 248
pulmonary edema in, 55
Heart rate, 16
age-related changes in, 16
in bradyarrhythmias, 16, 115, 117
in compensatory mechanisms, 65, 67
evaluation of, 115
postresuscitation, 199
in pulseless arrest, 115
in tachyarrhythmias, 16, 115, 126, 128, 130, 131
and tissue oxygen delivery, 64
Heart rhythm, 16
Helicopter transport, postresuscitation, 214

Hematologic system, postresuscitation assessment and management of, 209–210
Hemoglobin concentration
in anemic hypoxia, 63
in circulatory assessment, 31
in cyanosis, 20
in hypoxemia, 35
and pulse oximetry, 14
in respiratory assessment, 27, 28
and tissue oxygen delivery, 64
Hemorrhage
anemic hypoxia in, 63
hypovolemic shock in, 62, 69, 99–100
Herniation, cerebral, 57, 206
Histotoxic hypoxia, 35, 63
Hydrocephalus, disordered control of breathing in, 43, 57
Hydrocortisone, 239–240
in septic shock and adrenal insufficiency, 103, 105, 239–240
Hypercarbia, 34, 36–37
arterial blood gas analysis in, 27, 30
differentiated from hypoxemia, 37
in respiratory distress syndrome, acute, 56
Hyperglycemia, 96, 97
postresuscitation, 205
Hyperkalemia
albuterol in, 224
bicarbonate therapy in, 166, 252–253
bradycardia with pulse in, 123, 126
calcium therapy in, 166, 229–230
cardiac arrest in, 168, 178
in shock, 84
tachycardia with pulse in, 145, 147
terbutaline in, 255
Hypermagnesemia, calcium chloride therapy in, 229–230
Hypertension, nitroprusside therapy in, 253–254
Hyperthermia, postresuscitation management of, 205
Hypocalcemia
calcium therapy in, 166, 229–230
in shock, 84, 95
septic, 102
Hypoglycemia
cardiac arrest in, 168, 178
dextrose administration in, 232
postresuscitation, 205
in shock, 84, 96–97
septic, 102
tachycardia with pulse in, 145, 147
Hypokalemia
bradycardia with pulse in, 123
cardiac arrest in, 168, 178
tachycardia with pulse in, 145, 147
Hypomagnesemia, magnesium therapy in, 166, 244
Hypotension, 17–18
cardiac arrest in, 155–156
definition by blood pressure and age, 17, 68
in hypovolemic shock, 100
in neurogenic shock, 107
positioning of child in, 85
in septic shock, 68, 103, 104
Hypotensive shock, 5, 18, 66, 67–68
epinephrine in, 237
fluid deficit and therapy in, 94, 98
norepinephrine in, 249
postresuscitation management, 200, 201
Hypothermia
from blood product administration in shock, 95
bradycardia with pulse in, 123, 126
cardiac arrest in, 168, 178
in submersion and drowning accidents, 180, 181
postresuscitation management of, 205
tachycardia with pulse in, 145, 147
Hypoventilation
alveolar, hypoxemia in, 20, 36
central, 36
hypercarbia in, 36–37
Hypovolemia
bradycardia with pulse in, 123
cardiac arrest in, 168, 178
distributive shock in, 71
tachycardia with pulse in, 145, 147
urine output in, 21
Hypovolemic shock, 5, 21, 62, 69–70, 97–101
cardiogenic shock compared with, 77, 107
causes of, 69
compensated, 67, 69, 100
hemorrhagic, 62, 69, 99–100
management of, 83, 97–101
drug therapy in, 100
fluid therapy in, 83, 94, 97, 98–100, 101
neurogenic shock compared with, 75
nonhemorrhagic, 98–99
physiology of, 69
signs of, 69–70, 98, 100
Hypoxemia, 34–36, 62
arterial blood gas analysis in, 27
cyanosis in, 20
hypercarbia compared with, 37
in hypoxia, 35, 63

hypoxia compared with, 35
mechanisms of, 36
oxygen therapy in, 36, 250–251
pulse oximetry in, 14, 34
in respiratory distress syndrome, acute, 56
treatment of, 36
Hypoxia, 34–35, 62–63
anemic, 35, 63
bradycardia with pulse in, 123, 126
cardiac arrest in, 154, 168, 178
in trauma, 179
cerebral, 19
definition of, 62
histotoxic (cytotoxic), 35, 63
hypoxemia compared with, 35
hypoxemic, 35, 63
ischemic, 35, 63
oxygen therapy in, 250–251
physiology of shock in, 64–66
signs of, 34
tachycardia with pulse and poor perfusion in, 145, 147

I
Idioventricular escape rhythm, 118, 120
Ileus, postresuscitation, 209
Inamrinone, 89, 240–241
postresuscitation, 200, 202
Infections
postresuscitation transport in, 211, 216
septic shock in. *See* Septic shock
Inflammatory response syndrome, systemic, 73
Inotropic agents, 89
in septic shock, 74, 105
Inspiration
chest wall expansion in, 12
muscles in, 39, 40
signs of airway obstruction in, 42
Intercostal muscles in respiration, 39, 40
Intracranial pressure increase, 19
disordered control of breathing in, 57
postresuscitation assessment and management of, 204, 206
Intraosseous/intravenous access
in cardiac arrest advanced life support, 163–164
in shock, 86, 90
Ipratropium bromide, 241–242
in asthma, 53, 241–242
Ischemic hypoxia, 35, 63
Isotonic crystalloid solutions, 93, 94
in cardiogenic shock, 109
in hypovolemic shock, 98, 99, 100, 101
postresuscitation, 198
in septic shock, 102, 103, 104

J
Junctional ectopic tachycardia, 129
Junctional escape rhythm, 118, 120

K
Ketoacidosis, diabetic, 69, 94, 98
Kidneys
in hemorrhage and shock, 100
postresuscitation assessment and management, 206–207
signs of perfusion, 21
urine output, 21, 67, 100, 207

L
Laboratory tests
in postresuscitation assessment
cardiovascular, 197
gastrointestinal, 208
hematologic, 209
neurologic, 204
renal, 207
respiratory, 194
in shock, 87–88
in tertiary assessment, 26–32
cardiovascular, 30–31
respiratory, 26–29
Lactate, 30
in acidosis, 30, 84
in shock, 88
Lay rescuer basic life support, 161–162
Lidocaine, 242–243
in cardiac arrest, 166, 168, 174
in tachyarrhythmias, 139, 143, 166, 242–243
Life-threatening conditions
actions and interventions in, 25
general assessment in, 6
primary assessment in, 25
Light response, pupillary, 24
Liver failure, postresuscitation, 209
Lone rescuer CPR, 160–161, 162
Long QT syndromes, 133
Lung compliance, 39
Lung sounds, 12, 13–14
Lung tissue disease, 5, 43, 53–56
auscultation of air movement in, 12
causes of, 43, 53

lung and airway sounds in, 13, 14
management of, 53–56
in pneumonia, 43, 54
in pneumonitis, 55
in pulmonary edema, 3, 55–56
respiratory effort in, 11

M
Magnesium sulfate therapy, 140, 244
in asthma, 53, 244
in cardiac arrest, 166, 168, 174
in torsades de pointes, 140, 166, 244
Medical history, 26
Medications. *See* Drug therapy
Mental status, 21–24
in hypercarbia, 37
Metabolic disorders in shock, 84
Methemoglobinemia, 14, 27, 63
Methylprednisolone, 245
in anaphylactic shock, 106, 245
in asthma, 53, 245
Milrinone, 89, 246
in cardiogenic shock, 109
postresuscitation, 200, 202
in septic shock, 103, 105
Minute ventilation, 13
Mobitz type atrioventricular blocks, 118, 119, 121
Monitoring
postresuscitation
cardiovascular, 197
gastrointestinal, 208
neurologic, 204
renal, 207
respiratory, 194
in shock, 86–87, 90
advanced measures in, 91–92
cardiogenic, 108
in fluid therapy, 95
frequent reassessment in, 87, 90, 95
of glucose levels, 96
Motor response in Glasgow Coma Scale, 22, 23
Mottling of skin, 20
Muscles of respiration, 39–40
Myocardial dysfunction
inamrinone in, 240–241
milrinone in, 246
postresuscitation, 198
Myocarditis, 65

N
Naloxone, 247
Narcotic reversal with naloxone, 247
Nasal flaring and respiratory effort, 11
Neurogenic shock, 70, 75
differentiated from hypovolemic shock, 75
management of, 83, 107
physiology of, 75
signs of, 75
Neurologic system
assessment of
in disability evaluation, 21–24
postresuscitation, 204
signs of brain perfusion in, 19
in control of breathing, 40
infections affecting, 43, 57
in hemorrhage and shock, 100
postresuscitation, 204–206
shock in injury of, 70, 75, 83, 107
Neuromuscular blocking agents, postresuscitation, 195
Neuromuscular problems
disordered control of breathing in, 43, 57, 58
lung compliance in, 39
respiratory effort in, 12
Nitroglycerin, 89, 248
Nitroprusside, 89, 253–254
in septic shock, 103, 105
Norepinephrine, 89, 249
postresuscitation, 200, 201
in septic shock, 103, 104, 105
Normotensive shock
postresuscitation management of, 200, 202
septic, 103, 105

O
Obstruction of airway. *See* Airway obstruction
Obstructive shock, 5, 62, 78–80, 109–111
in cardiac tamponade, 78, 110
causes of, 78–80
central venous pressure in, 91
in ductal-dependent congenital heart disease, 78, 79, 111
management of, 83, 109–111
fluid therapy in, 94
objectives in, 110
physiology of, 78
in pulmonary embolism, 78, 80, 111
signs of, 83
in tension pneumothorax, 78, 79, 110
Oximetry, pulse, 14, 28

in hypercarbia, 37
in hypoxemia, 14, 34
indications for, 28
interpretation of, 14
postresuscitation, 194
Oxygen
arterial, 27, 28
postresuscitation, 193
in shock, 82, 90, 92
consumption in shock, 92
measures reducing, 84
delivery of, 64–66
hemoglobin saturation, 14, 27, 28, 64
in cyanosis, 20
in hypoxemia, 34, 35
hypoxemia. *See* Hypoxemia
hypoxia. *See* Hypoxia
therapy, 250–251
defibrillation in, 171
in hypoxemia, 36, 250–251
postresuscitation, 195, 198
in shock, 85
venous, 30
postresuscitation, 193, 195, 197, 198
in shock, 88, 92

P
P waves
in bradycardia, 117
in sinus tachycardia, 128
in supraventricular tachycardia, 130
in ventricular tachycardia, 132
Pacing, cardiac
in bradycardia with pulse, 123, 125
with implanted device, defibrillation in, 171
Pallor, 20
Peak expiratory flow rate, 29
in asthma, 29, 52
Pediatric advanced life support in cardiac arrest, 163–167
Pediatric assessment. *See* Assessment, pediatric
Pediatric assessment triangle, 4, 6
PEEP (positive end-expiratory pressure), postresuscitation, 196
Pericardiocentesis in cardiac tamponade, 110
PERRL (pupils equal round and reactive to light), 24
pH
in arterial blood gas analysis, 27
in venous blood gas analysis, 28
Pharmacology, 221–255. *See also* Drug therapy
Phosphodiesterase inhibitors, 89
in septic shock, 105
Physical examination
in general assessment, 6
in postresuscitation assessment
cardiovascular, 197
gastrointestinal, 208
hematologic, 209
neurologic, 204
renal, 207
respiratory, 194
in primary assessment, 7–24
cardiovascular, 15–21
exposure for, 24
neurologic, 21–24
respiratory, 7–14
in secondary assessment, 26
Platelet transfusions, postresuscitation, 210
Pneumonia, 43, 53, 54
Pneumonitis
aspiration, 55
chemical, 55
Pneumothorax, tension
bradycardia with pulse in, 123
cardiac arrest in, 168, 178
in trauma, 179
causes of, 79
central venous pressure in, 91
management of, 110
obstructive shock in, 78, 79, 110
signs of, 79
tachycardia with pulse and poor perfusion in, 145, 147
Poisoning
atropine in, 228
bradycardia with pulse in, 126
carbon monoxide, 14, 27, 63
cardiac arrest in, 182
disordered control of breathing in, 57, 58
epinephrine in, 237
fluid therapy in, 94
general assessment in, 6
histotoxic hypoxia in, 63
Positioning of child in shock, 85, 90
neurogenic, 107
Postresuscitation management, 191–217
algorithm on, 199–202
cardiovascular, 196–203
fluid therapy in, 198, 200, 201, 203
gastrointestinal, 208–209

hematologic, 209–210
learning objectives on, 191
neurologic, 204–206
primary goals in, 192
renal, 206–207
respiratory, 193–196
systematic approach in, 192
transport in, 210–217
Potassium chloride in postresuscitation fluid therapy, 203
Potassium serum levels
in bradycardia with pulse, 123, 126
in cardiac arrest, 168, 178
in hyperkalemia. *See* Hyperkalemia
in shock, 84, 88
in tachycardia with pulse and poor perfusion, 145, 147
PR interval
in sinus tachycardia, 128
in supraventricular tachycardia, 130
Preload, cardiac, 64, 65
in cardiogenic shock, 76, 107
central venous pressure as measure of, 65, 91
postresuscitation, 199
Primary assessment, 4, 7–25
ABCDE approach in. *See* ABCDE assessment
Procainamide, 251–252
in tachyarrhythmias, 139, 251–252
with pulse and adequate perfusion, 141, 143
with pulse and poor perfusion, 145, 147
Prostaglandin E_1, 225–226
in ductal-dependent lesions, 111, 225
Pulmonary artery catheterization, 92
in cardiogenic shock, 108
Pulse, 18
age-related changes in, 52
alternating, 91
in asthma, 18, 52
in bradycardia, 122–126
central, 18
checks in cardiopulmonary resuscitation, 172, 177
paradoxical, 18, 52
peripheral, 18
in shock, 67
cardiogenic, 77, 91
distributive, 72
in tachyarrhythmias, 134
and adequate perfusion, 141–144
and poor perfusion, 144–147
Pulse oximetry. *See* Oximetry, pulse
Pulseless arrest, 115
algorithm on management of, 167–178
development in bradycardia, 123, 125
epinephrine in, 168, 176, 236
Pulseless electrical activity, 158
algorithm on management of, 168, 175–177
outcome in, 183
Pupillary light response, 24
Purpura, 19

Q
QRS complex
in bradycardia, 117
in sinus tachycardia, 128
with pulse and adequate perfusion, 141, 142
with pulse and poor perfusion, 144, 145
in supraventricular tachycardia, 130
with pulse and adequate perfusion, 141, 142
with pulse and poor perfusion, 144, 145, 146
in ventricular tachycardia, 132, 133, 160
with pulse and adequate perfusion, 141, 142, 143
with pulse and poor perfusion, 144, 145, 146
Quiet tachypnea, 10

R
R-R interval
in sinus tachycardia, 128
in supraventricular tachycardia, 130
Radiography of chest. *See* Chest x-rays
Rales (crackles), 14
Red blood cells, packed, in postresuscitation therapy, 210
Renal system
in hemorrhage and shock, 100
postresuscitation assessment and management, 206–207
signs of perfusion, 21
urine output, 21, 67, 100, 207
Resistance
in airways, 38
vascular. *See* Vascular resistance
Respiratory arrest in asthma, 52
Respiratory assessment, 33, 46
arterial blood gas analysis in, 27
in bradycardia with pulse, 122
capnography in, 29
in cardiac arrest, 157
in cardiopulmonary failure, 156
categorization of type and severity problems in, 5, 40–43
chest x-rays in, 29, 194
exhaled carbon dioxide monitoring in, 28
general, 6

hemoglobin concentration in, 28
in hypercarbia, 37
in hypoxemia, 34
lung and airway sounds in, 13–14
peak expiratory flow rate in, 29
postresuscitation, 194
primary, 8–14, 25
pulse oximetry in, 14, 28
in respiratory distress and failure, 46
respiratory effort in, 10–12
respiratory rate in, 9–10
in supraventricular tachycardia, 130
tertiary, 26–29
tidal volume in, 12–13
venous blood gas in, 28
on work of breathing, 6, 10–12
Respiratory centers in brainstem, 40
Respiratory distress, 5, 40
cardiac arrest in, 33, 154
grunting sounds in, 13
in intracranial pressure increase, 57
management of, 45–58
oxygen therapy in, 250–251
in poisoning or drug overdose, 58
pulse oximetry in, 14, 28
signs of, 40
tachypnea in, 10, 40
Respiratory distress syndrome, acute, 43, 53, 56
Respiratory effort, 10–12
in airway obstruction, 42
in cardiogenic shock, 77
in respiratory failure, 41
Respiratory failure, 5, 41
arterial blood gas analysis in, 27
in asthma, 53
cardiac arrest in, 154, 155–156
prevention of, 3, 33, 41
in croup, 48, 49
grunting sounds in, 13
in intracranial pressure increase, 57
management of, 45–58
oxygen therapy in, 250–251
in poisoning or drug overdose, 58
postresuscitation, 195
pulse oximetry in, 28
signs of, 41
Respiratory problems, 33–58
in airway obstruction, 42, 47–53
cardiac arrest in, 154, 155–156
prevention of, 3, 33, 41
in disordered control of breathing, 43, 57–58
in hemorrhage and shock, 100
hypercarbia in, 36–37
hypoxemia in, 34–36
in lung tissue disease, 43, 53–56
management of, 45–58
learning objectives on, 45
physiology of, 34, 37–40
postresuscitation, 193–196
recognition of, 33–43
learning objectives on, 33
severity of, 5, 40–41
types of, 5, 41–43
Respiratory rate, 9–10
in airway obstruction, 42
in asthma, 52

S
SAMPLE mnemonic on secondary assessment, 25–26
Secondary assessment, 4, 25–26
Sedation, postresuscitation, 195
Seesaw (abdominal) breathing, 11–12
Seizures
disordered control of breathing in, 43, 57
postresuscitation management of, 206
Sepsis, 73–74
Septic shock, 63, 70, 72–74, 102–107
adrenal disorders in, 74, 102, 103, 105, 239–240
central venous pressure in, 91
cold, 103, 105
hypotension in, 68
importance of early recognition and treatment, 74
management of, 74, 83, 102–107
drug therapy in, 74, 88, 103, 104–105, 239–240
fluid therapy in, 94, 102, 103, 104
PALS algorithm on, 102, 103
therapeutic end points in, 105
normotensive, 103, 105
pathophysiology in, 72
signs of, 74
venous oxygen saturation in, 92
warm, 103, 104
Shock, 61–111, 81–111
accelerated progression of, 68, 82
advanced measures in, 91–92
anaphylactic, 70, 75, 83, 106
ancillary studies in, 87–88
cardiac arrest in, 62, 154

cardiogenic, 5, 76–78, 107–109. *See also* Cardiogenic shock
categorization by type and severity, 5, 66–80
causes of, 62
cold, 71, 103, 105
compensated, 5, 66, 67
in hemorrhage, 100
progression to hypotensive shock, 68
compensatory mechanisms in. *See* Compensatory mechanisms in shock
decompensated, 66
in hemorrhage, 100
definition of, 62
distributive, 5, 70–75, 101–107. *See also* Distributive shock
drug therapy in, 88–89. *See also* Drug therapy, in shock
end points of therapy in, 85
fluid therapy in, 86, 92–95. *See also* Fluid therapy, in shock
general measures in, 85–90
glucose levels in, 84, 87, 96–97, 102
hypotensive, 5, 18, 66, 67–68. *See also* Hypotensive shock
hypovolemic, 69–70, 97–101. *See also* Hypovolemic shock
metabolic disorders in, 84
monitoring in. *See* Monitoring, in shock
neurogenic, 70, 75, 83, 107
normotensive
postresuscitation management of, 200, 202
septic, 103, 105
obstructive, 5, 78–80, 109–111. *See also* Obstructive shock
oxygen content of blood in, 82
oxygen demand in, 84
physiology of, 64–66
postresuscitation management in, 199–202
pulse in, 18
recognition of, 61–80
learning objectives on, 61
septic, 72–74, 102–106. *See also* Septic shock
severity of, 5, 66–68
signs of, 67, 68
spinal, 75, 107
subspecialty consultations in, 89, 90
types of, 5, 68–80
warm, 71, 103, 104
warning signs in, 82
Shunting, hypoxemia in, 20, 36, 63
Sinus bradycardia, 117, 120
Sinus node arrest, 118, 120
Sinus tachycardia, 127–128
compared with supraventricular tachycardia, 131, 142
electrocardiography in, 127, 128, 131
with pulse and adequate perfusion, 141, 142
with pulse and poor perfusion, 144, 145, 146
signs and symptoms in, 131, 142, 144
Skin color and temperature
and cardiovascular function, 15
and end-organ perfusion, 19–21
in shock, 67
distributive, 72, 83
hypovolemic, 100
Spinal shock, 75, 107
Status asthmaticus, 42
magnesium therapy in, 244
methylprednisolone in, 245
terbutaline in, 255
Stomach distention, postresuscitation management of, 209
Stridor, 13
and chest retractions, 11
Stroke volume, 64–65, 66
in cardiogenic shock, 107
and systemic vascular resistance, 77
Submersion and drowning accidents, cardiac arrest in, 180–181
Subspecialty consultations in shock management, 89, 90
Sudden infant death syndrome, 155
Supraventricular tachycardia, 128–131
with aberrant conduction, 131, 146
cardioversion in, 136, 140, 144, 145, 146
causes of, 128–129
drug therapy in, 137–139, 140, 141, 143
adenosine, 137, 143, 145, 146, 222
amiodarone, 138, 226–227
procainamide, 139, 251–252
electrocardiography in, 130, 131, 140
narrow-complex, 130
with pulse and adequate perfusion, 141–143
with pulse and poor perfusion, 144–147
signs and symptoms in, 129–130, 131, 142, 144
sinus tachycardia compared with, 131, 142
vagal maneuvers in, 135, 140, 143, 145, 146
ventricular tachycardia compared with, 131
wide-complex, 131

T

T waves in ventricular tachycardia, 132
Tachyarrhythmias, 16, 65, 126–147. *See also specific arrhythmias*
atrial flutter, 132, 136, 139, 140
cardioversion in. *See* Cardioversion in tachyarrhythmias
classification of, 127
in compensatory mechanisms, 65, 67
drug therapy in, 137–140

in adequate perfusion, 141, 143
in poor perfusion, 145, 146, 147
emergency interventions in, 135–136
in hypovolemic shock, 69, 70
hemorrhagic, 100
initial management of, 134–135
narrow complex, 127, 134
pulse in, 134
and adequate perfusion, 141–144
and poor perfusion, 144–147
pulseless, 134
recognition of, 127–133
relative, 126
signs of, 127
sinus tachycardia, 127–128, 131
supraventricular tachycardia, 128–131
vagal maneuvers in, 135, 140, 141, 143, 145, 146
ventricular tachycardia, 132–133
wide complex, 127, 131, 134
Tachypnea, 10
and hypercarbia, 37
in hypovolemic shock, 69, 70, 100, 101
quiet, 10
in respiratory distress, 10, 40
Tamponade, cardiac, 78, 110
bradycardia with pulse in, 123
cardiac arrest in, 168, 178
in trauma, 179
causes of, 78
central venous pressure in, 91
management of, 110
obstructive shock in, 78, 110
signs of, 78
tachycardia with pulse in, 145, 147
Team members in postresuscitation transport, 215
Temperature
in hypothermia. *See* Hypothermia
postresuscitation management of, 205
of skin. *See* Skin color and temperature
Tension pneumothorax. *See* Pneumothorax, tension
Terbutaline, 255
in asthma, 53, 255
Termination of resuscitation, 182–183
Tertiary assessment, 4, 26–31
circulatory, 29–31
respiratory, 26–29
Thoracostomy in tension pneumothorax, 110
Thrombosis
bradycardia with pulse in, 123
cardiac arrest in, 168, 178
tachycardia with pulse in, 145, 147
Tidal volume, 12–13
Torsades de pointes, 133, 160
magnesium therapy in, 140, 166, 244
Toxic exposures
atropine in, 228
bradycardia with pulse in, 123, 126
cardiac arrest in, 168, 178, 182
chemical pneumonitis in, 55
epinephrine in, 237
tachycardia with pulse in, 145, 147
Tracheal intubation
in bradycardia with pulse, 123, 124, 125
in cardiac arrest, 164, 167
drug delivery in, 164, 174
exhaled carbon dioxide monitoring in, 28, 167
postresuscitation, 195
in transport, 212
Transdermal medication patch, defibrillation in, 171
Transfusion therapy
postresuscitation, 198, 210
in shock, 95
complications of, 95
hypovolemic, 99, 100, 101
indications for, 95
Transport, postresuscitation, 210–217
checklist on, 216–217
communication in, 211, 212–213, 216–217
with family, 213, 217
between hospitals, 211, 213, 216
between physicians, 212, 216
consent issues in, 212
coordination with receiving facility, 211, 216
documentation and follow-up in, 213, 217
infectious disease considerations in, 211, 216
modes of, 214, 216
preparations for, 212, 216
in advance, 211, 216
team members in, 215
triage in, 215
Trauma
bradycardia with pulse in, 123, 126
cardiac arrest in, 155, 168, 178, 179–180
of head. *See* Head injury
pulmonary contusion in, 43, 53
tachycardia with pulse and poor perfusion in, 145, 147
Trendelenburg position, 85
Triage in postresuscitation transport, 215

U

Urine output, 21
  age-related changes in, 21
  postresuscitation, 207
  in shock, 67
    hypovolemic, 100

V

Vagal maneuvers in tachyarrhythmias, 135, 140
  with pulse and adequate perfusion, 141, 143
  with pulse and poor perfusion, 145, 146
Vascular access
  for arterial blood pressure monitoring, 31, 91
  in cardiac arrest advanced life support, 163–164
  for central venous pressure monitoring, 31, 91
  in shock, 86, 90, 91
Vascular resistance
  splanchnic, 67
  systemic, 65, 66, 67
    in distributive shock, 70, 71, 83
    postresuscitation, 199
    and stroke volume, 77
Vasoactive agents, 88, 89
  in septic shock, 74, 88, 104–105
Vasodilator drugs, 89
  in cardiogenic shock, 109
  in septic shock, 105
Vasopressin, 89
  in cardiac arrest, 166
  in septic shock, 103, 104
Vasopressor drugs
  in cardiac arrest, 166
  in shock, 89
Venous blood gas analysis
  in circulatory assessment, 30
  in respiratory assessment, 28
  in shock, 88
Ventilation/perfusion imbalance, 20, 36, 63
Ventilatory support
  in hypoxemia, 36
  postresuscitation, 195, 196
Ventricular fibrillation, 133
  and cardiac arrest, 153, 154, 159
    algorithm on management of, 168–175
  conversion to organized rhythm, 172
  lidocaine in, 174, 242–243
  outcome in, 183
  persistence of, 173, 174
  termination of, 172, 174
  treatment sequence in, 175
Ventricular outflow tract obstruction, left, 79
Ventricular tachycardia, 132–133
  and cardiac arrest, 153, 154, 159–160
    algorithm on management of, 168–175
  cardioversion in, 136, 140, 141, 145, 146
  causes of, 132
  differentiated from supraventricular tachycardia, 131
  drug therapy in, 138–140, 141, 145, 147
    amiodarone, 166, 226–227
    lidocaine, 166, 242–243
    procainamide, 251–252
  electrocardiography in, 132–133, 160
  monomorphic, 133, 160
  outcome in, 183
  persistence of, 173, 174
  polymorphic, 133, 160
  with pulse and adequate perfusion, 141–143
  with pulse and poor perfusion, 144–147
  pulseless, 159–160, 168–175
  termination of, 172, 174
  treatment sequence in, 175
  wide complex, 131, 132, 141, 143, 146–147
Verapamil, 140
Verbal response in Glasgow Coma Scale, 22, 23
Vomiting, hypovolemic shock in, 69, 98

W

Warm shock, 71, 103, 104
Water
  and cardiac arrest in drowning accidents, 180–181
  defibrillation of victim in, 171
Wenckebach phenomenon in atrioventricular blocks, 118, 119, 121
Wheezing, 13
  in asthma, 13, 52
  and chest retractions, 11
Wolff-Parkinson-White syndrome, 128